ADOLESCENT MEDICINE: STATE OF THE ART REVIEWS

Nutrition and Physical Activity

GUEST EDITORS

Mary Story, PhD, RD

Nicole Larson, PhD, MPH, RD

December 2012 • Volume 23 • Number 3

ADOLESCENT MEDICINE:
STATE OF THE ART REVIEWS
December 2012
Editor: Carrie Peters
Marketing Manager: Marirose Russo
Production Manager: Shannan Martin
eBook Developer: Mark Ruthman
eBook Production Coordinator: Linda J. Atteo

Volume 23, Number 3
ISBN 978-1-58110-603-9
ISSN 1934-4287
MA0595
SUB1006

Adolescent Medicine: State of the Art Reviews is published three times per year by the American Academy of Pediatrics, 141 Northwest Point Blvd, Elk Grove Village, IL 60007-1019. Periodicals postage paid at Arlington Heights, IL.

POSTMASTER: Send address changes to American Academy of Pediatrics, Department of Marketing and Publications, Attn: AM:STARs, 141 Northwest Point Blvd, Elk Grove Village, IL 60007-1019.

Subscriptions: Subscriptions to *Adolescent Medicine: State of the Art Reviews* (AM:STARs) are provided to members of the American Academy of Pediatrics' Section on Adolescent Health as part of annual section membership dues. All others, please contact the AAP Customer Service Center at 866/843-2271 (7:00 am–5:30 pm Central Time, Monday–Friday) for pricing and information.

Adolescent Medicine: State of the Art Reviews

Official Journal of the American Academy of Pediatrics
Section on Adolescent Health

NUTRITION AND PHYSICAL ACTIVITY

EDITORS-IN-CHIEF

VICTOR C. STRASBURGER, MD, Distinguished Professor of Pediatrics, Division of Adolescent Medicine, University of New Mexico School of Medicine, Albuquerque, New Mexico

DONALD E. GREYDANUS, MD, Dr. HC (ATHENS), Professor & Chair, Department of Pediatric & Adolescent Medicine, Western Michigan University School of Medicine, Kalamazoo, Michigan

GUEST EDITORS

MARY STORY, PhD, RD, Professor, Division of Epidemiology and Community Health, Senior Associate Dean for Academic and Student Affairs, School of Public Health, University of Minnesota, Minneapolis, Minnesota

NICOLE LARSON, PhD, MPH, RD, Division of Epidemiology and Community Health, School of Public Health, University of Minnesota, Minneapolis, Minnesota

CONTRIBUTORS

CHRISA ARCAN, PhD, MHS, MBA, RD, Division of Epidemiology and Community Health, School of Public Health, University of Minnesota, Minneapolis, Minnesota

DAHEIA J. BARR-ANDERSON, PhD, MSPH, Department of Epidemiology and Biostatistics, Norman J. Arnold School of Public Health, University of South Carolina, Columbia, South Carolina

JERICA M. BERGE, PhD, MPH, LMFT, CFLE, Assistant Professor, Department of Family Medicine and Community Health, University of Minnesota Medical School, Minneapolis, Minnesota

CARMEN BYKER, PhD, Department of Health and Human Development, Montana State University, Bozeman, Montana

JORDAN A. CARLSON, MA, Doctoral Student in Public Health, University of California, San Diego and San Diego State University, San Diego, California

ISOBEL R. CONTENTO, PhD, Mary Swartz Rose Professor of Nutrition and Education, and Coordinator, Program in Nutrition, Department of Health and Behavior Studies, Teachers College Columbia University, New York, New York

SARAH E. CUSICK, PhD, Assistant Professor, Division of Global Pediatrics, University of Minnesota Medical School, Minneapolis, Minnesota

JEANNE DALEN, PhD, Oregon Research Institute, Eugene, Oregon

SALLY M. DAVIS, PhD, Department of Pediatrics, University of New Mexico School of Medicine, University of New Mexico, Albuquerque, New Mexico

CATHERINE M. GORDON, MD, MSc, Divisions of Adolescent Medicine and Endocrinology, Hasbro Children's Hospital, Warren Alpert Medical School of Brown University, Providence, Rhode Island

PATRICIA C. KEANE, MS, RD, Department of Pediatrics, University of New Mexico School of Medicine, University of New Mexico, Albuquerque, New Mexico

ALBERTA S. KONG, MD, MPH, Department of Pediatrics, University of New Mexico School of Medicine, University of New Mexico, Albuquerque, New Mexico

AMANDA E. KUCH, BA, Medical Student, University of Minnesota Medical School, Minneapolis, Minnesota

NICOLE LARSON, PhD, MPH, RD, Division of Epidemiology and Community Health, School of Public Health, University of Minnesota, Minneapolis, Minnesota

MELISSA N. LASKA, PhD, RD, Division of Epidemiology and Community Health, School of Public Health, University of Minnesota, Minneapolis, Minnesota

NINA S. MA, MD, Division of Endocrinology, Boston Children's Hospital, Harvard Medical School, Boston, Massachusetts

ALEXANDRA M. MIGNANO, BA, Department of Family and Preventive Medicine, University of California, San Diego, California

KATHERINE E. MURRAY, MD, MPH, Department of Pediatrics, University of Minnesota, Minneapolis, Minnesota

SYLVIA NEGRETE, MD, Department of Pediatrics, University of New Mexico School of Medicine, University of New Mexico, Albuquerque, New Mexico

DIANNE NEUMARK-SZTAINER, PhD, MPH, RD, Professor, Division of Epidemiology and Community Health, School of Public Health, University of Minnesota, Minneapolis, Minnesota

COURTNEY A. PINARD, PhD, Gretchen Swanson Center for Nutrition, Omaha, Nebraska, Department of Health Promotion, Social and Behavioral Health, University of Nebraska Medical Center, Omaha, Nebraska

BRIAN E. SAELENS, PhD, Department of Pediatrics and Psychiatry & Behavioral Sciences, University of Washington School of Medicine and Seattle Children's Hospital Research Institute, Seattle, Washington

JAMES F. SALLIS, PhD, Distinguished Professor of Family and Preventive Medicine, University of California, San Diego, California

SARAH G. SANDERS, MS, RN, Department of Pediatrics, University of New Mexico School of Medicine, University of New Mexico, Albuquerque, New Mexico

MARLENE B. SCHWARTZ, PhD, Deputy Director, Rudd Center for Food Policy and Obesity, Yale University, New Haven, Connecticut

SUSAN B. SISSON, PhD, CHES, Department of Nutritional Sciences, University of Oklahoma Health Sciences Center, Oklahoma City, Oklahoma

TERESA M. SMITH, MS, Gretchen Swanson Center for Nutrition, Omaha, Nebraska, Department of Health Promotion, Social and Behavioral Health, University of Nebraska Medical Center, Omaha, Nebraska

NICOLE A. VANKIM, MPH, Division of Epidemiology and Community Health, School of Public Health, University of Minnesota, Minneapolis, Minnesota

AMY L. YAROCH, PhD, Gretchen Swanson Center for Nutrition, Omaha, Nebraska, Department of Health Promotion, Social and Behavioral Health, University of Nebraska Medical Center, Omaha, Nebraska

NUTRITION AND PHYSICAL ACTIVITY

CONTENTS

Adolescence is characterized by dramatic developmental changes within the physical, cognitive, social-emotional, and spiritual/moral domains. This article provides an overview of these changes and implications for eating and physical activity behaviors. Adolescents' diets are low in important nutrients despite high nutritional demands for physical growth. Low levels of physical activity combined with high levels of electronic media use can have a negative impact on well-being, despite the potential benefits of media use in regards to pro-social behavior. Researchers and physicians need to consider developmental context when working with adolescents to support and guide improvements in eating and physical activity behaviors.

The family environment plays an important role in the development and maintenance of adolescents' dietary patterns and physical activity behaviors. Specifically, parenting style, behavior modeling by parents, family support and encouragement, and resources available in the home to support healthful eating and physical activity are key mechanisms through which families can promote or discourage adolescent healthful eating and physical activity. In this article, we review the empirical evidence regarding the role of family environment in adolescents' nutrition and physical activity and suggest corresponding cross-sector intervention strategies to improve adolescents' health behaviors.

Adolesc Med 23 (2012) xv

Preface

Adolescence (ages 11-21) and the transition to adulthood make up one of the most dynamic periods of human development, characterized by dramatic physical, cognitive, social, and emotional changes. The rapid growth that occurs during adolescence is second only to the growth that occurs during the first year of life and increases the body's demand for energy and nutrients. Total nutrient needs are greater during adolescence than at any other time in the lifecycle. Other changes include adolescents' growing independence, identity issues, experimentation, concerns about appearance, and need for social and peer acceptance, all of which can significantly affect their eating and physical activity behaviors, energy balance, and weight status.

Healthy eating and physical activity are essential for good health at every age, but adolescence is an especially critical stage for developing healthy patterns to carry into adulthood. Healthy eating during adolescence can help prevent problems such as iron deficiency, anemia, stunting, poor school performance, and dental caries, and can also promote optimal bone mineral accretion. Regular physical activity improves strength and endurance, builds healthy bones and lean muscle mass, increases cardiorespiratory fitness, reduces body fat, increases energy expenditure, promotes psychological well-being, and reduces feelings of depression and anxiety. Healthy eating and physical activity are both needed to maintain a healthy body weight and are especially important since obesity and overweight are major public health issues that currently affect one-third of adolescents in the United States and an increasing number of youth around the world. Over the long term, healthy eating and physical activity can reduce the risk of developing chronic conditions (eg, heart disease, certain cancers, type 2 diabetes, stroke, and osteoporosis) and reduce risk factors for diseases (eg, obesity, high blood pressure, and high cholesterol).

There is cause for concern because adolescents and young people making the transition to adulthood have dietary intakes that are among the poorest of any age group and have declining levels of physical activity, particularly among females. Physicians, non-physician clinicians, families, and communities can work together to improve the well-being of young people by promoting and creating opportunities for healthy eating and physical activity. Local, state, and federal policies need to be in place to create a supportive environment with accessible and affordable healthy food choices and opportunities for regular physical activity.

This volume of articles focuses on nutrition, eating, and physical activity issues and concerns of adolescents and offers strategies for improving the nutritional health of young people, increasing physical activity, and preventing and treating weight-related disorders.

Mary Story, PhD, RD
Professor, Division of Epidemiology and Community Health
Senior Associate Dean for Academic and Student Affairs
School of Public Health, University of Minnesota

Nicole Larson, PhD, MPH, RD
Division of Epidemiology and Community Health
School of Public Health, University of Minnesota

Adolesc Med 023 (2012) 411–423

The Intersection of Adolescent Development with Eating Behaviors and Physical Activity

Chrisa Arcan, PhD, MHS, MBA, RD[a*], Katherine E. Murray, MD, MPH[b]

[a]*Division of Epidemiology and Community Health, School of Public Health, University of Minnesota,* [b]*Department of Pediatrics, University of Minnesota*

INTRODUCTION

Proper nutrition and physical activity are key to maintaining health at all stages of adolescent development.[1] Thus, patterns of eating and physical activity behaviors among adolescents have been investigated in an effort to understand their association with a number of immediate and long-term health issues such as dental caries, eating disorders, obesity, depression, type 2 diabetes, and osteoporosis. Contextualizing eating and physical activity behavior patterns within a developmental framework is crucial to the design of this research and can help guide the design of effective interventions and strategies to promote healthful eating and physical activity. Adolescence is a particularly dynamic and vulnerable period for the development of unhealthy eating and physical activity behaviors. Despite this inherent developmental vulnerability, positive youth development theory posits the importance of aligning external influences with adolescents' internal strengths to target appropriate strategies and approaches to improve diet and physical activity at each stage.[2] This article aims to understand eating and physical activity behaviors among adolescents in the context of key developmental milestones within the physical, cognitive, social–emotional, and spiritual/moral domains.

DEVELOPMENTAL STAGES AND DOMAINS

Adolescence can be considered a developmental bridge because it is characterized by rapid changes in physical, cognitive, social–emotional, and spiritual/moral domains.[3] Therefore, eating and physical activity behaviors are best

*Corresponding author.
E-mail address: arca0021@umn.edu (C. Arcan).

 ISSN 1934-4287

understood when they are placed into the 3 developmentally distinct age periods (Table 1): early adolescence (11-14 years), middle adolescence (15-17 years), and late adolescence (18-21 years).[1]

Table 1
Psychosocial Processes and the Substages of Adolescent Development

Developmental Domains	Early Adolescence 11-14 years	Middle Adolescence 15-17 years	Late Adolescence 18-21 years
Emotionally Related			
Independence:	Emotional break from parents; decrease in family mealtime	Ambivalence about separation from parents and family	Integration of independence issues; establishment of personal sense of identity; further separation from parents
Body Image:	Adjustment to pubescent changes	"Trying on" different images to find real self	Integration of satisfying body image
Sexual Drives:	Adaptation to emerging sexuality; sexual curiosity	Sexual experimentation; emerging sexual interest in peers	Beginning of intimacy/caring
Cognitively Related			
Conceptualization:	Concrete thinking; inability to link healthy behaviors to future health outcomes	Concrete thinking and development of introspection and abstract thought; expansion of verbal abilities and conventional morality; adjustment to increased school demands	Abstract thinking
Value System:	Drop in superego; testing of moral system of parents	Self-centered	Self-centered idealism; rigid concepts of right and wrong; other oriented, asceticism
Socially Related			
Relationships:	Strong peer effect; unisex peer groups; adult "crushes" (friendships with adults outside the home); increasing exposure to media	Both males and females in the peer group; multiple adult role models; foods develop sociocultural meaning; eating outside the home with peers	Individual relationships more important than peer group; emerging social autonomy

Adapted from Stang J, Story M. Adolescent growth and development. In: *Guidelines for Adolescent Nutrition Services*. Stang J, Story M, eds. Minneapolis, MN: Center for Leadership, Education and Training in Maternal and Child Nutrition, Division of Epidemiology and Community Health, School of Public Health, University of Minnesota; 2005, and Felice ME. Adolescence. In: Levine MD, Carey WB, Crocker AC, eds. *Developmental-Behavioral Pediatrics*. 2nd ed. Philadelphia: WB Saunders, 1992.

During *early adolescence* concrete thinking that is focused on the present is the most dominant cognitive ability, resulting in the inability to link healthy behaviors to future health outcomes. For example, early adolescents tend to think of healthy eating as a short-term effort to meet goals relating to weight or shape weight gain.[4] Also, short-term gratification factors, such as taste preferences, tend to drive eating behavior at this age period. *Middle adolescence* is characterized by the development of abstract and future-oriented thinking. In addition, the quest for emotional autonomy leads to increased detachment from family and closer adherence to peer groups,[1,3,5,6] thus the need for peer acceptance can have a profound effect on adolescents' food choices and physical activity behaviors. *Late adolescence* is characterized by strong personal identity formation. Adolescents during this period continue to strengthen their ability for abstract thinking, are less likely to be influenced by peers, and more likely to be influenced by single individual relationships.[1] As adolescents develop more independence, family influences and conflicts over eating and physical activity diminish. Adolescents' new focus is on personal and vocational decisions.[5]

PHYSICAL GROWTH AND DEVELOPMENT

The rate of growth that occurs during adolescence is second only to the growth that occurs during infancy. The biological and physical transformations that occur over a period of several years place a high demand on the adolescent body for increased energy and nutrients. In fact, adolescence is the period with the greatest nutritional needs compared to any other time in the life cycle.[5]

The beginning of adolescence is marked by the onset of puberty and is characterized by numerous biological and physical changes, including sexual maturation, gains in height and weight, and the completion of skeletal growth.[1] About 80% of physical growth (attained height and weight) occurs between the ages 10 and 15 years, and 45% of skeletal mass is gained during adolescence.[7,8] Although all adolescents go through these stages, there is great variation in the onset, duration, and rate that these changes occur; thus, given the stage of physical development, adolescents of the same age can have vastly different nutritional needs.[1] The rapid physical growth that occurs especially during early adolescence increases energy requirements for all adolescents; however, because of differences in the body composition of males (higher proportion of muscle mass) and females (higher proportion of fat mass), there are gender differences in nutrient needs.[1] Females go through physical maturation at an earlier age than males, which increases their protein requirements more than males during early adolescence (10-14 years). However, during middle and late adolescence, males have higher protein needs than females because of higher gain in muscle and skeletal mass.[9]

The rapid rate of skeletal, muscular, and endocrine changes increases the demand for mineral intake (eg, iron, calcium). During periods of peak growth and sexual maturation, which occur in early adolescence, iron requirements are highest for both males and females. About a year after the peak growth period when menstruation begins, females also have increased iron requirements to replace losses, and it is recommended they consume 13 to 15 mg/day.[10] Iron-deficiency anemia as a result of inadequate iron intake is one of the most common diet-related deficiency diseases, and pregnant adolescents, vegetarians, and competitive athletes are particularly susceptible.[11]

Adequate intake of dietary calcium and vitamin D during adolescence reduces risk for fractures and promotes adult bone health and the prevention of osteoporosis, especially among females.[12] During the peak growth spurt, daily calcium deposition can be almost double that of the average deposition between the ages 10 and 20 years. Because up to 95% of total bone mass is gained by the end of late adolescence, it is important to maximize bone mineral content during this period to help prevent osteoporosis.[12] To support the development of peak bone mass, it is recommended that adolescents consume 1300 mg/day of calcium, which is the equivalent of 4 glasses of milk each day. However, in the past 4 decades, milk consumption among adolescents has declined by 50% to an average consumption of 1 glass per day.[13] During the same period, consumption of sugar-sweetened beverages has dramatically increased and replaced milk and water.[14] Soda consumption may also interfere with calcium absorption because of the high content of phosphorus in soda.[11] In a longitudinal study of adolescents 8 through 14 years of age, replacing milk intake with soft drink was correlated with lower bone mineral accrual, and increasing intake of fruit and vegetables resulted in higher bone mineral content among females only.[15]

Nutrient absorption may vary based on adolescents' weight status. For example, studies have shown that obese adolescents have lower mean serum levels of vitamin D than nonobese youth, and low levels of serum vitamin D were associated with insulin resistance among obese adolescents.[16] These findings indicate the importance of both healthy eating and optimal body weight for the maintenance of immediate health and prevention of chronic disease such as type 2 diabetes.

Because pubertal changes are characterized by a milieu of internal hormonal changes and significantly alter the outward appearance of the body, this creates a dynamic personal environment for the developing adolescent. Changes in body fat proportion, secondary sex characteristics, and muscle mass can intersect in dramatic ways with eating behaviors and physical activity patterns. Leptin communicates adequacy of energy stores to meet the demands of pubertal development.[17] Estrogen, growth hormone, and insulin-like growth factor-1 promote insulin resistance, which, in turn, increases circulating insulin levels and leads to increased adiposity during adolescence.[17] Overall, maturation leads to an increase in fat mass without commensurate increases in muscle or skeletal mass.[18]

Overweight and obesity rates in the United States continue to grow. In the past 3 decades, the rate of obesity among adolescents between the ages of 12 and 19 years has increased from 5% to 18.1%.[19] The effects of obesity extend beyond physical health and include social stigma that results in detrimental psychosocial consequences for the growing adolescent.[20] The social consequences of obesity are manifested through weight bias, teasing, and discrimination in various social environments, including schools, workplaces, health care settings, and even within the family home.[20] A large study of racially diverse adolescents found a high prevalence of weight teasing across all racial/ethnic groups; however, among girls who were teased, fewer black and mixed or other race females were bothered by peer teasing, compared to white females.

Pubertal changes may contribute to the declines in physical activity, particularly among females, during adolescence. The short- and long-term benefits of regular physical activity have been well documented.[21] Physical activity helps build and maintain healthy bones and muscles, helps reduce the risk of developing obesity and chronic diseases, and helps reduce feelings of depression and anxiety.[21,22] Although national guidelines recommend at least 60 minutes/day of moderate to vigorous physical activity, adolescents tend to reduce their physical activity levels as they age, and this is more profound among females.[23-26] Beginning as early as 10 years, adolescents reduce their physical activity levels by as much as 50%. A prospective study of white and black adolescent females found that by the age of 16 or 17 years, more than one-half of black and one-third of white females reported not engaging in leisure-time physical activity.[27] According to national data, a little more than one-third of high-school males and only 18.5% of high-school females engaged in moderate to vigorous physical activity for at least 60 minutes on each of the 7 days before the survey.[23] Proposed etiologies for the decline in physical activity include pubertal changes, fatigue, and body discomfort.[28] There is mixed evidence regarding the role of pubertal timing in the decline of physical activity, with some studies showing this decline to parallel the increase in biological age, especially in females,[24,28,29] while another study showed no correlation between pubertal timing and decline in physical activity.[18] However, due to variations in the measurement of pubertal development and timing and measures of physical activity, direct comparison of these studies is not possible.

Among early adolescent females, other possible etiologies that have been considered to explain declines in physical activity are low perceived competence, lack of opportunities, high perceived exertion, concern about physical appearance, and threats to females' gender identity; however, low perceived competence has been most frequently reported as the main reason for the decline of physical activity.[18,28] Other studies have found that physical activity was associated with self-efficacy, enjoyment, autonomous motivation, and need satisfaction.[26,30,31] Therefore, the internal belief about competence and likelihood of success along with strong internal motivation correlate with maintenance of physical activity. Internal motivation for physical activity for enjoyment or demonstration of competence is protective against other influences that may be corrosive to this activity. In one study, for example, girls who were participating in physical activity with a focus on appearance and fitness decreased their level of activity because of social evaluation of their physique with pubertal maturation. Girls who were participating for enjoyment and competence registered no such decline in physical activity.[32]

COGNITIVE DEVELOPMENT

One of the most dramatic areas of adolescent development is the neurodevelopmental change that occurs during the transition from childhood to adulthood. The emerging prefrontal cortex development is a lengthy process that continues throughout adolescence and into early adulthood.[33] Adolescents experience dramatic shifts in their ability to reason, understand, and recognize their personal identity.[10,34] In fact, the level of maturity is more important than age in predicting responsible decision making. It is found that during middle adolescence, the level of maturity of judgment may drop before it increases again in late adolescence.[34] These cognitive changes differentially influence adolescents' ability to comprehend the health benefits of nutrition and physical activity behaviors as well as to recognize the persuasive intent of marketing techniques. Because early adolescents have not fully developed their ability for abstract reasoning, they experience more challenges in overcoming barriers to behavior change and rarely link their current eating behaviors to future health outcomes.[9] Abstract thinking begins to develop during middle adolescence, which increases the ability to better appreciate future health consequences of current behavior. However, adolescents during this stage of development are mostly preoccupied with fitting in with a particular peer group, and thus peer pressure is a major determining factor of their eating behaviors.[9] With further development of abstract thinking skills, late adolescents are able to understand the long-term effects of their current behavior and more easily overcome barriers to behavior change.[9]

The different stages of cognitive development have a dramatic effect on the degree that children and adolescents are being influenced by marketing techniques and media messages. As marketers recognize that brand loyalty and product preference begins at an early age, they tailor their marketing techniques to fit the appropriate developmental stage.[35] Jean Piaget's theory of cognitive development—preoperational thought (2-7 years), concrete operational thought (7-11 years), and formal operational thought (12 years and older)—is widely used to explain age-based differences in the way children comprehend television and media content.[36] The development of *formal operational thought* begins at age 12 years with the advent of analytical thinking. Adolescents are able to clearly distinguish the multidimensional nature of products and are more familiar with advertising practices and brand names as their analytical reasoning skills develop.[35] However, despite clearly understanding product attributes and advertising motives, adolescents can be influenced to purchase certain products if they are appealing enough.

One of the characteristics consistent with adolescent development, especially during the early stages, is the binary manner in which adolescents perceive their environment. As a result, adolescents tend to dichotomize foods into "good" or "bad" and "tasty" or "tasteless" categories and fail to recognize the nuances of portion size, nutrient-to-calorie ratios, and individual rates of caloric expenditures.[4] What is lacking in this simplistic interpretation is the understanding of dynamism and the fluidity of concepts. For example, adolescents may fail to consider the caloric needs and the type of diet required by 2 individuals with extreme differences in physical activity. Physicians and nutrition educators need to be cognizant of adolescents' polar categorizations of foods and how this may affect eating patterns.

SOCIAL AND EMOTIONAL DEVELOPMENT

The dramatic biological changes that occur during puberty can have a profound effect on adolescents' emotional development and their preoccupation with their appearance and body image. The timing of the onset of puberty can be a source of emotional turmoil, especially for adolescents who experience a delay in their biological growth and development.[9] As peer groups gain center stage in the lives of adolescents, physical and biological growth become focal points for comparisons with peers.

Although increased body size may enhance males' body image, the opposite is true among females. A wide spectrum of body image disorders, including declines in perceived attractiveness and physical self-worth, and increases in disordered eating behaviors develop among females and early pubertal timing seems to be a risk factor.[18,37] Conversely, males with a slower rate of development tend to be at higher risk for negative body image disorders.

Identity Development

The process of *identity development* that begins during middle adolescence and continues through late adolescence is an integral force that influences teens' perceptions of food, eating, and physical activity behaviors. One of the developmental tenets of adolescence is the presence of teen "rebellion," or oppositionality and limit-testing. Despite these terms, such patterns of behavior suggest a need for an independent identity and an internal sense of control rather than outright rebellion against parental norms.[4] Perhaps this is pointing to a more nuanced understanding of the increasingly outmoded concepts of "rebellion" and its opposite "conformity." Conformity is a willingness to adhere to external norms without regard to internal wishes or influences. Current literature suggests conformity is balanced against a newer concept, "connectedness," that better captures a balance between self-determination and sensitivity to the influence of others. In a recent study, it was connectedness, rather than conformity, that protected adolescents from internalized negative body image.[38] Research suggests that individuals at this stage of development are best served by a sense of self-control and connectedness rather than obedience and conformity.

The Role of Peer Groups

During the period of dramatic emotional change and search for inner self, adolescents strive for acceptance and peer groups provide a sense of belongingness which helps attenuate feelings of alienation.[39] Starting in early adolescence, peer groups may have more influence than family in food choices of adolescents. Because food and eating occasions have multiple meanings, adolescents may use food to express independence, belongingness to a peer group, identity, or rebelliousness against the status quo. For adolescents, consumption of certain foods can help them project an identity, support an image, and express kinship with a desired peer group.[40] In qualitative studies, middle adolescents reported selecting food brands that are well known, popular, and socially acceptable to "fit in." Adolescents also reported that selecting healthy foods or "budget" foods would be socially risky as they would be teased as "geeky," "nerdy," or untrendy.[40]

Unfortunately, with the newly gained independence, including financial independence, adolescents tend to increase consumption of convenience and fast foods that are high in calories, fat, sugars, and sodium. A large study of ethnically diverse adolescents found the percentage of adolescents who ate at fast-food restaurants 3 times or more a week almost doubled to about 30% as they transitioned from early to middle adolescence.[41] The feelings of being accepted, being with their friends, and having fun are strong factors that determine adolescents' preferences for food and sources. As Newman and colleagues suggest, the feeling of belonging is positively correlated with overall health and happiness.[39] The challenge therefore of physicians and nonphysician clinicians is to help adolescents meet their nutritional needs and eat healthy while recognizing the power of food in building strong bonds and emotional well-being.[40]

Engaging in exercise with friends rather than with family becomes more important for adolescents.[42] Friends provide modeling, shared experiences, and introduction to new experiences,[26] as peer social support has been found to predict physical activity behaviors.[26,33,43,44] Identity development and peer relationships can sometimes be self-reinforcing; for example, obesity and body dissatisfaction have been prospectively associated with decreases in popularity.[33,45] Body image is also affected by direct feedback from peers through explicit teasing and negative feedback or comments made by a romantic partner.[37,46]

Adolescents use multiple venues to learn, communicate, and foster group and individual relationships. Electronic media has become a dominant form of communication, including instant and text messaging, and Internet sites such as blogs and social networks. In addition to helping adolescents stay connected with multiple peer groups, these communication media are used to share information about products and events. Food marketers in particular use multiple media venues to expose children and adolescents to repeated messages leading to the development of strong brand loyalty that is an integral part of peer connections. In addition to the persuasive nature of electronic media, its use has been associated with lower levels of physical activity, quality of life, and quality of family relationships among adolescents of all ages.[47,48] A systematic review found that watching TV for more than 2 hours per day was associated with decreased fitness and lowered scores for self-esteem, and lowering sedentary activities resulted in reductions in body mass index.[49] However, most studies indicated that electronic media use was positively associated with peer relationships or pro-social behavior.[48,49] As electronic media use becomes more ubiquitous, health interventions must include media literacy to effectively address the positive and negative influences of the new technologies on the overall health of children and adolescents.

Especially during middle adolescence, as the search for inner self grows and peer groups gain prominence, the influence of parents may appear diminished, but parents remain an important source of influence mostly through modeling, support in decision making, and setting and maintaining boundaries when necessary.[37,46] Parents can influence adolescents' body image and promote healthy lifestyles through modeling, establishing routines and rituals, and making healthful foods available at home.[37,50-52] In a study of middle school students, family meals were associated with fewer skipped meals, less fast food consumption in males, and improved nutrition 5 years later.[53] Parental support of physical activity was found to also increase the likelihood of being physically active among a large sample of high school students.[43]

MORAL AND SPIRITUAL DEVELOPMENT

Spirituality and religion are important aspects in the lives of adolescents. Adolescents in different stages of development try to explore the concepts of existence and the meaning of life.[54] In a study among adolescents and young adults (11-25 years), 90% reported religion was at least somewhat important in their lives.[55] In another study of freshmen in 236 colleges and universities in the United States, about 80% reported that they were "spiritual beings" or they had an interest in spirituality.[56] Both family and friends are strong influencing factors for spirituality among adolescents.[54] Although few studies exist that explore the association between spirituality and health behaviors, review studies have found spirituality to be associated with positive health outcomes and physical health.[57] In a large study of young adolescents, spiritual or religious beliefs were associated with a range of positive health behaviors, including greater intake of fruits and vegetables.[58]

As adolescents progress through the process of cognitive development, they develop their sense for moral reasoning, empathy, and volunteerism.[34] Morality refers to the way people choose to live their lives based on a set of values or principles.[34] With the growth of abstract thinking, adolescents begin to question the rules set by others and start making behavior choices based on their newly developed moral judgment. Because food and eating occasions take center stage as an expression of independence and social behavior, adolescents develop opinions based on moralistic notions when considering certain foods such as those sold at fast food restaurants.[59] With the worldwide increase in the prevalence of obesity and its association with eating behaviors and the larger food environment, consumption of convenience and fast food is often viewed as "unhealthy" or "bad."[59] This moralistic view of eating behavior has been found in studies with both adolescents and adults when evaluating and consuming ready-to-eat and fast food meals.[59,60] In a qualitative study, 13- to 19-year-old Canadian adolescents indicated that they either refrained from eating at fast-food restaurants because they considered it unhealthy or they continued consuming it despite feelings of guilt.[59] It is uncertain whether negative moral attitudes about consuming unhealthy foods that are developed during adolescence carry over into adulthood; however, studies among adults, including late adolescents, have shown that intentions to eat convenience meals were partially explained by moral attitudes.[61]

CONCLUSIONS

The importance of contextualizing eating and physical activity behaviors within the framework of adolescent development is supported by an expanding evidence base. Adolescents bridge key developmental milestones and are in an active stage of physical growth as well as cognitive and psychosocial development. These developmental contexts provide a framework for understanding the many factors that influence adolescent eating and physical activity behaviors. The process of identity formation and the quest for independence are 2 important characteristics of adolescent development that transcend many areas of youth behavior. For example, as young adolescents become aware of their social behavior, their food choices are more influenced by their peer groups than by their parents. Furthermore, adolescents—in their effort to communicate and foster new relationships—tend to embrace new communication methods. Therefore, the explosion of electronic media has a great effect, both positive and negative, on the way adolescents communicate, learn, and create. With the advent of abstract thinking, middle adolescents begin to question the rules set by others and start developing their moral view of their behavior and that of others. Thus, adolescents often select foods or refrain from eating certain foods considered "bad" or "unhealthy" based on their newly developed moral judgment. It is important that physicians and educators consider the specific developmental stage of adolescents when developing messages to improve dietary and physical activity behaviors.

References

1. Stang J, Story M. Adolescent growth and development. In: Stang J, Story M, eds. *Guidelines for Adolescent Nutrition Services*. Minneapolis, MN: Center for Leadership, Education and Training in Maternal and Child Nutrition, Division of Epidemiology and Community Health, School of Public Health, University of Minnesota; 2005:1
2. Lerner J, Phelps E, Forman Y, Bowers E. Positive youth development. In: Lerner R, Steinberg L, eds. *Handbook of Adolescent Psychology*. 3rd ed. Hoboken, NJ: John Wiley and Sons; 2009:524

3. Dixon S, Stein M. *Encounters with Children.* 4th ed. St. Louis, MO: Mosby; 2006
4. Stevenson C, Doherty G, Barnett J, Muldoon OT, Trew K. Adolescents' views of food and eating: Identifying barriers to healthy eating. *J Adolesc.* 2007;30(3):417-434
5. American Academy of Pediatrics. Adolescence. In: Holt I, Wooldridge N, Story S, Sofka D, eds. *Bright Futures: Nutrition.* 3rd ed. Elk Grove Village, IL: American Academy of Pediatrics; 2011
6. DiClementa RJ, Santelli JS, Crosby RA (eds). *Adolescent Health Understanding and Preventing Risk Behaviors.* San Francisco: San Francisco: Jossey-Bass; 2009.
7. World Health Organization (WHO). Adolescent nutrition: A neglected dimension. Available at: https://apps.who.int/nut/ado.htm. Accessed August 25, 2012
8. Story M. Nutritional requirements during adolescence. In: McAnarney E, Kreipe R, Orr D, Comerci G, eds. *Textbook of Adolescent Medicine.* Philadelphia, PA: W.B. Saunders; 1992:75-84
9. Story M, Stang J. Understanding adolescent eating behaviors. In: Stang J, Story M, eds. *Guidelines for Adolescent Nutrition Services.* Minneapolis, MN: Center for Leadership, Education and Training in Maternal and Child Nutrition, Division of Epidemiology and Community Health, School of Public Health, University of Minnesota; 2005:9
10. Story M, Stang J. Nutrition needs of adolescents. In: Stang J, Story M, eds. *Guidelines for Adolescent Nutrition Services.* Minneapolis, MN: Center for Leadership, Education and Training in Maternal and Child Nutrition, Division of Epidemiology and Community Health, School of Public Health, University of Minnesota; 2005:21
11. California Department of Public Health. California nutrition and physical activity guidelines for adolescents. Available at: http://www.cdph.ca.gov/HealthInfo/healthyliving/childfamily/Documents/MO-NUPA-01AdolescentNutrition.pdf. Updated 2012. Accessed August 20, 2012
12. Lytle LA. Nutritional issues for adolescents. *J Am Diet Assoc.* 2002;102(3 Suppl):S8-12
13. Sebastian R, Goldman J, Wilkinson E, LaComb R. Fluid milk consumption in the United States: What we eat in America, NHANES 2005-2006. September 2010; Dietary Data Brief No. 3 Available at: http://www.ars.usda.gov/SP2UserFiles/Place/12355000/pdf/DBrief/3_milk_consumption_0506.pdf. Accessed October 31, 2012.
14. Centers for Disease Control and Prevention (CDC). Beverage consumption among high school students—United States, 2010. *MMWR.* 2011;60(23):778-780
15. Whiting SJ, Vatanparast H, Baxter-Jones A, Faulkner RA, Mirwald R, Bailey DA. Factors that affect bone mineral accrual in the adolescent growth spurt. *J Nutr.* 2004;134(3):696S-700S
16. Olson ML, Maalouf NM, Oden JD, White PC, Hutchison MR. Vitamin D deficiency in obese children and its relationship to glucose homeostasis. *J Clin Endocrinol Metab.* 2012;97(1):279-285
17. Jasik CB, Lustig RH. Adolescent obesity and puberty: the "perfect storm." *Ann N Y Acad Sci.* 2008;1135:265-279
18. Knowles AM, Niven AG, Fawkner SG, Henretty JM. A longitudinal examination of the influence of maturation on physical self-perceptions and the relationship with physical activity in early adolescent girls. *J Adolesc.* 2009;32(3):555-566
19. Ogden C, Carroll C. Prevalence of obesity among children and adolescents: United states, trends 1963–1965 through 2007–2008. Division of health and nutrition examination surveys. CDC national center for health statistics. Available at: http://www.cdc.gov/nchs/data/hestat/obesity_child_07_08/obesity_child_07_08.pdf. Updated 2010. Accessed August 7, 2012
20. Washington RL. Childhood obesity: issues of weight bias. *Prev Chronic Dis.* 2011;8(5):A94
21. Warburton DE, Nicol CW, Bredin SS. Health benefits of physical activity: the evidence. *CMAJ.* 2006;174(6):801-809. Available at: http://www.health.gov/paguidelines/committeereport.aspx. Accessed October 31, 2012.
22. Physical Activity Guidelines Advisory Committee. *Physical Activity Guidelines Advisory Committee Report, 2008.* Available at: http://www.health.gov/paguidelines/committeereport.aspx. Accessed October 31, 2012.
23. Eaton DK, Kann L, Kinchen S, et al; Centers for Disease Control and Prevention (CDC). Youth risk behavior surveillance—United States, 2011. *MMWR* Surveill Summ. 2012;61(SS-4):1-162
24. Bradley RH, McRitchie S, Houts RM, Nader P, O'Brien M, NICHD Early Child Care Research Network. Parenting and the decline of physical activity from age 9 to 15. *Int J Behav Nutr Phys Act.* 2011;8:33

25. Wareham NJ, Corder K, van Sluijs EM. Decrease in activity from childhood to adolescence: potential causes and consequences. *Am J Prev Med.* 2008;35(6):604-605
26. Duncan SC, Duncan TE, Strycker LA, Chaumeton NR. A cohort-sequential latent growth model of physical activity from ages 12 to 17 years. *An of Behav Med.* 2007;33(1):80-89
27. Kimm SY, Glynn NW, Kriska AM, et al. Decline in physical activity in black girls and white girls during adolescence. *N Engl J Med.* 2002;347(10):709-715
28. Davison KK, Deane GD. The consequence of encouraging girls to be active for weight loss. *Soc Sci Med.* 2010;70(4):518-525
29. Baker BL, Birch LL, Trost SG, Davison KK. Advanced pubertal status at age 11 and lower physical activity in adolescent girls. *J Pediatr.* 2007;151(5):488-493
30. Gillison FB, Standage M, Skevington SM. Motivation and body-related factors as discriminators of change in adolescents' exercise behavior profiles. *J Adolesc Health.* 2011;48(1):44-51
31. Barr Anderson DJ, Young DR, Sallis JF, et al. Structured physical activity and psychosocial correlates in middle-school girls. *Prev Med.* 2007;44(5):404-409
32. Niven AG, Fawkner SG, Knowles AM, Stephenson C. Maturational differences in physical self-perceptions and the relationship with physical activity in early adolescent girls. *Pediatr Exerc Sci.* 2007;19(4):472-480
33. Esposito L, Fisher JO, Mennella JA, Hoelscher DM, Huang TT. Developmental perspectives on nutrition and obesity from gestation to adolescence. *Prev Chronic Dis.* 2009;6(3):A94
34. Gentry J, Campbell M. *Developing Adolescents: A Reference for Professionals.* Washington, DC: American Psychological Association; 2002. Available at: http://www.apa.org/pi/pii/develop.pdf. Accessed October 31, 2012.
35. Calvert SL. Children as consumers: Advertising and marketing. *Future Child.* 2008;18(1):205-234
36. Flavell J. *The Developmental Psychology of Jean Piaget.* Princeton, NJ: Van Nostrand; 1963
37. Markey CN. Invited commentary: why body image is important to adolescent development. *J Youth Adolesc.* 2010;39(12):1387-1391
38. Vartanian LR, Hopkinson MM. Social connectedness, conformity, and internalization of societal standards of attractiveness. *Body Image.* 2010;7(1):86-89
39. Newman BM, Lohman BJ, Newman PR. Peer group membership and a sense of belonging: their relationship to adolescent behavior problems. *Adolescence.* 2007;42(166):241-263
40. Stead M, McDermott L, Mackintosh AM, Adamson A. Why healthy eating is bad for young people's health: identity, belonging and food. *Soc Sci Med.* 2011;72(7):1131-1139
41. Bauer KW, Larson NI, Nelson MC, Story M, Neumark-Sztainer D. Fast food intake among adolescents: secular and longitudinal trends from 1999 to 2004. *Prev Med.* 2009;48(3):284-287
42. Dunton GF, Berrigan D, Ballard Barbash R, Perna FM, Graubard BI, Atienza AA. Adolescents' sports and exercise environments in a U.S. time use survey. *Am J Prev Med.* 2010;39(2):122-129
43. Williams SL, Mummery WK. Links between adolescent physical activity, body mass index, and adolescent and parent characteristics. *Health Educ Behav.* 2011;38(5):510-520
44. Craggs C, Corder K, van Sluijs EM, Griffin SJ. Determinants of change in physical activity in children and adolescents: a systematic review. *Am J Prev Med.* 2011;40(6):645-658
45. Rancourt D, Prinstein MJ. Peer status and victimization as possible reinforcements of adolescent girls' and boys' weight-related behaviors and cognitions. *J Pediatr Psychol.* 2010;35(4):354-367
46. Power TG, Bindler RC, Goetz S, Daratha KB. Obesity prevention in early adolescence: student, parent, and teacher views. *J Sch Health.* 2010;80(1):13-19
47. Marshall SJ, Biddle SJ, Gorely T, Cameron N, Murdey I. Relationships between media use, body fatness and physical activity in children and youth: a meta-analysis. *Int J Obes Relat Metab Disord.* 2004;28(10):1238-1246
48. Iannotti RJ, Kogan MD, Janssen I, Boyce WF. Patterns of adolescent physical activity, screen-based media use, and positive and negative health indicators in the U.S. and Canada. *J Adolesc Health.* 2009;44(5):493-499
49. Tremblay MS, LeBlanc AG, Kho ME, et al. Systematic review of sedentary behaviour and health indicators in school-aged children and youth. *Int J Behav Nutr Phys Act.* 2011;8:98

50. Merten MJ, Williams AL, Shriver LH. Breakfast consumption in adolescence and young adulthood: parental presence, community context, and obesity. *J Am Diet Assoc.* 2009;109(8):1384-1391
51. Hanson NI, Neumark-Sztainer D, Eisenberg ME, Story M, Wall M. Associations between parental report of the home food environment and adolescent intakes of fruits, vegetables and dairy foods. *Public Health Nutr.* 2005;8(1):77-85
52. Arcan C, Neumark-Sztainer D, Hannan P, van den Berg P, Story M, Larson N. Parental eating behaviours, home food environment and adolescent intakes of fruits, vegetables and dairy foods: longitudinal findings from project EAT. *Public Health Nutr.* 2007;10(11):1257-1265
53. Burgess Champoux TL, Larson N, Neumark-Sztainer D, Hannan PJ, Story M. Are family meal patterns associated with overall diet quality during the transition from early to middle adolescence? *J Nutr Educ Behav.* 2009;41(2):79-86
54. Shek DT. Spirituality as a positive youth development construct: a conceptual review. *ScientificWorldJournal.* 2012;2012:458953 Epub 2012 Apr 24.
55. Holder DW, DuRant RH, Harris TL, Daniel JH, Obeidallah D, Goodman E. The association between adolescent spirituality and voluntary sexual activity. *J Adolesc Health.* 2000;26(4):295-302
56. Astin A, Astin H, Lindholm J, Bryant A, Szelenyi K, Calderone S. The spiritual life of college students: A national study of college students' search for meaning and purpose, 2005, Los Angeles: Higher Education Research Institute, UCLA. Available at: http://spirituality.ucla.edu/docs/reports/Spiritual_Life_College_Students_Full_Report.pdf. Accessed August 25, 2012
57. Powell LH, Shahabi L, Thoresen CE. Religion and spirituality. Linkages to physical health. *Am Psychol.* 2003;58(1):36-52
58. Lytle LA, Varnell S, Murray DM, et al. Predicting adolescents' intake of fruits and vegetables. *J Nutr Educ Behav.* 2003;35(4):170-175
59. McPhail D, Chapman GE, Beagan BL. "Too much of that stuff can't be good": Canadian teens, morality, and fast food consumption. *Soc Sci Med.* 2011;73(2):301-307
60. Arvola A, Vassallo M, Dean M, et al. Predicting intentions to purchase organic food: the role of affective and moral attitudes in the theory of planned behaviour. *Appetite.* 2008;50(2-3):443-454
61. Olsen NV, Sijtsema SJ, Hall G. Predicting consumers' intention to consume ready-to-eat meals: the role of moral attitude. *Appetite.* 2010;55(3):534-539

Adolesc Med 023 (2012) 424–439

Familial Influences on Adolescents' Eating and Physical Activity Behaviors

Jerica M. Berge, PhD, MPH, LMFT, CFLE*[a], Brian E. Saelens, PhD[b]

[a]*Department of Family Medicine and Community Health, University of Minnesota Medical School, Minneapolis, MN 55455*

[b]*Department of Pediatrics and Psychiatry & Behavioral Sciences, University of Washington School of Medicine and Seattle Children's Hospital Research Institute, Seattle, WA 98121*

Research suggests that the family environment plays a key role in the development and maintenance of adolescent dietary intake and physical activity behaviors. Specifically, parenting style, family support and encouragement, behavior modeling by parents, and resources available in the home are important mechanisms through which families promote, or discourage, physical activity and healthful eating.[1,2] Healthful dietary intake (eg, consuming 5 fruits and vegetables per day) and physical activity (eg, engaging in 60 minutes of moderate-to-vigorous physical activity per day) are part of the overall energy balance that shapes adolescent weight status and long-term health.[3,4] Given that approximately one-third of adolescents in the United States are overweight or obese,[5] and the negative physical[4,6] and mental[7-9] health concerns associated with obesity, it is important to understand how familial factors influence dietary and physical activity behaviors in adolescents to achieve a healthy energy balance.

Identifying familial factors that contribute to, or are barriers to, adolescents' physical activity and eating behaviors can inform strategies to improve these behaviors. In this article we review evidence about familial influences on adolescents' weight and weight-related behaviors; highlight areas of needed research; and discuss strategies that parents, physicians, and policy makers should consider implementing to improve familial support for adolescents to engage in healthy eating and physical activity behaviors.

*Corresponding author.
E-mail address: mohl0009@umn.edu (J. M. Berge).

 ISSN 1934-4287

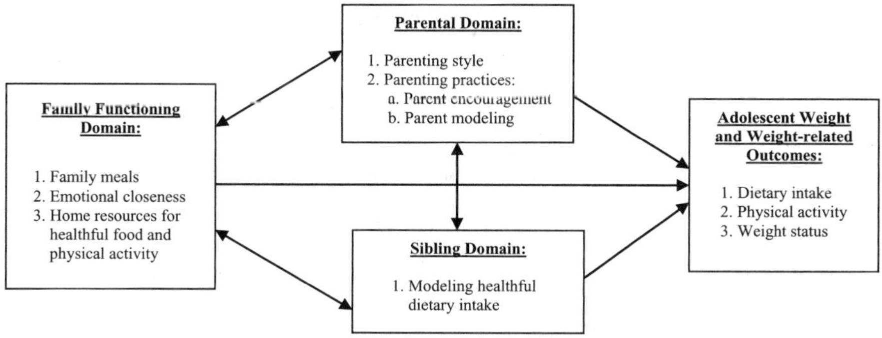

Fig 1. Potential pathways between domains in the family home environment and adolescent dietary intake, physical activity, and weight status. From Berge JM. A review of familial correlates of child and adolescent obesity: what has the 21st century taught us so far? *Int J Adolesc Med Health.* 2009; 21(4):457-483

FAMILY SYSTEMS THEORY

Family systems theory posits that families live in complex systems in which multiple reciprocal interactions occur simultaneously,[10-12] such that each family member is shaping and being shaped by other family members' actions all of the time. For example, health behaviors occur within a family system that either supports and models them, or downplays their importance. Figure 1 depicts multiple domains within the family system and potential relationships between familial weight-related behaviors and adolescent weight and these behaviors.

FAMILIAL INFLUENCES ON ADOLESCENTS' DIETARY INTAKE AND PHYSICAL ACTIVITY

Parent Domain

Parenting style and parenting practices are parental characteristics that can shape adolescent dietary and physical activity behaviors. Parenting style is considered a stable characteristic of parenting and contributes to the daily environmental and emotional context for child rearing (Fig 2). The 4 classic parenting styles are: authoritative, authoritarian, permissive, and neglectful.[13] Parenting style is defined by 2 dimensions: (a) the degree of responsiveness; and (b) the degree of demandingness of the parent.[14] Responsiveness is the extent to which a parent fosters individuality, self-regulation, and self-assertion in their child by being attuned to meeting their child's needs and demands. Whereas, demandingness is the extent to which parents cultivate self-control and responsibility in their child through parental supervision, rules/structure, and disciplinary efforts. For example, an authoritative parent balances high levels of demandingness with high levels of responsiveness.

	High Demandingness	Low Demandingness
High Responsiveness	**Authoritative** Empathic and respectful of child's opinions, but maintains clear boundaries/expectations	**Permissive** Empathic, but indulgent without discipline
Low Responsiveness	**Authoritarian** Low warmth and strict discipline	**Neglectful** Emotionally uninvolved and does not set rules or have expectations

Fig 2. Parenting styles. Adapted from Baumrind D. Rearing competent children. In Damon W (ed). *Child development today and tomorrow.* San Francisco: Jossey-Bass; 1989:349-378

Across a variety of behaviors, an authoritative parenting style is believed to provide the structure and support needed for children to internalize and maintain positive behaviors, whereas authoritarian, permissive, and neglectful parenting styles may interfere with children's ability to learn self-regulation, including regulation of eating and physical activity behaviors.[14]

Parenting practices are considered state dependent, changing based on the context, and include specific strategies used by parents to socialize their children through direct (eg, encouraging) and indirect (eg, modeling) behaviors. Parental practices related to health behaviors include verbal encouragement, logistical support, modeling behaviors, and participating in behaviors with the adolescent. For example, when families eat meals or are active together, parents are providing a time and place where adolescents can eat healthful (or unhealthful) foods or be active and thus are encouraging, supporting, and reinforcing adolescents' food and physical activity choices.

Parenting Style Cross-sectional studies in adolescents consistently find that authoritative parenting style is associated with lower body mass index (BMI); greater availability of fruit and vegetables in the home; higher consumption of fruits, vegetables, and dairy products; and lower consumption of sugar-sweetened beverages.[1,15-18] In contrast, authoritarian and neglectful parenting styles are more often associated with higher adolescent BMI, higher availability of sweets and unhealthy foods in the home, and lower vegetable consumption.[1,17-22]

Longitudinal studies have found that, compared to youth of authoritative mothers, those with authoritarian mothers had an increased risk of overweight, and adolescents of permissive and neglectful mothers were twice as likely to be overweight.[23-25] Additionally, longitudinal studies have shown that authoritative parenting style predicted higher fruit and vegetable intake and family meal consumption in adolescents 5 years later.[25,26] Few studies have looked simultaneously at the influence of mothers' and fathers' parenting style on adolescent weight and weight-related behaviors. Berge et al looked at both the independent and combined relationships between mothers' and fathers' parenting style and adolescent BMI. They found a negative association between authoritative parenting style and adolescent boys' BMI and a positive interaction between maternal authoritarian parenting style and paternal neglectful parenting style that predicted higher BMI in boys.[1]

Findings are more limited and inconsistent regarding parenting style and adolescent physical activity.[2,15,17] However, consistent with authoritative parenting style, parent rules around limiting TV and other screen time is related to lower adolescent sedentary behavior.[27]

In summary, several cross-sectional and longitudinal studies have indicated that adolescents who have parents that are both warm/responsive and demanding/set limits (ie, authoritative parenting style) have a higher intake of healthful foods, lower intake of unhealthful foods, reduced risk of overweight/obesity, and lower levels of sedentary behavior. The relationship between parenting style and adolescents' physical activity remains unclear.

Parenting Practices

Parent Support and Encouragement for Healthful Dietary Intake and Physical Activity Adolescents' fruit and vegetable consumption has been closely linked to parental support and encouragement to make healthful food choices.[28-31] For example, Larson et al[32] found that adolescent-reported parental support for healthful eating was associated with increases in adolescents' intake of fruits and vegetables as they moved into young adulthood. However, another recent study found that parental support for healthful eating was accompanied by parent modeling of healthful eating behaviors, but parental support was not associated with girls' fruit and vegetable intake after accounting for parental modeling.[33] These findings highlight the need to understand how factors in the family environment co-occur and which factors are especially influential on adolescents' eating behaviors.

Studies examining parental support for healthful eating and adolescents' soft drink intake have shown mixed findings. One study found that social support for healthful eating from significant others, including parents, was not associated with middle school girls' soft drink intake.[34] However, a Dutch study found that parents who restricted their adolescents' soft drink intake, as well as adolescents' perception that their parents wanted them to reduce soft drink intake, was associated with lower intake.[35] Thus, encouragement focused toward a specific dietary habit, not general healthful eating, may be critical in influencing adolescents' behavior.

Parents can support their adolescents' physical activity through verbal encouragement, providing transportation to physical activity locations, and paying for sports team participation or memberships to exercise facilities. Cross-sectional studies have consistently found that parental support for physical activity was related to adolescents' participation in regular physical activity.[36-43] A recent study documented that parental support and encouragement of physical activity was also related to less adolescent screen time (eg, TV watching).[44] A few longitudinal studies have further suggested that parental support is associated with changes in adolescents' physical activity over time.[43,47] For example, Dowda et al[41] found that girls who reported low family support had more rapid declines in physical activity between 8th and 12th grade. Additionally, among participants in Project EAT-II, a 5-year longitudinal[32] population-based study, parental support for physical activity was associated with increases in adolescents' physical activity as they moved from middle school to high school.[45] However, research also suggests that there may be differences by race/ethnicity in the relationship between parents' encouragement and adolescents' physical activity. One study found that parental encouragement was positively related to white and black boys' physical activity, but was unrelated to Asian and Hispanic boys' physical activity, suggesting in these latter populations the need for other positive influences on physical activity.[46]

Parent Modeling of Healthful Dietary Intake and Physical Activity Several studies have found consistent relationships between parental consumption of fruits, vegetables, and soft drinks and adolescents' consumption of these foods.[28,33,47-52] A recent qualitative study found that many of the parents who reported they stopped drinking soft drinks as part of diabetes treatment had children who modeled this behavior by switching to water or 100% fruit juice.[53] Interestingly, a recent longitudinal study by Pearson et al[54] found that mothers' healthful eating patterns, but not fathers' eating patterns, were associated with increases in adolescents' fruit intake over time. Maternal versus paternal influence requires further research to understand why mothers' dietary behaviors may be particularly influential for adolescents' dietary habits.

A comprehensive review in 2007 noted that the evidence regarding the role of parental modeling (ie, parent being active) on adolescents' physical activity habits was mixed,[55,56] but more recent studies have consistently reported positive associations between parents' physical activity and adolescents' physical activity.[42,45,57,58] Kahn and colleagues found that mother's physical activity, as well as the level of importance a mother placed on physical activity, was positively related to their adolescent's physical activity.[42] In addition, Anderssen et al[57] observed that adolescents whose mothers were active exhibited less of a decline in physical activity over time. Two recent studies that looked simultaneously at parental modeling of and support for physical activity found that modeling was the stronger predictor of adolescents' physical activity.[33,59]

Although less often examined, there is emerging evidence that parents' sedentary behavior is related to adolescents' sedentary behavior, including parents' TV viewing time being positively related to adolescent girls' TV viewing time.[33,60] There are inconsistencies in the strength and even direction of the relationship between parents' TV viewing time and adolescent boys' TV viewing time based on race/ethnicity.[61]

Taken together, research evidence suggests that parental behavior modeling, rather than encouragement alone, seems important both to adolescents' dietary habits and physical activity. Berge et al[1] found that adolescents whose parents encouraged healthful behavior but did not model it had a higher BMI than adolescents whose parents modeled healthful behavior but didn't actively encourage it. Indeed, parental behavior modeling offers an ideal way for parents to help their child be healthier (and themselves) without having to actively encourage them, which may be perceived as nagging.

Overall Family Functioning

Family functioning consists of reciprocal interactions among all family members and includes the ability to manage daily routines (eg, family meals, providing healthful food options in the home), communicate, problem-solve, and be supportive, as well as being emotionally responsive to each other.

Family Meals The frequency and quality of family meals is a mechanism through which families can support healthier diet quality among adolescents.[62] Both Gillman et al[63] and Neumark-Sztainer et al[64] found that greater frequency of family meals was associated with lower intake of soft drinks, and Larson et al observed that adolescents who reported eating family meals during high school increased their vegetable intake into the young adult years.[65] A meta-analysis found that children and adolescents who ate meals regularly with family members were more likely to consume healthful foods and less likely to consume unhealthful foods such as soft drinks, fast food, and fried food. Children and adolescents in families that shared at least 3 family meals per week had a 20% lower odds of eating unhealthful foods than those in families that had fewer than 3 family meals together.[66] These findings clearly suggest the importance of family meals.

Family Emotional Closeness/Connection Cross-sectional studies investigating family closeness/connection in relation to adolescent weight and weight-related behaviors have found that high family connectedness predicts lower BMI, more frequent breakfast consumption, more frequent family meals, lower family conflict, and lower parent–child conflict specific to eating habits in youth.[1,16,67-71] Additionally, better overall family functioning involving high closeness/communication has been found to be associated with less sedentary behavior and more physical activity in adolescent boys, but not in girls.[72]

Home Resources Having fruits and vegetables available and accessible at home is consistently and positively related to adolescents' fruit and vegetable intake.[29,34,52,73,74] Home availability of fruits and vegetables may also interact with other support for healthy eating.[74] For example, Young et al[75] found that when fruit and vegetable availability was high, parental modeling had a stronger effect on adolescents' intake than when there were few fruits and vegetables available in the home.

Similarly, soft drink consumption is higher with greater home availability and accessibility.[49-51,76] Bere et al[50] found that having high soft drink accessibility in the home and the frequency of serving soft drinks at dinner was associated with a 5-fold higher odds of adolescents consuming 2 or more soft drinks per day. Hanson et al[52] found that home soft drink availability was also associated with lower consumption of dairy in adolescents.[77] Displacement of healthy foods by unhealthy foods was similarly observed by Pearson et al[54] in that home availability of less healthy, energy-dense food was associated with decreases in consumption of healthier foods over a 2-year period. Findings emphasize the importance of not only having healthy foods available in the home, but also minimizing the presence of unhealthy food as adolescents seem to be more likely to select the unhealthy option when both choices are available.

Cross-sectional studies examining the relationship between resources in the home and adolescents' physical activity levels demonstrate consistent findings, although longitudinal results are mixed.[78-81] Specifically, studies conducted with adolescents have found that the presence of exercise equipment in the home was cross-sectionally, but not longitudinally, associated with self-reported physical activity.[79-81] More recent evidence has also confirmed cross-sectional relationships between home equipment availability and adolescents' physical activity as measured by accelerometers.[82] However, reverse causality may be operating as adolescents who engage in more physical activity may also choose to purchase (or have their parents purchase) more sports-related equipment.

The evidence exploring possible associations between overall media device availability in the home and adolescents' physical activity or sedentary behavior is also mixed. Some studies have found that adolescents with screen-based equipment (eg, television) in their bedroom have higher screen-based sedentary behavior,[33,83] although this is not uniformly observed and the association may differ by gender.[82] Specifically, Sirard et al found that a higher ratio of activity-to-media equipment in the home was related to lower accelerometry-measured sedentary behavior among adolescents.[82]

In summary, availability and accessibility of healthful foods in the home were consistently associated with more healthful dietary intake in adolescents. In addition, some evidence suggests that more frequent family meals and higher emotional connectedness in the family are associated with more healthful dietary intake, higher breakfast consumption, and lower BMI. There is some emerging evidence that availability of physical activity equipment at home is associated with more physical activity in adolescents, while there is inconsistent evidence regarding the effect of home media equipment on adolescents' sedentary time.[79-82]

Siblings

Relationships in the sibling domain are important because they tend to be the longest lasting relationship among family members—even longer than parent-child or husband–wife relationships.[84] Family systems theory posits that siblings have an effect, whether positive or negative, on each other's health-related behaviors. For example, if a brother or sister teases their sibling about their weight or body shape/size it may result in restrained eating behaviors or decreased physical activity. Alternately, existing evidence in the child development literature indicates that siblings have a beneficial effect on one another's cognitive, social, and emotional development.[84] Most sibling research related to adolescent weight-related behaviors has focused on dietary intake patterns.[85-87] These studies have shown mixed findings, with 1 study showing that siblings have similar dietary intake patterns (eg, fruit and vegetables, sugar-sweetened beverages),[85] another study indicating that siblings have different energy intake patterns,[86] and a third study showing that siblings have similar restrained eating behaviors (ie, dieting) over time.[87] Thus, research looking at the influence of siblings' weight-related behaviors on adolescent dietary intake and physical activity is limited, but the existing literature suggests that siblings may have an influence on adolescents' dietary intake.

RECOMMENDATIONS FOR FUTURE RESEARCH

Numerous cross-sectional and several longitudinal studies highlight the importance of authoritative parenting style, parental support, behavioral modeling, frequent family meals, and the presence of healthful home resources for adolescents' healthful dietary intake and physical activity. Additional research is needed to: (1) provide clarity regarding the areas in which current evidence is mixed; (2) better understand the temporal relationships between family environment factors and adolescents' behaviors (eg, some evidence suggests that a parent's physical activity is related to younger children's physical activity, is less related to early adolescents' physical activity, but then re-emerges as related to older adolescents' physical activity);[88,89] (3) determine how family environment factors co-occur and interact to provide optimal support for adolescents' healthful behavior; (4) identify which family factors most affect adolescents' sedentary behavior; and (5) identify whether family factors are more related to specific types of adolescents' physical activity (eg, recreational vs. transportation-related physical activity). Many of these questions could be addressed with randomized controlled trials and other experimental designs in which specific family factors are or are not modified and state-of-the-art measures of intervention process/fidelity are completed to assess familial factor change.

SPECIFIC STRATEGIES TO IMPROVE ADOLESCENT HEALTHFUL EATING AND PHYSICAL ACTIVITY

More evidence is also needed about the effectiveness of intervention strategies focused on changing family factors in order to change adolescents' dietary and physical activity behaviors. Fewer than one-quarter of the studies (n = 7 of 35 studies) in a review of studies on parent encouragement of youth to increase physical activity focused on adolescents.[90] None of these adolescent–focused studies explicitly focused on training or counseling around parenting to increase adolescents' physical activity, instead focusing on parent-adolescent co-participation[91] and education of parents.[90,92] Findings from other recent reviews of adolescent obesity treatment and prevention interventions are also mixed regarding the needed amount and type of parental involvement to optimize adolescent health behaviors.[93,94] These inconsistencies in the literature suggest that more research is needed to identify the best way(s) to include parents and families in interventions regarding adolescent dietary intake and physical activity. Nevertheless, observational research has identified potentially modifiable familial environment factors that parents, providers, and policy makers can address to improve or sustain adolescents' dietary intake and involvement in physical activity.

Recommendations for Families

Although it may be difficult to change parenting style, it may be possible to teach specific parenting practices to parents to make the family environment more healthful, including:

Parent modeling and encouraging healthful dietary intake and frequent physical activity. Parents should be particularly aware of their own dietary intake and physical activity attitudes and behaviors. According to family systems theory[12] and observational research, parents who model healthful eating habits[28,33,47,52] (eg, eating fruits and vegetables) and engage in frequent physical activity[36-42] are more likely to have children, even older adolescents, who engage in these same behaviors.

Healthful food availability and accessibility in the home. Having healthful foods available and accessible (eg, cut-up and ready to eat) in the home increases the likelihood that adolescents eat more fruits and vegetables and reduce intake of sugar-sweetened beverages.[29,34,52,73,74] Parents should make a concerted effort to keep healthful foods available/accessible and limit the availability of unhealthy food and beverages at home.

Frequent family meals. Having frequent family meals has been associated with more healthful eating patterns in children,[95-97] adolescents,[32,98-102] and parents.[103-105] For example, several studies showed a significant positive association between 5 or more family meals a week and adolescent healthful dietary intake.[27,106]

Create home environments that support physical activity and discourage sedentary behavior. Parents who support adolescent physical activity, including participating in activities with their adolescent, have adolescents who report more physical activity.[78-81] Thus, parents should consider looking for opportunities to be active as a family and to create a home environment that rewards physical activity and discourages sedentary behavior.

Set specific rules around screen time and limit access to screen-based equipment in the home. Parents who have rules about screen time limits have adolescents who report fewer hours of sedentary behavior.[83] The American Academy of Pediatrics (AAP) recommends: (a) no more than 2 hours of screen time per day for children and adolescents; and (b) parents should not allow televisions (and perhaps other "screens") in bedrooms.[107]

More than one or all of these recommendations likely need to be implemented to help sustain or change adolescents' behavior to be more healthful. Many of these recommendations are likely to be most effective and easier to sustain if implemented before children enter adolescence, but this should not discourage parents and other caregivers from modifying their home environments, improving their eating and physical activity behaviors, and establishing expectations of their adolescents for healthy eating and physical activity.

Recommendations for Physicians

Physicians and other health care providers working with families can be involved with family-based prevention efforts. Physicians may consider utilizing time during well-child visits and other opportunities to provide recommendations about adolescent health behavior (eg, recommended levels of physical activity and limits on sedentary behavior). Recommendations for parents, such as the parenting practices listed previously, may be useful for providers to share with parents because research has shown that parents of adolescents have become increasingly more concerned about adolescent weight and weight-related behaviors.[108]

Policy Recommendations

Implementing broader environmental and policy improvements in neighborhoods, schools, and within social networks to reduce the structural barriers that many families face when trying to improve their health is an important step to improving adolescent health behaviors.

One specific example of a policy and larger environmental intervention to help parents to be more physically active with their adolescents would be to develop public recreation spaces that encourage multi-generational physical activity. Creating space for parents/adults and children/adolescents to be active together or at least co-located in the community promotes more adolescent physical activity and community ownership of the youth obesity problem.

In addition, another policy recommendation to consider is allowing changes in workplace policies and procedures that allow for parents to have more flexible hours, benefits for less than full time employment, and greater flexibility in regards to where and when their work is completed.[109] These alterations may increase the likelihood that parents will be able to create healthier home environments, such as having more frequent family meals because parents could more easily be home for the dinner hour.

CONCLUSIONS

Research suggests that families have the potential to positively influence adolescents' dietary and physical activity behaviors. Specifically, strengthening parenting practices that support adolescents' participation in healthful behavior and making healthful food and physical activity resources more available and accessible in the home are strategies likely to play important roles in promoting healthful eating and physical activity. That said, research findings on associations between the family environment and adolescent behaviors have not always been consistent or as strong as expected, and further research is needed to clarify the picture and to better guide recommendations for parents.

References

1. Berge JM, Wall M, Bauer KW, Neumark-Sztainer D. Parenting characteristics in the home environment and adolescent overweight: a latent class analysis. *Obesity.* 2010;18(4):818-825
2. Berge JM. A review of familial correlates of child and adolescent obesity: what has the 21st Century taught us so far? *Int J Adolesc Med Health.* 2009;21(4):457-483
3. Story M, Neumark-Sztainer D, French S. Individual and environmental influences on adolescent eating behaviors. *J Am Diet Assoc.* 2002;102:S40-51
4. Daniels SR. Complications of obesity in children and adolescents. *Int J Obes (Lond).* 2009;33(Suppl 1):S60-S65
5. Ogden CL, Carroll MD, Curtin LR, Lamb MM, Flegal KM. Prevalence of high body mass index in US children and adolescents, 2007-2008. *JAMA.* 2010;303(3):242-249
6. Ogden C, Carroll M, Curtin L, Lamb M, Flegal K. Prevalence of high body mass index in US children and adolescents, 2007-2008. *JAMA.* 2010;303(3):8
7. Must A, Strauss RS. Risks and consequences of childhood and adolescent obesity. *Int J Obes Relat Metab Disord.* 1999;23(Suppl 2):S2-S11
8. Daniels SR. The consequences of childhood overweight and obesity. *Future Child.* 2006;16(1):47-67
9. Daniels SR, Arnett DK, Eckel RH, et al. Overweight in children and adolescents: pathophysiology, consequences, prevention, and treatment. *Circulation.* 2005;111(15):1999-2012

10. Minuchin S. *Families and Family Therapy*. Cambridge, MA: Harvard University Press; 1974
11. Bertalanffy LV. Theoretical models in biology and psychology. In: Krech D, Klein GS, eds. *Theoretical models and personality*. Durham, NC: Duke University Press; 1952:24-38
12. Whitchurch GG, Constantine LL. Systems theory. In: Boss PG, Doherty WJ, LaRossa R, Schumm WR, Steinmetz SK, eds. *Sourcebook on family theories and methods: A contextual approach*. New York, NY: Plenum Press; 1993
13. Baumrind D, ed. *Rearing Competent Children*. In: Damon, ed. *Child Development Today and Tomorrow.* San Francisco: Jossey-Bass; 1989
14. Story M, Neumark-Sztainer D, French S. Individual and environmental influences on adolescent eating behaviors. *J Am Diet Assoc.* 2002;102(Journal Article):S40-51
15. Arredondo EM, Elder JP, Ayala GX, Campbell N, Baquero B, Duerksen S. Is parenting style related to children's healthy eating and physical activity in Latino families? *Health Educ Res.* 2006;21(6): 862-871
16. Chen J, Kennedy C. Family functioning, parenting style, and Chinese children's weight status. *J Fam Nurs.* 2004;10:262-279
17. Gable S, Lutz, S. Household, parent and child contributions to childhood obesity. *Family Relations.* 2000;49(3):293-300
18. Kremers SP, Brug J, deVries H, Engels, RC. Parenting style and adolescent fruit consumption. *Appetite.* 2003;41(1):43-50
19. Moens E, Braet C, Soetens B. Observation of family functioning at mealtime: a comparison between families of children with and without overweight. *J Pediatr Psychol.* 2007;32(1):52-63
20. Mellin AE, Neumark-Sztainer D, Story M, Ireland M, Resnick MD. Unhealthy behaviors and psychosocial difficulties among overweight adolescents: the potential impact of familial factors. *J Adolesc Health.* 2002;31:145-153
21. van der Horst K, Kremers S, Ferreira I, Sign A, Oenema A, Brug J. Perceived parenting style and practices and the consumption of sugar-sweetened beverages by adolescents. *Health Educ Res.* 2007;22(2):295-304
22. Schmitz KH, Lytle LA, Phillips GA, Murray DM, Birnham AS, Kubik MY. Psychosocial correlates of physical activity and sedentary leisure habits in young adolescents: the Teens Eating for Energy and Nutrition at School study. *Prev Med.* 2002;34:266-278
23. Rhee KE, Lumeng JC, Appugliese DP, Kaciroti N, Bradley RH. Parenting styles and overweight status in first grade. *Pediatrics.* 2006;117:2047-2054
24. Rhee KE. Childhood overweight and the relationship between parent behaviors, parenting style, and family functioning. *The Annals of the American Academy of Political and Social Science.* 2008;615:11-37
25. Berge J, Wall M, Loth K, Neumark-Sztainer D. Parenting style as a predictor of adolescent weight and weight-related behavior. *J Adolesc Health.* 2010;46(4):331-338
26. Berge JM. Parenting style and family meals: cross-sectional and 5-year longitudinal associations. *J Am Diet Assoc.* 2010;110:1036-1042
27. Norman GJ, Schmid BA, Sallis JF, Calfas KJ, Patrick K. Psychosocial and environmental correlates of adolescent sedentary behaviors. *Pediatrics.* Oct 2005;116(4):908-916
28. Pearson N, Biddle SJ, Gorely T. Family correlates of fruit and vegetable consumption in children and adolescents: a systematic review. *Public Health Nutr.* 2008(Journal Article):1-17
29. Granner ML, Sargent RG, Calderon KS, Hussey JR, Evans AE, Watkins KW. Factors of fruit and vegetable intake by race, gender, and age among young adolescents. *J Nutr Educ Behav.* 2004; 36(4):173-180
30. Sanchez A, Norman GJ, Sallis JF, Calfas KJ, Cella J, Patrick K. Patterns and correlates of physical activity and nutrition behaviors in adolescents. *Am J Prev Med.* 2007;32(2):124-130
31. Neumark-Sztainer D, Wall M, Perry C, Story M. Correlates of fruit and vegetable intake among adolescents. Findings from Project EAT. *Prev Med.* 2003;37(3):198-208
32. Larson NI, Neumark-Sztainer D, Harnack L, Wall M, Story M, Eisenberg ME. Fruit and vegetable intake correlates during the transition to young adulthood. *Ame J Prev Med.* 2008;35(1):33-37

33. Bauer KW, Neumark-Sztainer D, Fulkerson J, Hannan P, Story M. Familial correlates of adolescent girls' physical activity, television use, dietary intake, weight, and body composition. *Int J Behav Nutr Phys Act.* 2011;8:25-31
34. Haerens L, Craeynest M, Deforche B, Maes L, Cardon G, De Bourdeaudhuij I. The contribution of psychosocial and home environmental factors in explaining eating behaviours in adolescents. *Eur J Clin Nutr.* 2008;62(1):51-59
35. de Bruijn GJ, Kremers SP, de Vries H, van Mechelen W, Brug J. Associations of social-environmental and individual-level factors with adolescent soft drink consumption: results from the SMILE study. *Health Educ Res.* 2007;22(2):227-237
36. Heitzler CD, Martin SL, Duke J, Huhman M. Correlates of physical activity in a national sample of children aged 9-13 years. *Prev Med.* 2006;42(4):254-260
37. Kuo J, Voorhees CC, Haythornthwaite JA, Young DR. Associations between family support, family intimacy, and neighborhood violence and physical activity in urban adolescent girls. *Am J Public Health.* 2007;97(1):101-103
38. Trost SG, Sallis JF, Pate RR, Freedson PS, Taylor WC, Dowda M. Evaluating a model of parental influence on youth physical activity. *Am J Preventive Med.* 2003;25(4):277-282
39. Springer AE, Kelder SH, Hoelscher DM. Social support, physical activity and sedentary behavior among 6th-grade girls: a cross-sectional study. *Int J Behav Nutr Phys Act.* 2006;3(Journal Article):8
40. Neumark-Sztainer D, Story M, Hannan PJ, Tharp T, Rex J. Factors associated with changes in physical activity: a cohort study of inactive adolescent girls. *Arch Pediatr Adolesc Med.* 2003;157:803-810
41. Dowda M, Dishman R, Pfeiffer K, Pate RR. Family support for physical activity in girls in 8th to 12th grade in South Carolina. *Preventive Medicine.* 2007;44:153-159
42. Kahn JA, Huang B, Gillman MW. Patterns and determinants of physical activity in U.S. adolescents. *J Adolesc Health.* 2008;42(4):369-377
43. Williams SL, Mummery WK. Links between adolescent physical activity, body mass index, and adolescent and parent characteristics. *Health Educ Behav.* 2011;8(5):510-520
44. Leatherdale ST, Faulkner G, Arbour-Nicitopoulos K. School and student characteristics associated with screen-time sedentary behavior among students in grades 5-8, Ontario, Canada, 2007-2008. *Prev Chron Dis.* 2010;7(6):A128
45. Bauer KW, Nelson MC, Boutelle KN, Neumark-Sztainer D. Parental influences on adolescents' physical activity and sedentary behavior: longitudinal findings from Project EAT-II. *Int J Behav Nutr Phys Act.* 2008;5:12
46. McGuire MT, Hannan PJ, Neumark-Sztainer D, Falkner Crossrow, NH, Story M. Parental correlates of physical activity in a racially/ethnically-diverse adolescent sample. *J Adolesc Health.* 2002;30(4):253-261
47. Elfhag K, Tholin S, Rasmussen F. Consumption of fruit, vegetables, sweets and soft drinks are associated with psychological dimensions of eating behaviour in parents and their 12-year-old children. *Public Health Nutr.* 2008;11(9):914-923
48. van der Horst K, Oenema A, Ferreira I, et al. A systematic review of environmental correlates of obesity-related dietary behaviors in youth. *Health Educ Res.* 2006;22(2):203-226; article first published online 2006 Jul 21
49. Campbell KJ, Crawford DA, Salmon J, Carver A, Garnett SP, Baur LA. Associations between the home food environment and obesity-promoting eating behaviors in adolescence. *Obesity (Silver Spring).* 2007;15(3):719-730
50. Bere E, Glomnes ES, te Velde SJ, Klepp KI. Determinants of adolescents' soft drink consumption. *Public Health Nutr.* 2008;11(1):49-56
51. Bauer KW, Neumark-Sztainer D, Fulkerson JA, Hannan PJ, Story M. Familial correlates of adolescent girls' physical activity, television use, dietary intake, weight, and body composition. *Int J Behav Nutr Phys Act.* 2011;8:25
52. Hanson NI, Neumark-Sztainer D, Eisenberg ME, Story M, Wall M. Associations between parental report of the home food environment and adolescent intakes of fruits, vegetables, and dairy foods. *Public Health Nutr.* 2005;8(Journal Article):77-85

53. Laroche HH, Heisler M, Forman J, Anderson M, Davis MM. When adults with diabetes attempt to drink less soda: resulting adult-child interactions and household changes. *J Natl Med Assoc.* 2008;100(9):1004-1011
54. Pearson N, Biddle SJ, Gorely T. Family correlates of fruit and vegetable consumption in children and adolescents: a systematic review. *Public Health Nutr.* Feb 2009;12(2):267-283
55. Van der Horst K, Paw MJ, Twisk JW, Van Mechelen W. A brief review on correlates of physical activity and sedentariness in youth. *Med Sci Sports Exerc.* 2007;39(8):1241-1250
56. Ferreira I, van der Horst K, Wendel-Vos W, Kremers S, van Lenthe FJ, Brug J. Environmental correlates of physical activity in youth - a review and update. *Obes Rev.* 2007;8(2):129-154
57. Anderssen N, Wold B, Torsheim T. Are parental health habits transmitted to their children? An eight year longitudinal study of physical activity in adolescents and their parents. *J Adolesc.* 2006;29(4):513-524
58. Davison KK. Activity-related support from parents, peers, and siblings and adolescents' physical activity: are there gender differences? *J Phys Act Health.* 2004;1:363-376
59. Heitzler CD, Lytle L, Erickson DJ, Barr-Anderson D, Sirard JR, Story M. Evaluating a model of youth physical activity. *Am J Health Behav.* 2010;34(5):593-606
60. Uijtdewilligen L, Nauta J, Singh AS, et al. Determinants of physical activity and sedentary behaviour in young people: a review and quality synthesis of prospective studies. *Br J Sports Med.* 2011;45:896-905
61. McGuire M, Hannan P, Neumark-Sztainer D, Falkner-Cossrow N, Story M. Parental correlates of physical activity in a racially/ethnically-diverse adolescent sample. *J Adolesc Health.* 2002;30(4): 253-261
62. Hammons AJ, Fiese BH. Is frequency of shared family meals related to the nutritional health of children and adolescents? *Pediatrics.* 2011;127(6):e1565-1574
63. Gillman MW, Rifas-Shiman SL, Frazier AL, et al. Family dinner and diet quality among older children and adolescents. *Arch Fam Med.* 2000;9(3):235-240
64. Neumark-Sztainer D, Hannan PJ, Story M, Croll J, Perry C. Family meal patterns: associations with sociodemographic characteristics and improved dietary intake among adolescents. *J Am Diet Assoc.* 2003;103(3):317-322
65. Larson NI, Neumark-Sztainer D, Hannan PJ, Story M. Family meals during adolescence are associated with higher diet quality and healthful meal patterns during young adulthood. *J Am Diet Assoc.* 2007;107(9):1502-1510
66. Hammons AJ, Fiese BH. Is frequency of shared meals related to the nutritional health of children and adolescents? *Pediatrics.* 2011;127(6):e1565-1574
67. Zeller MH, Reiter-Purtill J, Modi AC, Gutzwiller J, Vannatta K, Davies WH. Controlled study of critical parent and family factors on the obesigenic environment. *Obesity.* 2007;15:126-136
68. Lamerz A, Kuepper-Nybelen J, Wehle C, Bruning N, Trost-Brinkhues G, Brenner H, Hebebrand J, Herpertz-Dahlman B. Social class, parental education, and obesity prevalence in study of 6-year old children in Germany. *Int J Obes (Lond).* 2005;29:373-380
69. Turner HM, Rose KS, Cooper MJ. Schema and parental bonding in overweight and nonoverweight female adolescents. *Int J Obes (Lond).* 2005;29:381-387
70. Vieweg VR, Johnston CH, Lanier JO, Fernandez A, Pandurangi AK. Correlation between high risk obesity groups and low socioeconomic status in school children. *South Med J.* 2007;100(1):8-13
71. Taylor CB, Bryson S, Doyle AAC, Luce KH, Cunning D, Abascal LB, Rockwell R, Field, AE, Striegel-Moore R, Winselberg AJ, Wilfley, DE. The adverse effect of negative comments about weight and shape from family and siblings on women at high risk for eating disorders. *Pediatrics.* 2006;118:731-738
72. Berge JM, Wall M, Larson N, Loth K, Neumark-Sztainer D. Family functioning: associations with weight status, eating behaviors and physical activity in adolescents. *J Adolesc Health.* In press
73. Cullen KW, Baranowski T, Owens E, Marsh T, Rittenberry L, de Moor C. Availability, accessibility, and preferences for fruit, 100% fruit juice, and vegetables influence children's dietary behavior. *Health Educ Behav.* 2003;30(5):615-626

74. Befort C, Kaur H, Nollen N, et al. Fruit, vegetable, and fat intake among non-Hispanic black and non-Hispanic white adolescents: associations with home availability and food consumption settings. *J Am Diet Assoc.* 2006;106(3):367-373
75. Young EM, Fors SW, Hayes DM. Associations between perceived parent behaviors and middle school student fruit and vegetable consumption. *J Nutr Educ Behav.* 2004;36(1):2-8
76. Grimm GC, Harnack L, Story M. Factors associated with soft drink consumption in school-aged children. *J Am Diet Assoc.* 2004;104(8):1244-1249
77. Nelson MC, Neumark-Sztainer D, Hannan PJ, Story M. Five-year longitudinal and secular shifts in adolescent beverage intake: findings from project EAT (Eating Among Teens)-II. *J Am Diet Assoc.* 2009;109(2):308-312
78. Sallis JF, Johnson MF, Calfas KJ, Caparosa S, Nichols JF. Assessing perceived physical environmental variables that may influence physical activity. *Res Q Exerc Sport.* 1997;68(4):345-351
79. Motl RW, Dishman RK, Ward DS, et al. Perceived physical environment and physical activity across one year among adolescent girls: self-efficacy as a possible mediator? *J Adolesc Health.* 2005;37(5):403-408
80. Motl RW, Dishman RK, Saunders RP, Dowda M, Pate RR. Perceptions of physical and social environment variables and self-efficacy as correlates of self-reported physical activity among adolescent girls. *J Pediatr Psychol.* 2007;32(1):6-12
81. Dowda M, Pate RR, Sallis JF, et al. Agreement between student-reported and proxy-reported physical activity questionnaires. *Pediatr Exerc Sci.* 2007;19:310-318
82. Sirard JR, Laska MN, C.D. P, Farbakhsh K, Lytle L. Adolescent physical activity and screen time: associations with the physical home environment. *Int J Behav Nutr Phys. Act.* 2010;7:82
83. Ramirez ER, Norman GJ, Rosenberg DE, et al. Adolescent screen time and rules to limit screen time in the home. *J Adolesc Health.* 2011;48:379-385
84. Noller P. Sibling relationships in adolescence: learning and growing together. *Personal Relationships.* 2005;12:1-22
85. de Leeuw RN, Snoek HM, van Leeuw JFJ, van Strien T, Engels RCME. Similarities and reciprocal influences in eating behavior within sibling pairs: a longitudinal study. *Eat Behav.* 2007;8:464-473
86. Roemmich JN, White TM, Paluch R, Epstein LH. Energy intake, parent control of children's eating, and physical activity in siblings discordant for obesity. *Appetite.* 2010;55(2):325-331
87. Snoek HM, van Strien T, Janssens JM, Engels RC. Longitudinal relationships between fathers', mothers', and adolescents' restrained eating. *Appetite.* 2009;52(2):461-468
88. Madsen KA, McCulloch CE, Crawford PB. Parent modeling: perceptions of parents' physical activity predict girls' activity throughout adolescence. *J Pediatr.* 2009;154:278-283
89. Wiley AR, Flood TL, Andrade FCD, Aradillas C, Cerda EM. Family and individual predictors of physical activity for older Mexican adolescents. *J Adolesc Health.* 2011;49:222-224
90. O'Connor TM, Jago R, Baranowski T. Engaging parents to increase youth physical activity: a systemic review. *Am J Prev Med.* 2009;37(2):141-149
91. Ransdell LB, Taylor A, Oakland D, Schmidt J, Moyer-Mileur L, Shultz B. Daughters and mothers exercising together: effects of home and community-based programs. *Med Sci Sport Exerc.* 2003;35(2):286-296
92. Patrick K, Calfas K, Norman G, Zabinski M, Sallis J, Rupp L. Randomized controlled trial of a primary care and home-based intervention for physical activity and nutrition behaviors: PACE+ for adolescents. *Arch Pediatr Adolesc Med.* 2006;160(2):128-136
93. Golley RK, Hendrie GA, Slater A, Corsini N. Interventions that involve parents to improve children's weight-related nutrition intake and activity patterns—What nutrition and activity targets and behaviour change techniques are associated with intervention effectiveness? *Obes Rev.* 2011;12:114-130
94. van Sluijs EMF, Kriemler S, McMinn AM. The effect of community and family interventions on young people's physical activity levels: a review of reviews and updated systematic review. *Br J Sports Med.* 2011;45(11):914-922
95. Jacobs MP, Fiese BH. Family mealtime interactions and overweight children with asthma: Potential for compounded risks? *J Pediatr Psychol.* 2007;32(1):64-68

96. Ackard D, Neumark-Sztainer D. Family mealtime while growing up: associations with symptoms of bulimia nervosa. *Eat Disord.* 2001;9:239-249
97. Moens E, Braet C, Soetens B. Observation of family functioning at mealtime: a comparison between families of children with and without overweight. *J Pediatr Psychol.* 2007;32(1):52-63
98. Larson NI, Story M, Wall M, Neumark-Sztainer D. Calcium and dairy intakes of adolescents are associated with their home environment, taste preferences, personal health beliefs, and meal patterns. *J Am Diet Assoc.* 2006;106:1816-1824
99. Larson NI, Neumark-Sztainer D, Hannan PJ, Story M. Family meals during adolescence are associated with higher diet quality and healthful meal patterns during young adulthood. *J Am Diet Assoc.* 2007;107:1502-1510
100. Neumark-Sztainer D, Wall MM, Hannan PJ, Story M, Croll J, Perry C. Correlates of fruit and vegetable intake among adolescents: findings from Project EAT. *Prev Med.* 2003;37(3):198-208
101. Gillman MW, Rifas-Shiman SL, Frazier AL, et al. Family dinner and diet quality among older children and adolescents. *Arch Fam Med.* 2000;9(3):235-240
102. Videon TM, Manning CK. Influences on adolescent eating patterns: the importance of family meals. *J Adolesc Health.* 2003;32:365-373
103. Sobal J, Hanson K. Family meals and body weight in US adults. *Public Health Nutr.* 2011; article first published online February 28, DOI:10.1017/S1368980011000127
104. Boutelle K, Fulkerson JA, Neumark-Sztainer D, Story M, French SA. Fast food for family meals: relationships with parent and adolescent food intake, home food availability and weight status. *Public Health Nutr.* 2007;10:16-23
105. Boutelle KN, Birnbaum AS, Lytle LA, Murray DM, Story M. Associations between perceived family meal environment and parent intake of fruit, vegetables, and fat. *J Nutr Educ Behav.* 2003;35(1):24-29
106. Neumark-Sztainer D, Hannan PJ, Story M, Croll J. Family meal patterns: associations with sociodemographic characteristics and improved dietary intake among adolescents. *J Am Diet Assoc.* 2003;103:317-322
107. Schor EL; American Academy of Pediatrics Task Force on the Family. Family Pediatrics: Report of the Task Force on The Family. *Pediatrics.* 2003;111:1541-1571
108. Berge JM, Arikian A, Neumark-Sztainer D, Doherty W. Healthful eating and physical activity in the home environment: results from multi-family focus groups. *J Nutr Educ Behav.* 2012;44(2): 123-131
109. Breaugh JA, Frye NK. Work–family conflict: the importance of family-friendly employment practices and family-supportive supervisors. *J Bus Psychol.* 2008;22(4):345-35

Adolesc Med 023 (2012) 440–456

Determinants of Undernutrition and Overnutrition among Adolescents in Developing Countries

Sarah E. Cusick, PhD*[a], Amanda E. Kuch, BA[b]

[a]*Assistant Professor, Division of Global Pediatrics, University of Minnesota Medical School, 717 Delaware Street SE, Room 365, Mail Code 1932, Minneapolis, MN 55414*

[b]*Medical Student, University of Minnesota Medical School, 717 Delaware Street SE, Room 365, Mail Code 1932, Minneapolis, MN 55414*

Adolescence, defined by the World Health Organization (WHO) as the period of life between 10 and 19 years,[1] is a period of remarkable growth. The rate of physical growth during adolescence is second only to that during the first year of life, and this physical growth occurs concomitantly with dramatic cognitive and psychosocial changes.[2] Approximately 85% of the 1.2 billion adolescents worldwide live in developing countries, as defined by the country classifications of the United Nation's Children's Fund (UNICEF).[3] For the purpose of this article, the term "developing countries" includes both "developing countries" and "least-developed countries" according to the UNICEF classification scheme. In many of these countries, stunting, underweight, and micronutrient deficiencies among adolescents frequently result from inadequate nutrition and infections during early childhood combined with a diet insufficient to meet the intense nutritional demands of rapid growth during adolescence. Adolescent pregnancy, which is common in many developing countries, exacts an additional nutritional toll. However, this undernutrition increasingly coexists with burgeoning overweight and obesity, necessitating a complex, multifactorial approach to alleviating the public health burden of worldwide adolescent malnutrition.

This article describes the magnitude of adolescent undernutrition in developing countries and highlights areas for intervention to prevent the harmful cycle of intergenerational undernutrition in which poor nutritional status in adolescence

*Corresponding author.
E-mail address: scusick@umn.edu (S. E. Cusick).

 ISSN 1934-4287

plays a pivotal role. The growing problem of overnutrition in developing countries is also described, with case studies from 2 countries serving as examples.

THE NUTRITIONAL STATUS OF ADOLESCENTS: AN OVERLOOKED PROBLEM

With a mortality rate lower than any other age group and relatively little morbidity, adolescents are typically not prioritized for public health interventions.[3] As a group, adolescents also have less undernutrition than infants and preschool-aged children, historically making the establishment of standardized anthropometric definitions less of a pressing concern for young people this age.[4] The rapidity of the adolescent growth spurt, differences in the timing of sexual maturation, and genetic factors all impose tremendous variability on adolescent height and weight, making maturational age and chronological age discordant and establishment of international standards for adolescent growth difficult.[4] The consequent use of different definitions of underweight and overweight in studies evaluating adolescent nutritional status complicates assessment of the magnitude of adolescent malnutrition in developing countries and impairs meaningful comparisons.

A relationship between anthropometric cutoffs and functional consequences in adulthood, particularly with regard to cutoffs for overweight and obesity, has yet to be established, necessitating the use of statistically derived cutoffs. The 2 most used sets of anthropometric definitions and cutoffs for adolescent growth are (1) the 1995 WHO cutoffs for stunting, thinness, at risk for overweight, and obesity[4] that were based on data collected by the National Center for Health Statistics (NCHS) in adolescents from the United States (Table 1), and (2) a series of age-specific cutoffs defined by the International Obesity Task Force (IOTF) in 2000 and 2007[5,6] that were based on data collected in Brazil, Great Britain, Hong Kong, the Netherlands, Singapore, and the United States. The IOTF cutoffs reflect centile curves that at age 18 years pass through the widely

Table 1
Recommended cut-off values and original sources of reference data for adolescents[4]

Indicator	Anthropometric variable	Cut-off values
Stunting or low height-for-age	Height-for-age	$<$3rd percentile or <-2 Z-scores
Thinness or low BMI-for-age	BMI-for-age	$<$5th percentile
At risk for overweight	BMI-for-age	$\geq$85th percentile
Obese	BMI-for-age	$\geq$85th percentile BMI *and*
	TRSKF-for-age	$\geq$90th percentile TRSKF *and*
	SSKF-for-age	$\geq$90th percentile SSKF

SSKF, subscapular skinfold thickness; TRSKF, triceps skinfold thickness

used adult body mass index (BMI) cutoffs of 25 and 30 to define overweight and obesity,[5] respectively, or drawn through BMI cutoffs of 16, 17, and 18.5 to define thinness of grade 1, 2, and 3.[6] These centile curves were averaged for each survey to produce gender and age-specific cutoffs for children aged 2 to 18 years.

UNDERNUTRITION

A series of 11 cross-sectional studies coordinated by the International Center for Research on Women (ICRW) between 1990 and 1994 highlighted key issues in adolescent nutrition in developing countries.[7] These studies—conducted in Ecuador, Mexico, Guatemala (2 studies), Jamaica, Nepal, India, Philippines (2 studies), Benin, and Cameroon—revealed that stunting, underweight, and iron deficiency anemia were widespread among adolescents.

Stunting

Stunting, or impaired linear growth, in adolescents represents long-term nutritional deficiency. The consequences of stunting in adolescence include greater risk of obstetric complications, including obstructed labor in females, and diminished physical capacity among adolescents of both sexes.[7]

The prevalence of stunting, defined in the ICRW studies as height-for-age less than the 5th percentile of the NCHS/WHO 1995 reference data, was high in 9 of the 11 studies, ranging from 26%-65%.[7] Kurtz reports that the pattern of height-for-age was remarkably similar among girls in the 9 countries in which stunting was prevalent, in that the mean height of girls did not improve across the 8 years of adolescence for which data were collected.[7] Data from Nepal[8] and Ecuador[9] typify this pattern (Fig 1). In Nepal, the mean height of girls was near the 5th

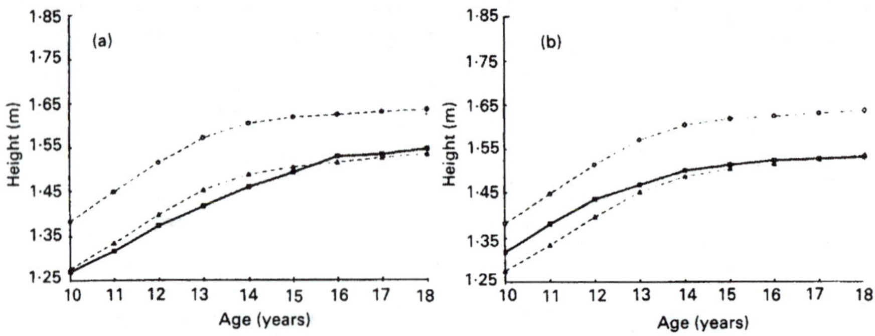

Fig 1. Height of adolescent girls by age in the (a) Nepal and (b) Ecuador studies within the Nutrition of Adolescent Girls Research Program of the International Center for Research on Women. (●), 50th Percentile of the National Center for Health Statistics (NCHS) reference data (Hammill et al. 1979); (■), adolescent data from Nepal or Ecuador; (▲), 5th percentile of the NCHS reference data. From Kurtz K. Adolescent nutritional status in developing countries. *Proc Nut Soc.* 1996;55:321-331. Reprinted with permission.

percentile of the NCHS curve at 10 and 18 years of age and less than the 5th percentile slightly between ages 11 and 15 years. The mean height of adolescent girls in Ecuador was slightly greater than the 5th percentile at age 10, but dropped to the 5th percentile by age 18 years.

More recent surveys suggest that stunting remains prevalent in developing countries throughout the world, with a prevalence of 12.1% among Kenyan schoolgirls ages 12 to 16 years,[10] approximately 15% among Pakistani boys and girls 11 to 14 years of age,[11] and 67.3% and 57.8% among Nigerian boys and girls aged 15 to 18 years,[12] respectively. All of these studies defined stunting as height-for-age less than 2 standard deviations less than the 1995 WHO/NCHS reference median, a more stringent definition than that used in the ICRW studies. In contrast to the findings in the ICRW studies in Nepal and Ecuador, the prevalence of stunting apparently declines with age across the adolescent years in some recent studies without intervention.[10,13] For example, the cross-sectional study in Kenyan schoolgirls revealed that the prevalence of stunting declined from approximately 20% among 12-year-olds to 2% among 16-year-olds, as the mean height-for-age z-score converged toward the US reference median (Fig 2).[10] Similarly, the mean height of a cohort of Senegalese children aged 1 to 5 years who had a nearly 30% prevalence of stunting came within 2 cm of the WHO/NCHS reference median for height when that cohort reached early adulthood (18-23 years), with no formal intervention.[13]

The decline in stunting prevalence in the Kenyan survey was concurrent with an average delay in menarche of 1.5 to 2 years compared to the NCHS/US reference curve.[10] This finding led researchers to conclude that although stunting was common among young adolescent girls, the maturational delay permitted prolonged growth and eventual attainment of greater height. The debate over whether stunted young adolescents can regain linear height and "catch up" to their optimal height is not resolved, but the proposed mechanism for catch-up

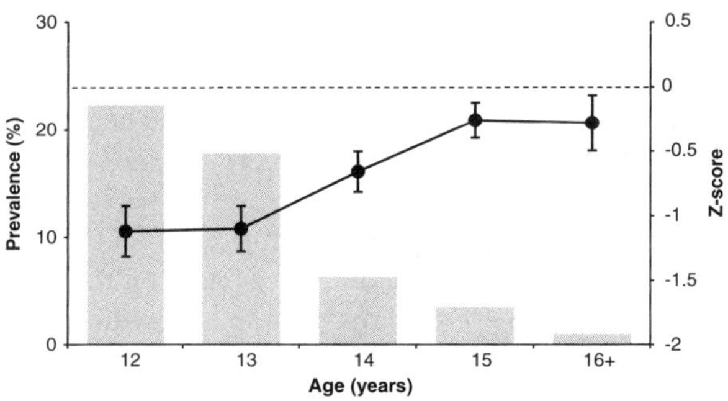

Fig 2. Measures of linear growth by age in 934 adolescent schoolgirls from western Kenya. From Leenstra T, Petersen L, Kariuki S, Oloo A, Kager P, ter Kuile F. Prevalence and severity of malnutrition and age at menarche; cross-sectional studies in adolescent schoolgirls in western Kenya. *Eur J Clin Nutr*. 2005;59:41-48. Reprinted with permission from Macmillan Publishers Ltd.

growth is that which the authors of the Kenyan study proposed.[14,15] Approximately 20% of adult height is gained during adolescence, with the most gained at a rapid rate during a period of 1 to 2 years preceding the early stages of sexual maturation, typically marked by menarche in females or attainment of adult voice in males,[4] at which time the growth rate slows. In undernourished populations, menarche or the onset of puberty is often delayed, permitting a longer period of growth and perhaps more time for "catch-up growth."[14,16] Conversely, when the environment of the stunted individual changes, as when families migrate from rural to urban areas[13] or in the case of internationally adopted children,[17] catch-up growth may be so rapid as to hasten the onset of puberty, thus shortening the period of most rapid growth and limiting adult height.

Food interventions aimed at alleviating adolescent stunting may not spur height gain beyond increases that occur naturally during the adolescent growth spurt and may in fact promote excess weight gain in populations in which concurrent underweight is not prevalent.[14] Instead, the prevention of adolescent stunting ideally begins with intervention much earlier in development, as stunting among adolescents reflects chronic undernourishment, likely beginning with inadequate nutrition during the first 2 to 3 years of life.[14] At this age, food scarcity and inadequate nutrient intake limit growth, and frequent infections and diarrhea cause malabsorption of critical nutrients. Young children respond well to food interventions, which serve to optimize not only height, but also permit full cognitive development and attainment of complete physical capacity.[14] Aside from food interventions, promotion of breastfeeding and the intake of nutrient-dense weaning foods and prevention of infectious diseases through the use of clean water are key in optimizing the nutritional status and growth of young children,[14] with this optimized early growth critical for the prevention of impaired linear growth in adolescence.

Thinness or Underweight

The 1995 WHO expert committee identified BMI-for-age less than the 5th percentile as the best indicator for thinness in adolescence.[4] Although the term "underweight" is often used to describe thinness in adolescents with low BMI-for-age, the indicator of weight-for-age that is typically used to define underweight in young children is not meaningful in this age group because weight changes dramatically with height during adolescence and height is largely determined by genetic factors. The use of various definitions makes assessment of the public health burden and targeting of interventions challenging. However, patterns of thinness among adolescents in developing countries can be described based on the ICRW studies and other more recent research. These patterns include a declining prevalence of thinness and increasing BMI throughout adolescence in both boys and girls, although boys typically have a greater prevalence of thinness than girls.

The ICRW studies found thinness (BMI-for-age <5th percentile defined by NCHS/WHO reference data) to be highly prevalent in only 3 countries: India

(53%), Nepal (36%), and Benin (23%).[7] Observed patterns in mean BMI in Nepal and Ecuador are illustrative of the gender differences often found in developing countries. The mean BMI of girls in Nepal was at approximately the 5th percentile of the reference curve at age 10, but increased to the 50th percentile between ages 15 and 18 years (Fig 3).[8] In Ecuador, the mean BMI of girls was at the 50th percentile of the reference at age 10 and increased well above that by age 18.[9] These increases in BMI across adolescence occurred despite the absence of concurrent gains in girls' height-for-age relative to the reference (see Fig 1). Boys' mean BMI remained lower in relation to the reference curve in Nepal and Ecuador, staying at the 5th percentile from 10 to 16 years and then rising in late adolescence (Fig 4). Ecuadorian boys tracked at the 50th percentile throughout adolescence (see Fig 4).

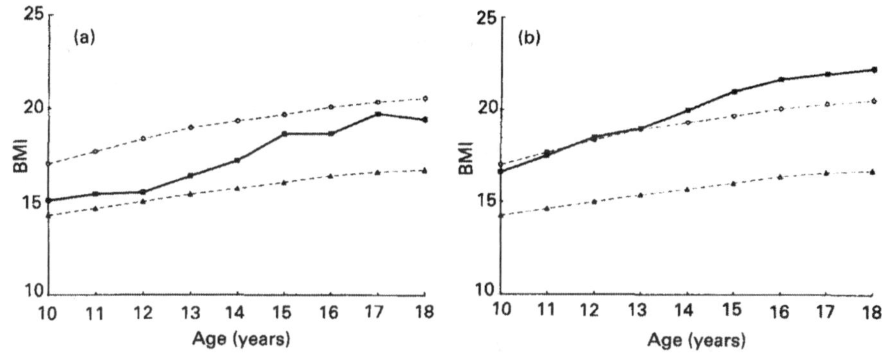

Fig 3. BMI of adolescent girls by age in the (a) Nepal and (b) Ecuador studies within the Nutrition of Adolescent Girls Research Program of the International Center for Research on Women. (●), 50th Percentile of the National Center for Health Statistics (NCHS) reference data (Hammill *et al.* 1979); (■), adolescent data from Nepal or Ecuador; (▲), 5th percentile of the NCHS reference data. From Kurtz K. Adolescent nutritional status in developing countries. *Proc Nut Soc.* 1996;55:321-331. Reprinted with permission.

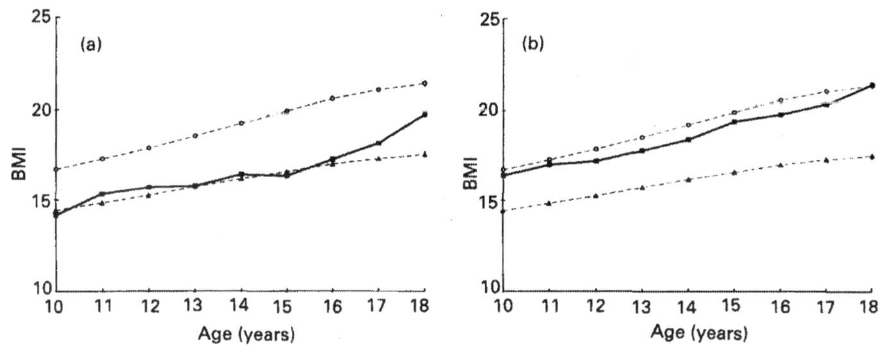

Fig 4. BMI of adolescent boys by age in the (a) Nepal and (b) Ecuador studies within the Nutrition of Adolescent Girls Research Program of the International Center for Research on Women. (●), 50th Percentile of the National Center for Health Statistics (NCHS) reference data (Hammill et al. 1979); (■), adolescent data from Nepal or Ecuador; (▲), 5th percentile of the NCHS reference data. From Kurtz K. Adolescent nutritional status in developing countries. *Proc Nut Soc.* 1996;55:321-331. Reprinted with permission.

The declining prevalence of thinness with age among adolescent girls is in part the result of the gain in body fat that occurs after menarche. Data from the study of Kenyan schoolgirls clearly demonstrates this relationship, finding that the prevalence of thinness among Kenyan schoolgirls aged 12 to 18 years was 15.6%, but this prevalence declined significantly with age and degree of sexual maturation.[10] The odds of thinness decreased significantly with increases in maturity rating, as assessed by the Tanner scale for breast development, and post-menarchal girls were 85% less likely than pre-menarchal girls to be thin.

Despite the reported low prevalence of thinness among adolescents in the ICRW studies, recent surveys suggest that thinness or underweight persists as a public health problem among adolescents in developing countries. The wide range of definitions for adolescent thinness again makes assessment of patterns difficult, but recent Demographic and Health Surveys (DHS, 2002-2007) revealed that "underweight" (BMI < 18.5) was prevalent among adolescent girls in sub-Saharan Africa and South Asia. Among the countries that participated in this survey, the prevalence of underweight in girls aged 15 to 19 years ranged from 27% to 47% (Fig 5).[3] Using the same definition, Ogechi et al found that more than 20% of Nigerian boys and girls were underweight.[12]

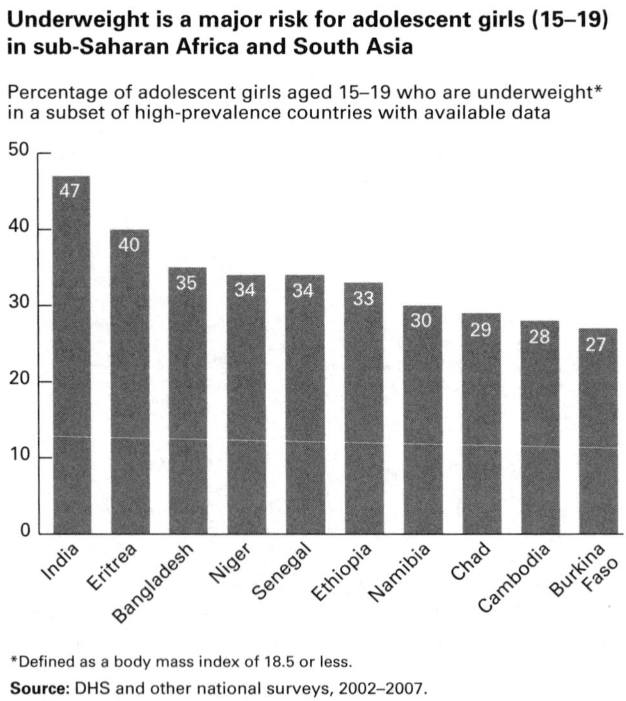

Fig 5. UNICEF. Adolescence: An age of opportunity. *State of the World's Children*. February 2011

Ogechi et al further found that underweight was associated with diets high in carbohydrates, low in fat, and inadequate in protein, particularly among boys.[12] Protein-rich foods are expensive in developing countries, and their frequent consumption is often limited to adolescents from the wealthiest families, as demonstrated in a recent study of the nutritional status and intake of adolescent Bangladeshi girls.[18] Using a 7-day food frequency questionnaire, Alam et al found that girls of the highest asset quintile ate fish or meat 2.1 days per week more than girls in the lowest asset quintile and consumed eggs/milk 2 days per week more. Indeed, food insecurity (lack of access to food to meet nutritional demands) at both the household and individual levels is an important determinant of adolescent undernutrition in many developing countries and has been linked with other adverse outcomes, including psychological stress, impaired cognition, and increased school absenteeism.[19,20]

Finally, infection with intestinal helminths, which is associated with unclean water and unhygienic living conditions, also contributes to underweight in adolescents. Studies of government schools in Ogun State, Nigeria, revealed that in many schools tap water was not available, sanitation of latrines was poor, soap for hand washing was not present, and garbage was lying around school grounds.[21] Such unsanitary conditions contributed to the high prevalence of helminth infections, with 54.9% of school children in the urban government school and 63.5% of children in the rural government school infected with *Ascaris lumbricoides*, *Trichuris trichiura*, *Taenia* species, and/or hookworm. These helminths can affect nutritional status through several mechanisms, including impairment of appetite and growth and, in the case of hookworm, via intestinal blood loss leading to iron deficiency.[22]

The link between intestinal helminths and poor nutritional status has been shown in several studies, including a recent study in Nigeria in which 32.9% of malnourished pupils (experiencing stunting, wasting, and/or underweight) versus 25.4% of nonmalnourished students attending public primary schools in Osun State were found to be infected with intestinal helminths.[23] Hookworm infection, in particular, was significantly associated with underweight, wasting, and stunting, whereas *Trichuris* was a risk factor for stunting. Similarly, in a cross-sectional sample of 1113 individuals from Brazil,[24] hookworm and *Ascaris* infections were prevalent among individuals aged 10 to 19 years, impacting 76.4% and 57.8% of adolescents, respectively. In combined multivariate regression analysis including children and adolescents aged 6 months to 19 years, *Ascaris* infection was associated with greater odds of stunting, low lean mass, and low fat mass.

Iron Deficiency

Iron deficiency is the most common nutritional deficiency worldwide.[25] The rapid growth of the adolescent period, and the accompanying increases in lean body mass, blood volume, and red cell mass, exact a large toll on iron stores, making adolescence a period of peak risk for iron deficiency in both boys and girls. Adequate iron is critical in adolescence because it helps ensure full cognitive function and optimal physical performance and better prepares girls for future pregnancy.[26] A recent *Lancet* article highlighted the long-term consequences of iron deficiency in adolescence, identifying iron-deficiency anemia as the 8th leading cause of disability-adjusted life years (DALYs) among boys aged 10 to 14 years and the 7th leading cause among girls aged 10 to 14 years.[27]

Because iron deficiency is the most common cause of anemia, the prevalence of anemia is typically used at the population level as an indicator of iron deficiency. The prevalence of anemia among adolescent girls aged 15 to 19 ranged from 49% to 68% in representative countries of sub-Saharan Africa and South Asia included in recent DHS and national surveys conducted between 2003 and 2009 (Fig 6),[3] indicating that little has affected anemia prevalence among adolescents on a global scale since the ICRW studies (1990-1994). Anemia was in fact found to be the most significant nutritional problem experienced by adolescents in ICRW countries, with a prevalence of 55% in India, 58% in Guatemala, 55% in India, 42% in Nepal, and 32% in Cameroon.[7]

Both boys and girls are at risk for iron deficiency during adolescence. In boys, the iron requirement climbs rapidly from 10 to 15 mg/day during the adolescent

Anaemia is a significant risk for adolescent girls (15–19) in sub-Saharan Africa and South Asia

Prevalence of anaemia among adolescent girls aged 15–19 in a subset of high-prevalence countries with available data

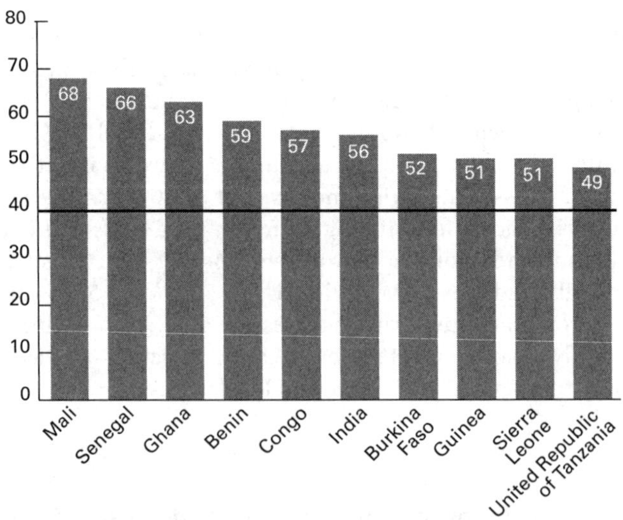

*The horizontal line at the 40% mark represents the threshold at which anaemia is considered a severe national public health issue.

Source: DHS and national surveys, 2003–2009.

Fig 6. UNICEF. Adolescence: An age of opportunity. *State of the World's Children*. February 2011

growth spurt, but any iron deficiency during this period of rapid growth and sexual maturation can be quickly corrected as the rate of growth slows and the need for iron diminishes.[28] Iron requirements also increase during adolescent growth in girls from 8 to 15 mg/day, but in contrast to boys, this increased need does not diminish following the period of rapid growth as menstruation necessitates additional dietary iron.[28]

In addition to the increased physiologic requirements for iron exacted by growth and menstruation, infectious diseases such as malaria and hookworm can also affect iron absorption, use, and loss in adolescents, and frequently contribute to iron deficiency in this age group. Malaria-related inflammation downregulates iron absorption at the gut level and also impairs its flux out of storage compartments, hindering its incorporation into red blood cells.[29] Iron deficiency resulting from hookworm typically results from direct intestinal blood loss caused by this parasite.[30]

Although adolescents often don't receive intervention priority, iron supplementation is an effective strategy for reducing anemia in this age group. The WHO recommends 3 months of preventative iron supplementation of 60 mg iron per day be given to adolescents living in areas where the population prevalence of anemia is greater than 40%.[31] Daily dietary iron supplementation of adolescent girls has been shown to improve mood and the ability to concentrate in school.[32] Perhaps more logistically feasible, weekly iron supplementation has also proven to be effective in reducing anemia prevalence in many developing countries.[33,34] Many recent studies have further found that multiple micronutrient supplementation of adolescent girls may improve not only iron status and reduce anemia prevalence,[35] but may have beneficial effects on the status of other micronutrients, including riboflavin, vitamin A, and vitamin C.[36]

OVERNUTRITION

Along with the problems of adolescent undernutrition, many developing countries also struggle with increasing adolescent overweight and obesity. In contrast to the more gradual process of urbanization in industrialized Western nations, the growth of large cities has occurred more rapidly in developing countries.[37] In 2009, around 50% of the world's 1.2 billion adolescents lived in urban areas, and this proportion is predicted to grow to 70% by 2050, with the most rapid increases in developing countries (Fig 7).[3] The impetus for this massive move to urban areas varies by country, but the driving forces can be dichotomized into "push factors" (eg, natural disasters, war, economic disasters, famine) and "pull factors" (eg, marriage, desire for better education or housing, job opportunities).[37] The nutritional effect of this large-scale urbanization, often coined the "nutrition transition," is that as people assume a more sedentary lifestyle, have more ready access to snack or street foods, and reduce consumption of more traditional foods, the prevalence of overweight and obesity increases substantially. Although

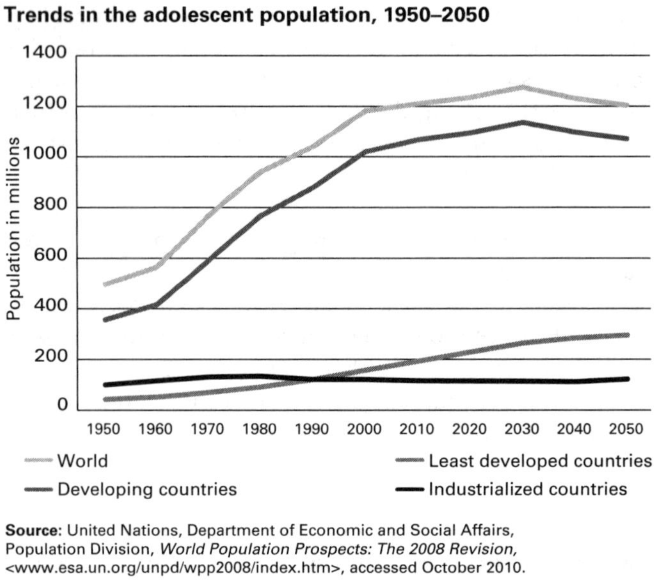

Fig 7. UNICEF. Adolescence: An age of opportunity. *State of the World's Children*. February 2011

the rise in overweight and obesity among adolescents in developing countries undergoing rapid urban growth has been described in several countries, including Brazil,[38] China,[39] Vietnam,[40] Sudan,[41] and Botswana,[42,43] the phenomenon is particularly well exemplified in South Africa[44-46] and India.[47-50]

South Africa

South Africa has undergone rapid urbanization since the 1950s and struggles with the dual problem of coexisting undernutrition and overnutrition. The 2002 South African Youth Risk Behaviour Survey documented a combined prevalence of overweight and obesity of 21% among 13- to 19-year-olds, with a much higher prevalence among girls (25%) than boys (7%).[51] National electrification of South Africa in the past few years, an increased number of televisions in homes, and a resulting reduction of physical activity among youth, have likely contributed to this prevalent overnutrition, which has recently been observed in both urban and rural areas of the country.[44]

In the Agincourt area of rural northeast South Africa, prevalent stunting among young children coexists with the growing problem of overnutrition among adolescents. Among youth aged 13 to 19 years in this area, the prevalence of combined overweight and obesity presented in a 2010 study was 16% among girls and 4% among boys.[44] Similarly, 16% of girls and 1% of boys had a high waist circumference, potentially indicating increased risk of metabolic disease. Because this study took place in a rural, impoverished area, the setting is not identical to that typically observed in nutrition transition countries undergoing rapid urbanization. However, some components are similar. The study site was a former apartheid homeland area with plots too small for subsistence agriculture. Consequently, people in the region rely on purchased food, which may lead to less food and undernutrition among those with limited financial resources, or cheaper energy-dense food and overnutrition among those with a bit more money.

A 2011 follow-up study of predictors of weight status and central obesity among adolescents aged 10 to 20 years living in the Agincourt area identified key child, maternal, and household factors.[45] Obesity increased with age and pubertal development and was much higher in girls than in boys. Potential explanations for this gender difference include more physical activity among boys and physiologic differences in fat and muscle gain. Further, cultural differences may play a role, as a larger body was observed as more beautiful among South African female adolescents in one study.[52] Maternal age was associated with central obesity among adolescents. The authors postulated that this relationship may be the result of less knowledge of the adverse effects of obesity among older mothers or the possibility that older mothers may monitor their child's behavior less, potentially affecting eating and physical activity patterns. Finally, socioeconomic status of the household, as assessed by an asset survey, was related to the odds of overweight and obesity, with a 2-fold higher odds observed among participants of the highest versus lowest socioeconomic status tertile.[45]

India

Extremes of undernutrition and overnutrition in India parallel the country's extremes of poverty and wealth. Numerous studies have found that overweight and obesity are significantly more prevalent among adolescents of higher socioeconomic status and among those in urban versus rural areas.[47-50] Various definitions and cutoffs for overweight and obesity further complicate assessment of the problem. Using Indian-specific BMI cutoffs, Gupta et al[47] tracked secular trends in the prevalence of obesity and overweight among Indian adolescents aged 14 to 17 living in urban areas and found that the prevalence of obesity rose significantly from 9.8% in 2006 to 11.7% in 2007. In accordance with other studies, the authors reported that high socioeconomic status, predominantly assessed as attendance at private versus government-funded school, was associated with an increasing trend in overweight and obesity. However, unlike other studies, adolescent males rather than females were more likely to be overnourished. The authors pose that this finding may be because of a heightened concern over appearance among female, but not among male, adolescents.

Further exploring the predictors of adolescent overweight and obesity in 12- to 17-year-old urban adolescents in Hyderabad, India, Laxmaiah et al[48] found that adolescents who watched more than 3 hours per day of television were nearly twice as likely, and those of high socioeconomic were more than 4 times as likely, to be overweight or obese. Regularly playing outdoor games for more than

6 hours per week or doing household activities for more than 3 hours per day were associated with a lower prevalence of overweight and obesity.

Finally, a literature review of 11 studies evaluating the nutritional status of Indian school children (6-18 years) from middle- and high-income households highlighted the fact that micronutrient undernutrition can coexist with obesity and overweight.[49] In these 11 studies, which utilized various cut-offs to define overnutrition, the prevalence of overweight ranged widely from 8.5% to 29.0% and the prevalence of obesity ranged between 1.5% to 7.5%. Concurrent with this overnutrition, the prevalence of anemia ranged from 19% to 88%, and deficiencies of folate (nearly 100%), riboflavin, niacin, vitamin C, vitamin A, and vitamin B12 were also reported to be common (40-60% prevalence for each) in one study included in the review.

A LINK BETWEEN UNDERNUTRITION AND OVERNUTRITION?

In addition to environmental factors contributing to the increasing prevalence of overweight and obesity in many countries undergoing the nutrition transition, it is possible that childhood undernutrition, prevalent in many of these countries, may predispose individuals to obesity and associated chronic diseases later in life. A wide body of literature describes how poor fetal and childhood developmental programming, including intrauterine growth restriction and childhood stunting, can lead to obesity and chronic disease later in life, particularly if an individual shifts from an environment of deprivation to one of relatively more wealth and abundance.

Although seemingly unrelated, the nutritional problems of undernutrition and overnutrition among adolescents in developing countries are intricately woven together in an intergenerational cycle of malnutrition. As described by a United Nations Standing Committee on Nutrition in 2000 and depicted in Figure 8,[28] a malnourished mother is more likely to have inadequate pregnancy weight gain, contributing to inadequate fetal nutrition and a low birth weight infant. Low birth weight infants in developing countries are often born into environments where proper nutrition, health care, and sanitation are lacking and infectious disease is prevalent. Consequently the young child experiences stunted growth and, remaining in the same environment, becomes a stunted adolescent. If an adolescent who is stunted or consumes an inadequate diet becomes pregnant, she is at higher risk of delivering a low birth weight infant, and the cycle begins again. However, if the environment of the child who was low birth weight or experienced stunted growth changes to one with more ready access to food, greater wealth, and less physical activity, the risk of obesity and associated chronic disease later in life may be elevated.

CONCLUSIONS

Several intervention points exist where this cycle of intergenerational malnutrition could be disrupted. One is to promote growth and improve nutritional status in

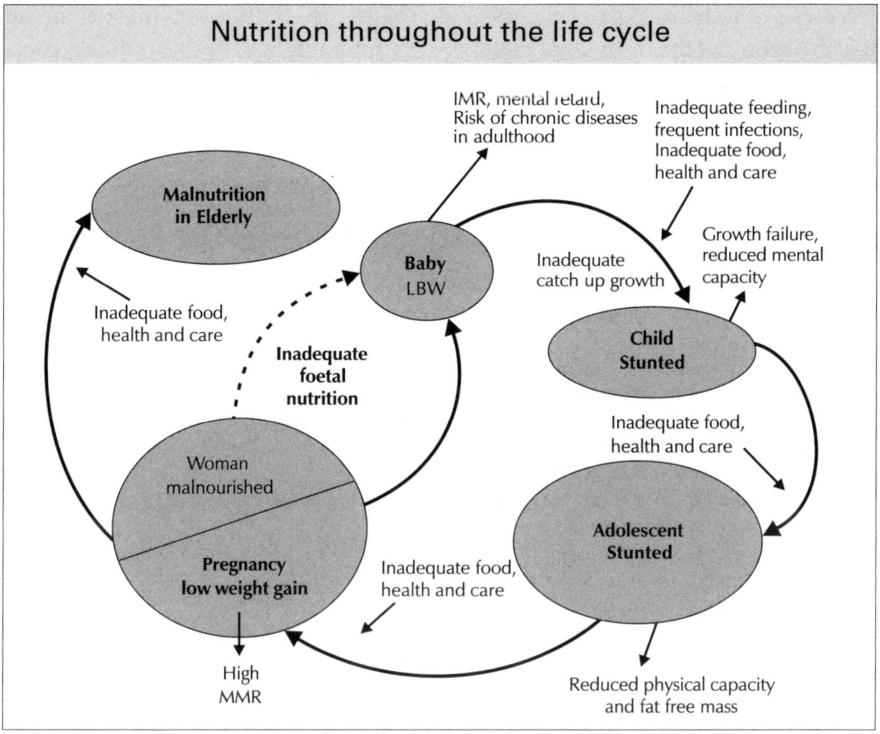

Fig 8. World Health Organization. Adolescent nutrition: a review of the situation in selected South-East Asian countries. 2006. Available at: http://www.searo.who.int/EN/Section13/Section38_11624.htm. Accessed April 14, 2012

early childhood, through food supplementation programs, breastfeeding promotion, and nutritional guidance during weaning, along with control of infectious disease. Another is to increase awareness of the benefits of postponing the age of marriage so that women enter into pregnancy with optimal nutritional status and have a lower risk of pregnancy complications. Roughly 16 million adolescent girls aged 15 to 19 years give birth each year, representing about 11% of all births worldwide.[53] Ninety-five percent of these births to adolescent mothers occur in low- and middle-income countries.[53] Pregnancy exacts a profound nutritional toll on an adolescent girl, increasing her requirement for both macronutrients and micronutrients. The increased nutritional needs of the mother are in direct competition with those of the fetus, particularly if the mother is still growing herself.[54] Increasing evidence also suggests that intrauterine growth restriction can increase the risk for obesity and chronic disease in adulthood,[55] while maternal hemoglobin can affect infant hemoglobin concentration for up to 12 months after birth.[56]

Intervention at any of these generational stages would result in improved nutritional status and health of adolescents. Improving the nutritional status of adolescents not only breaks the vicious cycle of intergenerational malnutrition, but it also optimizes the individual talents, skills, and potential of this critical group, increasing quality of life and the productivity of nations.

References

1. World Health Organization. Maternal, newborn, child and adolescent health. Adolescent development page. Available at: http://www.who.int/maternal_child_adolescent/topics/adolescence/dev/en/index.html. Accessed April 13, 2012
2. Cordeiro L, Lamstein S, Mahmud Z, Levinson F. Adolescent malnutrition in developing countries: a close look at the problem and at two national experiences. *SCN News*. Late 2005-Early 2006; issue 31
3. UNICEF. Adolescence: an age of opportunity. *State of the World's Children*. February 2011. Available at: www.unicef.org/sowc2011/index.php. Accessed October 31, 2012.
4. WHO Expert Committee. Adolescents. In: WHO, *Physical status: The use and interpretation of anthropometry*. Geneva, Switzerland; 1995:263-311. Available at: http://whqlibdoc.who.int/trs/WHO_TRS_854.pdf. Accessed October 31, 2012.
5. Cole T, Bellizzi M, Flegal K, Dietz W. Establishing a standard definition for child overweight and obesity worldwide: international survey. *BMJ*. 2000;320:1240-1243
6. Cole T, Flegal K, Nicholis D, Jackson A. Body mass index cut offs to define thinness in children and adolescents: international survey. *BMJ*. 2007;335:194; article first published online Jun 25
7. Kurtz K. Adolescent nutritional status in developing countries. *Proc Nut Soc*. 1996;55:321-331
8. Regmi S, Adhikari R. A study on the factors influencing nutritional status of adolescent girls in Nepal. *Nutrition of Adolescent Girls Research Program*. 1994; 6. Washington, D.C.: International Center for Research on Women
9. de Grijalva Y, de Grijalva I. Improving nutritional practices of Ecuadorian adolescents. *Nutrition of Adolescent Girls Research Program*. 1994; 11. Washington, D.C.: International Center for Research on Women
10. Leenstra T, Petersen L, Kariuki S, Oloo A, Kager P, ter Kuile F. Prevalence and severity of malnutrition and age at menarche; cross-sectional studies in adolescent schoolgirls in western Kenya. *Eur J Clin Nutr*. 2005;59:41-48
11. Jafar T, Qadri Z, Islam M, Hatcher J, Bhutta Z, Chaturvedi N. Rise in childhood obesity with persistently high rates of undernutrition among urban school-aged Indo-Asian children. *Arch Dis Child*. 2008;93:373-378
12. Ogechi P, Akhakhia I, Ugwunna A. Nutritional status and energy intake of adolescents in Umuahia Urban, Nigeria. *Pakistan J Nutr*. 2007;6:641-646
13. Coly A, Milet J, Diallo A et al. Preschool stunting, adolescent migration, catch-up growth, and adult height in young Senegalese men and women of rural origin. *J Nutr*. 2006;136:2414-2420
14. Kurtz K. Adolescent Growth. UN system archives. Available at: http://www.unsystem.org/SCN/archives/scnnews11/ch04.htm. Accessed April 14, 2012
15. Delisle H, Chandra-Mouli V, de Benoist B. Should adolescents be specifically targeted for nutrition in developing countries? To address which problems and how? Available at: http://www.idpas.org/pdf/1803ShouldAdolescentsBeTargeted.pdf. Accessed April 14, 2012
16. Kulin H, Bwibo N, Mutie D, Santner B. The effect of chronic childhood malnutrition on pubertal growth and development. *Am J Clin Nutr*. 1982;36:527-536
17. Proos L. Growth and development of Indian children adopted in Sweden. *Indian J Med Res*. 2009;130:646-650
18. Alam N, Roy S, Ahmed T, Ahmed A. Nutritional status, dietary intake, and relevant knowledge of adolescent girls in rural Bangladesh. *J Health Popul Nutr*. 2010;28:86-94
19. Belachew T, Hadley C, Lindstrom D, Gebremariam A, Lachat C, Kolsteren P. Food insecurity, school absenteeism and educational attainment of adolescents in Jimma Zone Southwest Ethiopia: a longitudinal study. *Nutr J*. 2011;10:29

20. Hamelin A, Habicht J, Beaudry M. Food insecurity: consequences for the household and broader social implications. *J Nutr.* 1999;129:525S-528S
21. Ekpo U, Odoemene S, Mafina C, Sam-Wobo S. Helminthiasis and hygiene conditions of schools in Ikenne, Ogun State, Nigeria. *PLoS Neglected Tropical Diseases.* 2008;2:e146
22. World Bank Publications. Adolescent nutrition. Available at: http://web.worldbank.org/WBSITE/EXTERNAL/TOPICS/EXTHEALTHNUTRITIONANDPOPULATION/EXTNUTRITION/0,,contentMDK:20206757~menuPK:483704~pagePK:148956~piPK:216618~theSitePK:282575,00.html. Accessed April 14, 2012
23. Oninla S, Onayade A, Owa J. Impact of intestinal helminthiasis on the nutritional status of primary-school children in Osun State, south-western Nigeria. *Ann Trop Med Parasitol.* 2010;104:583-594
24. Jardim-Botelho A, Brooker S, Geiger S. Age patterns in undernutrition and helminth infection in a rural area of Brazil. *Trop Med Int Health.* 2008;13:454-467
25. World Health Organization. Micronutrient deficiencies: iron deficiency anaemia. Available at: http://www.who.int/nutrition/topics/ida/en/. Accessed April 14, 2012
26. Lynch S. The potential impact of iron supplementation during adolescence on iron status in pregnancy. *J Nutr.* 2000;130(Suppl 2S):448S-451S
27. Gore F, Bloem P, Patton G, et al. Global burden of disease in young people aged 10-24 years: a systematic analysis. *Lancet.* 2011;277:2093-2102
28. World Health Organization. Adolescent nutrition: a review of the situation in selected South-East Asian countries. 2006. Available at: http://www.searo.who.int/EN/Section13/Section38_11624.htm. Accessed April 14, 2012
29. Nweneka C, Doherty C, Cox S, Prentice A. Iron delocalisation in the pathogenesis of malarial anaemia. *Trans R Soc Trop Med Hyg.* 2010;104:175-184
30. Stephenson L. Helminth parasites, a major factor in malnutrition. *World Health Forum.* 1994;15:169-172
31. World Health Organization. Iron deficiency anaemia: assessment, prevention, and control. A guide for programme managers. 2001. Available at: http://whqlibdoc.who.int/hq/2001/WHO_NHD_01.3.pdf. Accessed April 14, 2012
32. Ballin A, Berar M, Rubinstein U, Kleter Y, Hershkovitz A, Meytes D. Iron state in female adolescents. *Am J Dis Child.* 1992;146:803-805
33. Deshmukh P, Garg B, Bharambe M. Effectiveness of weekly supplementation of iron to control anemia among adolescent girls of Nashik, Maharashtra, India. *J Health Popul Nutr.* 2008;26:74-78
34. Kotecha P, Nirupam S, Karkar P. Adolescent girls' anaemia control programme, Gujarat, India. *Indian J Med Res.* 2009;130:584-589
35. Ahmed F, Khan M, Akhtaruzzaman M, et al. Effect of long-term intermittent supplementation with multiple micronutrients compared with ion-and-folic acid supplementation on Hb and micronutrient status of non-anaemic adolescent schoolgirls in rural Bangladesh. *Br J Nutr.* 2012;16:1-10
36. Ahmed F, Khan M, Akhtaruzzaman M, et al. Long-term intermittent multiple micronutrient supplementation enhances hemoglobin and micronutrient status more than iron+folic acid supplementation in Bangladeshi rural adolescent girls with nutritional anemia. *J Nutr.* 2010;140:1879-1886
37. Godfrey R, Julien M. Urbanisation and health. *Clin Med.* 2005;5:137-141
38. Kac G, Velasquez-Melendez G, Schlussel M, Segall-Correa A, Silva A, Perez-Escamilla R. Severe food insecurity is associated with obesity among Brazilian adolescent females. *Public Health Nutr.* 2012;17:1-7
39. Cui Z, Dibley M. Trends in dietary energy, fat, carbohydrate and protein intake in Chinese children and adolescents from 1991 to 2009. *Br J Nutr.* 2012;16:1-8
40. Tang H, Dibley M, Sibbritt D. Gender and socio-economic differences in BMI of secondary high school students in Ho Chi Minh City. *Asia Pac J Clin Nutr.* 2007;16:74-83
41. Nagwa M, Elhussein A, Azza M, Abdulhadi N. Alarming high prevalence of overweight/obesity among Sudanese children. *Eur J Clin Nutr.* 2011;65:409-411

42. Wrotniak B, Malete L, Maruapula S, et al. Association between socioeconomic status indicators and obesity in adolescent students in Botswana, an African country in rapid nutrition transition. *Pediatr Obes.* 2012;7:e9-e13
43. Maruapula S, Jackson J, Holsten J, et al. Socio-economic status and urbanization are linked to snacks and obesity in adolescents in Botswana. *Public Health Nutr.* 2011;14:2260-2267
44. Kimani-Murage E, Kahn K, Pettifor J, et al. The prevalence of stunting, overweight and obesity, and metabolic disease risk in rural South African children. *BMC Public Health.* 2010;10:158
45. Kimani-Murage E, Kahn K, Pettifor J, Tollman S, Klipstein-Grobusch K, Norris S. Predictors of adolescent weight status and central obesity in rural South Africa. *Public Health Nutr.* 2011;14:1114-1122
46. Kruger R, Kruger H, MacIntyre U. The determinants of overweight and obesity among 10- to 15-year-old school children in the North West Province, South Africa – the THUSA BANA (Transition and Health during Urbanisation of South Africans; BANA, children) study. *Public Health Nutr.* 2005;9:351-358
47. Gupta D, Shah P, Misra A, et al. Secular trends in prevalence of overweight and obesity from 2006-2009 in urban Asian Indian adolescents aged 14-17 years. *PLoS One.* 2011;6:e17221
48. Laxmaiah A, Nagalla B, Vijayaraghavan K, Nair M. Factors affecting prevalence of overweight among 12- to 17-year-old urban adolescents in Hyderabad, India. *Obesity.* 2007;6:1384-1390
49. Srihari G, Eilander A, Muthayya S, Kurpad A, Seshadri S. Nutritional status of affluent Indian school children: what and how much do we know? *Indian Pediatr.* 2007;44:204-213
50. Stigler M, Arora M, Dhavan P, Shrivastav R, Reddy K, Perry C. Weight-related concerns and weight-control behaviors among overweight adolescents in Delhi, India: a cross-sectional story. *Int J Behav Nutr Phys Act.* 2011;8:9
51. Reddy S, Resnicow K, James S, Kambaran N, Omardien R, Mbewu A. Underweight, overweight and obesity among South African adolescents: results of the 2002 National Youth Risk Behaviour Survey. *Public Health Nutr.* 2008:1-5
52. McHiza Z, Goedecke J, Lambert E. Intra-familial and ethnic effects on attitudinal and perceptual body image: a cohort of South African mother-daughter dyads. *BMC Public Health.* 2011;11:433
53. World Health Organization. Maternal, newborn, child and adolescent health. Adolescent pregnancy. Available at: http://www.who.int/maternal_child_adolescent/topics/maternal/adolescent_pregnancy/en/index.html. Accessed April 14, 2012
54. Stang J. Physical and Psychosocial Growth and Development of Adolescents. In: *Guidelines for Adolescent Nutrition Services.* M Story, J Stang, I Alton, eds. Minneapolis, MN: Center for Leadership, Education and Training in Maternal and Child Nutrition, Division of Epidemiology and Community Health, School of Public Health, University of Minnesota; 2005
55. Barker D. The origins of the developmental origins theory. *J Intern Med.* 2007;261:412-417
56. Miller MF, Stoltzfus RJ, Mbuya N. Total body iron in HIV-positive and HIV-negative Zimbabwean newborns strongly predicts anemia throughout infancy and is predicted by maternal hemoglobin concentration. *J Nutr.* 2003;133:3461-3468

Adolesc Med 023 (2012) 457–470

The Truth about Vitamin D and Adolescent Skeletal Health

Nina S. Ma, MD*[a], Catherine M. Gordon, MD, MSc[b]

[a]*Division of Endocrinology, Boston Children's Hospital, Harvard Medical School, USA*

[b]*Divisions of Adolescent Medicine and Endocrinology, Hasbro Children's Hospital, Warren Alpert Medical School of Brown University, USA*

Vitamin D plays a critical role in skeletal homeostasis. This is illustrated by severe deficiency resulting in profound skeletal abnormalities such as rickets in growing children, and osteomalacia in adults.

In the past, vitamin D deficiency was a major health problem. However, after the discovery that sun exposure and vitamin D fortification of common dietary sources could cure and prevent rickets, the skeletal health consequences of vitamin D deficiency were eradicated from healthy populations. Vitamin D deficiency rickets is now uncommon in industrialized countries except among high-risk groups such as those with end-stage liver or kidney disease, malabsorption, or dark skin and low dietary calcium intake.[1,2]

The discussion about vitamin D has changed over time and now focuses on identifying optimal intake levels that yield maximal health benefits beyond simply preventing rickets and osteomalacia. For example, the adolescent skeleton accumulates a considerable amount of bone mass during pubertal growth, and adult osteoporosis prevention begins during the pediatric and adolescent years.[3-6] While mildly low vitamin D levels may not cause rickets or osteomalacia, there are concerns that chronic vitamin D insufficiency contributes to subtle bone mineralization defects and low bone density during a vulnerable window of skeletal growth.

The vitamin D receptor has been identified in more than 30 tissues, and it is involved in the regulation of more than 200 genes.[2,7] The role of vitamin D in the

*Corresponding author.
E-mail address: nina.ma@childrens.harvard.edu (N. S. Ma).
Catherine M. Gordon, MD, MSc, is a consult for the Pfizer-sponsored Mobility Advisory Board. Nina S. Ma, MD, does not have financial disclosures or conflicts of interest to report.

 ISSN 1934-4287

regulation of cell proliferation, differentiation, and apoptosis has broadly implicated this nutrient in the treatment and prevention of cancers, autoimmune disorders, infection, cardiovascular disease, and other maladies.[7] There is an evolving complexity to vitamin D and its newfound interactions beyond its role in calcium, phosphorous, and skeletal homeostasis.

Research in the nonclassical benefits of vitamin D is ongoing, but, currently, there is insufficient evidence to recommend the evaluation and treatment of vitamin D deficiency for extraskeletal effects. So, the focus of this article is the relationship between vitamin D and skeletal health outcomes only. The specific aims are to present (1) the multiple forms and functions of vitamin D, (2) the prevalence and correlates of vitamin D deficiency in adolescents, (3) the identification of an optimal serum level, and (4) the evaluation and treatment of hypovitaminosis D in adolescent youth.

FORMS AND FUNCTIONS OF VITAMIN D

Vitamin D is synthesized in the skin (D_3) or ingested through the diet or supplements (D_2 or D_3). D_2 and D_3 are biologically inert and require 2 additional steps for activation. The first step occurs in the liver where the 25-hydroxylase enzyme hydroxylates carbon-25 to form 25-hydroxyvitamin D (25-OH-D). The half-life of 25-OH-D approximates 2 to 3 weeks.[1,2] Because of its longer half-life, a serum 25-OH-D level is the most accurate measure of vitamin D stores and reflects total exposure through sunlight, diet, and supplements.[8] There are assays that discriminate D_2 from D_3, and these may be helpful to assess consumption of plant-and-animal-derived sources of vitamin D, respectively. However, knowing the total 25-OH-D (D_2 plus D_3) level is usually sufficient for the care of most patients. 25-OH-D is also the biomarker that is used most often to examine relationships between vitamin D status and health outcomes.

The second activation step occurs in the kidneys where the 1α-hydroxylase enzyme converts 25-OH-D to 1,25-dihydroxyvitamin D (calcitriol). Calcitriol is the biologically active form of vitamin D and exerts its action on the small intestine and bone to raise serum calcium and phosphorus concentrations. The half-life of calcitriol is only 4 hours. Also, its activation is tightly regulated. Thus, the concentration of calcitriol may be normal or even elevated in the setting of vitamin D deficiency. Therefore, checking a 1,25-dihydroxyvitamin D level typically offers little clinical value except in specialized circumstances.[1-3]

PREVALENCE OF VITAMIN D DEFICIENCY

There is a high prevalence of vitamin D deficiency among adolescents. Approximately 31% to 33% of US youth ages 12 to 19 years have serum 25-OH-D levels less than 20 ng/mL (50 nmol/L) and 75% to 79% have levels less than 30 ng/mL (75 nmol/L).[9] Residence at northern geographic latitudes further increases the risk for vitamin D deficiency.[10,11] In Boston, Massachusetts, up to 42% of healthy adolescents have 25-OH-D levels at or less than 20 ng/mL and in Cleveland, Ohio, 54% of healthy, post-menarchal girls have levels at or less than 20 ng/mL.[12,13]

When specific seasonal and racial/ethnic differences are considered, the highest prevalence of deficiency occurs during the colder months and among black youth.[12,13] These observations may be explained by decreased sunlight exposure and cutaneous vitamin D synthesis, especially in dark-skinned persons. Also, there are racial/ethnic differences in beverage consumption. Lower average milk intake among black youth may account further for their lower 25-OH-D levels when compared to white and Hispanic youth.[14]

There is an even higher prevalence of vitamin D deficiency in obese adolescents. Among adolescents with a body mass index (BMI) greater than the 95th percentile at an urban center in the US Northeast, 72% of girls and 69% of boys had 25-OH-D levels less than 20 ng/mL. An alarming 100% of girls and 91% of boys had levels at or less than 30 ng/mL.[15] Similar findings were observed in Poland, where 86% of obese adolescents had 25-OH-D levels less than 20 ng/mL.[16]

Debate exists as to whether vitamin D deficiency is a modern subclinical disorder of pandemic proportions or an over-diagnosis due to a paradigm shift in the definition of what constitutes "deficiency." According to a recent report from the Institute of Medicine (IOM), a serum 25-OH-D level of 20 ng/mL covers the requirement of at least 97.5% of the population.[17] The Endocrine Society guideline views 30 ng/mL as a minimum 25-OH-D level for individuals at risk for vitamin D deficiency.[8] Regardless of how "sufficiency" is defined by a serum 25-OH-D level of 20 ng/mL or 30 ng/mL, vitamin D deficiency is common in adolescents.

CORRELATES OF VITAMIN D DEFICIENCY

There are several possible explanations for a high prevalence of vitamin D deficiency in adolescents. A few of these risk factors may also explain the 15% to 16% decline in vitamin D status during the past 2 decades in US adolescents (Fig 1).[9] Between 1988 to 1994 and 2001 to 2006, the population mean serum 25-OH-D level decreased from 26 ng/mL to 22 ng/mL among those ages 12 to 19 years (Fig 2).[9]

Nutrition

It is estimated that less than 10% of vitamin D is gleaned through the diet.[2,18] Natural food sources rich in vitamin D include cod liver oil and fatty fish (wild salmon, tuna, mackerel, and sardines).[7] For most adolescents, these sources of vitamin D have always been unpopular food choices.

There are conflicting reports on whether changes in milk consumption help to explain the recent decline in 25-OH-D in the United States.[9,12,19,20] As forti-

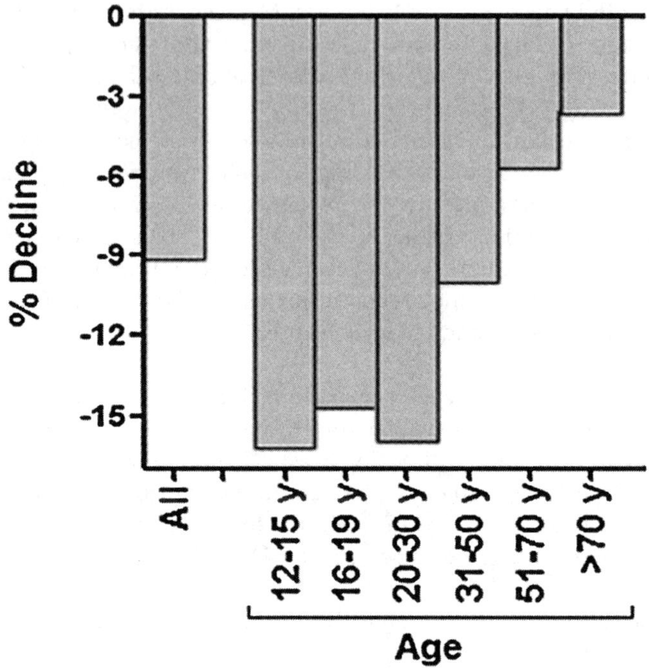

Fig 1. Decline in vitamin D status from NHANES 1988 to 1994 to NHANES 2001 to 2006 by age. Adapted with permission from Ganji V, Zhang X, Tangpricha V. Serum 25-hydroxyvitamin D concentrations and prevalence estimates of hypovitaminosis D in the U.S. population based on assay-adjusted data. *J Nutr*. 2012;142:498-507.

fication practices have not changed significantly in recent years and US fortified milk contains only 100 international units (IU) of vitamin D per 8-ounce serving, marked shifts in milk consumption would be necessary to lower serum 25-OH-D levels. Therefore, although low consumption of vitamin D enriched foods and beverages contribute to low systemic levels of vitamin D in adolescents, it is reasonable to surmise that there are other factors besides nutrition that have contributed to the decline in vitamin D status over time (Fig 3).

Sunscreen

Increased sun protection is advocated to prevent premature aging and some skin cancers. However, the use of sunscreen effectively blocks solar ultraviolet B radiation and abrogates greater than 90% of cutaneous vitamin D synthesis.[21] When the skin's capacity to make vitamin D is hampered, the body relies heavily on nutritional sources of vitamin D. As already discussed, adolescents consume few foods rich in vitamin D.

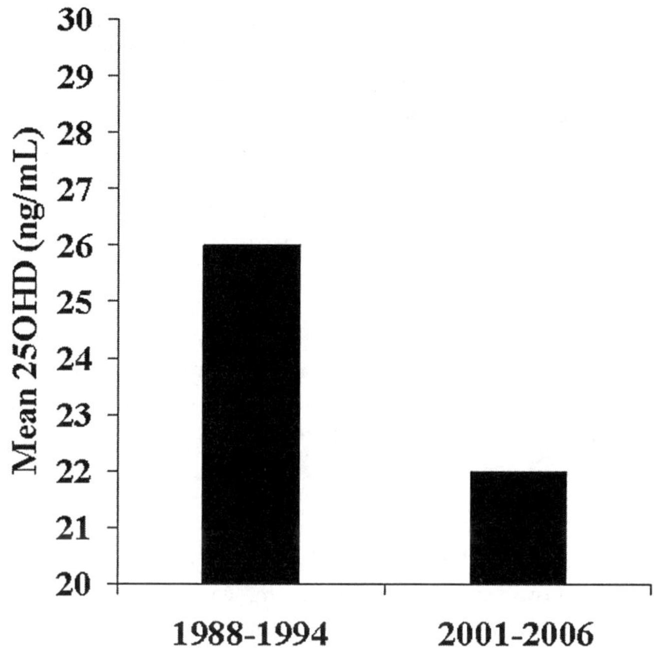

Fig 2. Mean serum 25-OH-D concentrations decreased from 26 ng/mL to 22 ng/mL among adolescents ages 12 to 19 years between 1988 to 1994 and 2001 to 2006.

Obesity

There is a high prevalence of obesity in adolescents. Current estimates are 18.4% for obese and 33.6% for overweight or obese among the 12- to 19-year-old age group.[22] The decline in serum 25-OH-D levels in the US population has been linked to increasing BMI trends.[9,20]

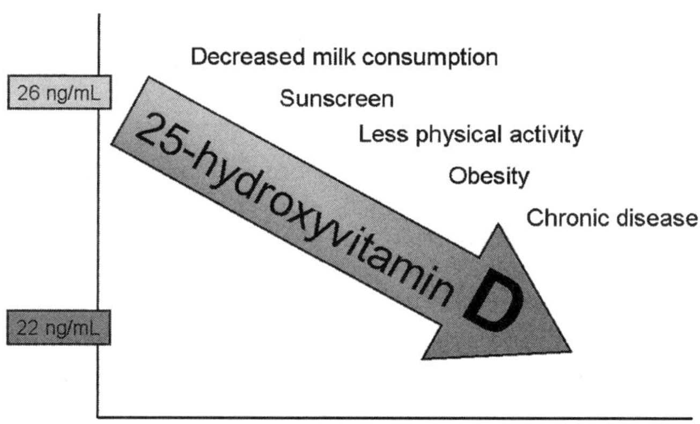

Fig 3. Risk factors for vitamin D deficiency in adolescents.

Wortsman et al[23] examined the mechanism leading to the association of subnormal vitamin D levels with obesity and demonstrated that after the same ultraviolet B radiation exposure, obese subjects increased their serum 25-OH-D levels 57% less than those who were not obese. These data suggest that obese individuals readily sequester cutaneous vitamin D into adipose tissue rendering it less bioavailable. Wortsman et al also demonstrated that after an oral dose of vitamin D, peak serum 25-OH-D levels inversely correlated with BMI.[23] Thus, larger doses of vitamin D intake are necessary in obesity.

Obese adolescents also typically engage in fewer athletic activities, and low physical activity is an independent predictor of hypovitaminosis D.[12] Decreased physical activity as a surrogate for sunlight exposure and cutaneous vitamin D synthesis combined with decreased bioavailability of vitamin D render obese adolescents at very high risk for deficiency.

Chronic Disease

Vitamin D deficiency is well documented among young people with cystic fibrosis, inflammatory bowel disease, and other malabsorption syndromes.[24-29] The explanation for this finding is specific to the underlying disease pathophysiology and the presence of a chronic illness.

Cystic fibrosis has been referred to as the "perfect storm" for vitamin D deficiency.[24] Inadequate intake, impaired intestinal absorption, reduced hepatic hydroxylation of vitamin D, and decreased levels of vitamin D-binding protein are all potential causes of deficiency in those with cystic fibrosis. Other chronic disease models mimic to varying degrees the different causes of low vitamin D seen in individuals with cystic fibrosis.

The long-term use of medications such as corticosteroids and antiepileptic drugs also increase vitamin D catabolism and further exacerbate the severity of vitamin D deficiency.[7,30-32] In addition, chronically ill patients often spend less time in the sunlight because of frequent hospitalizations or intentional avoidance of exposure because of photosensitivity from antibiotics or immunosuppressive therapies.[7]

The etiology for vitamin D deficiency in chronic illness is multifactorial. It is possible that the longer survival of individuals with chronic disease is contributing to the prevalence and decline in vitamin D.

Anorexia Nervosa

It is intriguing that female adolescents with anorexia nervosa and low fat mass have a low prevalence of vitamin D deficiency. In one study, only 2% of female adolescents had serum 25-OH-D levels lower than 20 ng/mL.[33] The low prevalence of vitamin D deficiency in anorexia nervosa is in contrast to the very high rates seen in obese adolescent youth. The reason for this finding is uncertain, but it is conjectured that females with anorexia nervosa compensate for poor nutritional intake with diligent adherence to low-caloric nutrient supplementation.[33] The bioavailability of vitamin D in adolescents with low fat mass was examined and shown to be similar to normal weight controls.[34]

OPTIMAL SERUM 25-OH-D IN ADOLESCENTS

An IOM committee carefully integrated the evidence on 25-OH-D concentrations and bone health outcomes. They concluded that 25-OH-D levels of 16 ng/mL would meet the needs of approximately one-half of the population, and 20 ng/mL would cover the requirement of at least 97.5% of the population. The IOM committee did not find that 25-OH-D levels greater than 20 ng/mL were consistently associated with greater benefits at a population level.[17]

However, when considering the needs of an individual, particularly if an adolescent is afflicted with chronic disease, vitamin D experts recommend aiming for a serum 25-OH-D level greater than 30 ng/mL. This recommendation is based on adult studies that demonstrate more efficient intestinal calcium absorption, a plateau in parathyroid hormone (PTH), and hip and nonvertebral fracture prevention when 25-OH-D concentrations are greater than 30 ng/mL.[8] Whether these data can be generalized to younger patient populations is uncertain. To explore what is the optimal serum 25-OH-D level for adolescents, studies have examined bone mineral density (BMD), inflection points for maximal PTH suppression, and fracture risk outcomes.

Bone Density

There are a fair number of studies that show positive associations between 25-OH-D and BMD.[10,35-37] In females 14 to 16 years, a vitamin D level at or less than 16 ng/mL was found to correspond with low forearm bone density.[10] In healthy, peripubertal girls ages 9 to 15 years, research has also shown a significant association between baseline 25-OH-D and 3-year change in BMD at the lumbar spine and femoral neck.[37] Girls in the highest tertile of mean baseline 25-OH-D (17.8 ng/mL) had 26% greater BMD gains over 3 years at the lumbar spine compared to girls in the lowest tertile (7.6 ng/mL).[37] In a recent meta-analysis of 6 randomized controlled trials of vitamin D supplementation, the studies with low baseline vitamin D levels (<14 ng/mL) demonstrated significant changes in total body bone mineral and lumbar spine BMD. However, a statistically significant effect of vitamin D supplementation on BMD was not found in healthy children and adolescents when serum 25-OH-D levels were greater than 20 ng/mL.[38]

PTH Suppression

Vitamin D deficiency causes secondary hyperparathyroidism and in many adult studies, serum 25-OH-D is negatively correlated with PTH.[39] The elevation in PTH is the proposed mechanism through which vitamin D deficiency contributes to fracture risk in adults, potentially through increased bone resorption.[40] Identifying an inflection point for maximal PTH suppression is, therefore, another strategy to estimate optimal serum 25-OH-D levels.

Previous studies in children and adolescents suggested, as in adults, a similar inverse relationship between serum 25-OH-D and PTH. However, until recently, those studies were small and nongeneralizable.[10,12,41,42] To elucidate the relationship between serum 25-OH-D and PTH in young patients, Hill et al analyzed pooled data for 735 subjects ages 7 to 18 years from 3 separate study sites. The results of this study indicated an absence of a clearly defined inflection point.[43] The interplay of different mechanisms regulating PTH in growing skeletons compared to adults is a plausible explanation for these results. More research is needed to determine if PTH suppression should be used to help define vitamin D sufficiency in children and adolescents.

Fracture Risk

With regard to vitamin D status and fracture risk outcomes in adolescents, the evidence is limited.[44] In a cross-sectional analysis of girls ages 11 to 17 years from the Growing Up Today Study, vitamin D intake was unrelated to stress fracture.[45] However, a prospective study conducted by Sonneville et al demonstrated that vitamin D intake was predictive of lower stress fracture risk in 9- to 15-year-old adolescent females who participated in at least 1 hour per day of high-impact activity (eg, running, basketball, soccer, tennis, cheerleading, volleyball). Girls in the highest quintile of vitamin D intake (mean = 663 IU/day) were shown to have an approximately 50% lower risk of stress fracture compared to those in the lowest quintile (mean = 107 IU/day).[46]

In a different study that examined obese children and adolescents, youth with vitamin D levels less than 16 ng/mL were 7.33 times more likely to have Blount disease than those with higher vitamin D levels. No association was shown between vitamin D status and slipped capital femoral epiphysis or fracture in obese adolescents.[47]

Limitations

There is fair evidence that clinically significant bone health benefits may be seen with 25-OH-D levels at approximately 20 ng/mL. The evidence to support higher vitamin D levels is less consistent. However, the data available to determine an optimal serum 25-OH-D threshold for adolescents is heterogeneous and may be difficult to interpret.[48] Across studies, there are differences in baseline characteristics, as well as outcome measures. Multiple competing and confounding factors among vitamin D studies also exist, including age, gender, race/ethnicity, BMI, calcium intake, physical activity, season, and geographical location. Also, inherent to the study of adolescents are unique patterns of growth and puberty.

Moreover, the laboratory assays for 25-OH-D are not standardized, and there may be up to 32% inter-laboratory imprecision.[49] Vitamin D intoxication is extremely rare and 25-OH-D levels approaching 100 ng/mL have not been associated with harm.[2] Hypercalcemia and hyperphosphatemia are not typically seen until 25-OH-D levels reach closer to 150 ng/mL.[7] There is minimal risk in aiming for 25-OH-D levels around 30 ng/mL.

EVALUATION OF VITAMIN D STATUS

Individuals at risk for vitamin D deficiency or who may benefit from optimizing their vitamin D status should be screened with a serum 25-OH-D level. Those at risk for metabolic bone disease from vitamin D deficiency include individuals with heritable disorders of vitamin D metabolism, malabsorption, or chronic ailments affecting organs involved in the synthesis and activation of vitamin D (ie, skin, liver, kidney). The Endocrine Society guideline outlines a detailed list of candidate risk groups that would benefit from screening (Table 1).[8]

Also, there are seasonal variations in vitamin D status. Screening for vitamin D deficient states may be of highest yield during the colder months. Accounting for this, the timing of an adolescent's evaluation of vitamin D status usually defaults to when other blood tests are checked or when the patient is already in the office. Healthy adolescents that are not at risk for vitamin D deficiency do not require and are not recommended for routine screening.

TREATMENT OF VITAMIN D DEFICIENCY

The amount of vitamin D required to raise serum 25-OH-D levels varies depending on the risk profile of the adolescent. For youth ages 1 to 18 years who are not obese, the Endocrine Society recommends treatment of vitamin D deficiency with daily 2000 IU supplements of either D_2 or D_3, or weekly 50,000 IU supplements of D_2 for 6 weeks.[8] These recommendations were guided by a randomized controlled trial in a sample of healthy infants and toddlers living in Boston. Each 6-week treatment regimen resulted in therapeutic increases in median 25-OH-D from 17 to 36 ng/mL.[50]

Higher treatment doses of vitamin D have been examined and healthy adolescents ages 10 to 17 years may be safely given a weekly dose of 14,000 IU of D_3 (average daily dose of 2000 IU) for 1 year. In a long-term study, this regimen increased mean 25-OH-D concentrations from 15 ng/mL to 36 ng/mL.[51]

Table 1
Candidates for screening with a serum 25-OH-D level.

Rickets
Osteomalacia
Osteoporosis
Chronic kidney disease
Hepatic failure
Malabsorption syndromes
Cystic fibrosis
Inflammatory bowel disease
Crohn disease
Bariatric surgery
Radiation enteritis
Hyperparathyroidism
Medications
Antiseizure medications
Glucocorticoids
AIDS medications
Antifungals (eg, ketoconazole)
Cholestyramine
Black and Hispanic children and adults
Pregnant and lactating women
Older adults with history of falls
Older adults with history of nontraumatic fractures
Obese children with adults (BMI >30 kg/m^2)
Granuloma-forming disorders
Sarcoidosis
Tuberculosis
Histoplasmosis
Coccidiomycosis
Berylliosis
Some lymphomas

Adapted with permission from Holick MF, Binkley NC, Bischoff-Ferrari HA, et al. Evaluation, treatment, and prevention of vitamin D deficiency: an Endocrine Society Clinical Practice Guideline. *J Clin Endocrinol Metab.* 2011;96:1911-1930.

Although higher doses of vitamin D may be safe and also raise vitamin D levels into a desirable range, there may not be a greater yield compared to the short-term regimens recommended by the Endocrine Society guideline.

When vitamin D treatment regimens are compared in children and adolescents with inflammatory bowel disease, 2000 IU of D_2 daily for 6 weeks is inferior to 2000 IU of D_3 daily and 50,000 IU of D_2 weekly for 6 weeks. In one study, the latter 2 regimens were successful at raising serum 25-OH-D levels greater than 20 ng/mL in 95% of subjects and the highest 25-OH-D levels were achieved by those taking 50,000 IU of D_2 for 6 weeks. However, if a serum 25-OH-D level greater than 30 ng/mL was used to define sufficiency in this risk group, 62% of participants who received 2000 IU of D_3 and 25% of subjects who received

50,000 IU of D_2 weekly remained vitamin D deficient after treatment.[29] These data show that even higher doses of vitamin D than the ones studied may be necessary to replete vitamin D stores in children and adolescents with malabsorption syndromes, at least in northern geographic latitudes. This is also consistent with the Endocrine Society guideline that patients with obesity, malabsorption, or on medications that increase vitamin D metabolism (anticonvulsants, glucocorticoids, antifungals, and antirejection or AIDS treatment) may require 2 to 3 times higher doses of vitamin D to treat deficient states compared to healthy cohorts.[7,8]

There are conflicting data in the literature on whether D_3 is more effective than D_2 in treating vitamin D deficiency.[52,53] Yet, harmonious with the previously discussed study in inflammatory bowel disease by Pappa et al, patients with cystic fibrosis have been shown to respond more robustly to D_3 compared to D_2 as well.[29,54] These data indicate use of D_3 supplements may be preferable in high risk groups, but more evidence is needed to inform this recommendation. Clinical care guidelines by the Cystic Fibrosis Foundation recommend that all individuals with cystic fibrosis be treated with vitamin D_3, but currently the Endocrine Society supports the use of either D_2 or D_3 for treatment of vitamin D deficiency.[8,25]

Professional groups and experts in the vitamin D field have published various strategies to treat and prevent vitamin D deficiency.[2,7,8,17,25] Choosing a particular treatment plan may be swayed by the cause of deficiency, cost, and level of patient adherence. Whichever treatment plan is undertaken, monitoring serum 25-OH-D levels is important and the only way to reassess vitamin D status. There is value in rechecking the serum 25-OH-D level in approximately 3 months (steady state) following initiation of treatment to ensure there is an adequate therapeutic response.

Also, the adolescent's adherence to a maintenance vitamin D regimen to prevent recurrent deficient states is equally important as treating low vitamin D levels at the outset. For youth ages 1 to 18 years with chronic disease and predisposed to vitamin D deficiency, the Endocrine Society recommends daily vitamin D intake of 600-1000 IU.[8] The recommended dietary allowance for vitamin D is 600 IU daily for healthy individuals ages 1 to 70 years.[17]

CONCLUDING REMARKS

Vitamin D deficiency is common and adolescents are at risk for deficiency during a critical window of bone mass acquisition. Patients and physicians are encouraged to maximize bone health where safely possible. Although we acknowledge that there is insufficient evidence to recommend higher vitamin D intake at a population level, to view vitamin D too simplistically may be regrettable, especially in individuals already at risk for low systemic vitamin D and low bone mineral density. There is minimal risk associated with maintaining higher serum 25-OH-D levels and the potential for significant benefits. It is our opinion that physicians should aim to keep serum 25-OH-D levels greater than 30 ng/mL in their adolescent patients until further data are available to indicate otherwise.

References

1. Holick MF. Resurrection of vitamin D deficiency and rickets. *J Clin Invest.* 2006;116:2062-2072
2. Misra M, Pacaud D, Petryk A, Collett-Solberg PF, Kappy M; Drug and Therapeutics Committee of the Lawson Wilkins Pediatric Endocrine Society. Vitamin D deficiency in children and its management: review of current knowledge and recommendations. *Pediatrics.* 2008;122:398-417
3. Bailey DA, Martin AD, McKay HA, Whiting S, Mirwald R. Calcium accretion in girls and boys during puberty: a longitudinal analysis. *J Bone Miner Res.* 2000;15:2245-2250
4. Osteoporosis prevention, diagnosis, and therapy. *NIH Consensus Statement.* 2000;17:1-45
5. Bishop N, Braillon P, Burnham J, et al. Dual-energy X-ray absorptiometry assessment in children and adolescents with disease that may affect the skeleton: the 2007 ISCD Pediatric Official Positions. *J Clin Densitom.* 2008;11:29-42
6. Bianchi ML. Osteoporosis in children and adolescents. *Bone.* 2007;41:486-495
7. Holick MF. Vitamin D deficiency. *N Engl J Med.* 2007;357:266-281
8. Holick MF, Binkley NC, Bischoff-Ferrari HA, et al. Evaluation, treatment, and prevention of vitamin D deficiency: an Endocrine Society Clinical Practice Guideline. *J Clin Endocrinol Metab.* 2011;96:1911-1930
9. Ganji V, Zhang X, Tangpricha V. Serum 25-hydroxyvitamin D concentrations and prevalence estimates of hypovitaminosis D in the U.S. population based on assay-adjusted data. *J Nutr.* 2012;142:498-507
10. Outila TA, Karkkainen MU, Lamberg-Allardt CJ. Vitamin D status affects serum parathyroid hormone concentrations during winter in female adolescents: associations with forearm bone mineral density. *Am J Clin Nutr.* 2011;74:206-210
11. Lehtonen-Veromaa M, Mottonen T, Irjala K, et al. Vitamin D intake is low and hypovitaminosis D common in healthy 9- to 15-year-old Finnish girls. *Eur J Clin Nutr.* 1999;53:746-751
12. Gordon CM, DePeter KC, Feldman HA, Grace E, Emans SJ. Prevalence of vitamin D deficiency among healthy adolescents. *Arch Pediatr Adolesc Med.* 2004;158:531-537
13. Harkness LS, Cromer BA. Vitamin D deficiency in adolescent females. *J Adolesc Health.* 2005;37:75
14. Centers for Disease Control and Prevention (CDC). Beverage consumption among high school students – United States, 2010. *MMWR Morb Mortal Wkly Rep.* 2011;60:778-780
15. Harel Z, Flanagan P, Forcier M, Harel D. Low vitamin D status among obese adolescents: prevalence and response to treatment. *J Adolesc Health.* 2011;48:448-452
16. Garanty-Bogacka B, Syrenicz M, Goral J, et al. Serum 25-hydroxyvitamin D (25-OH-D) in obese adolescents. *Pol J Endocrinol.* 2011;62:506-511
17. IOM (Institute of Medicine). Dietary reference intakes for calcium and vitamin D. Washington DC: The National Academies Press; 2011
18. Norris JM. Can the sunshine vitamin shed light on type 1 diabetes? *Lancet.* 2001;358:1476-1478
19. Nielsen SJ, Popkin BM. Changes in beverage intake between 1977 and 2001. *Am J Prev Med.* 2004;27:205-210
20. Looker AC, Pfeiffer CM, Lacher DA, Schleicher RL, Picciano MF, Yetley EA. Serum 25-hydroxyvitamin D status of the US population: 1988-1994 compared with 2000-2004. *Am J Clin Nutr.* 2008;88:1519-1527
21. Matsuoka LY, Ide L, Wortsman J, MacLaughlin JA, Holick MF. Sunscreens suppress cutaneous vitamin D3 synthesis. *J Clin Endocrinol Metab.* 1987;64:1165-1168
22. Ogden CL, Carroll MD, Kit BK, Flegal KM. Prevalence of obesity and trends in body mass index among US children and adolescents, 1999-2010. *JAMA.* 2012;307:483-490

23. Wortsman J, Matsuoka LY, Chen TC, Lu Z, Holick MF. Decreased bioavailability of vitamin D in obesity. *Am J Clin Nutr.* 2000;72:690-693
24. Hall WB, Sparks AA, Aris RM. Vitamin D deficiency in cystic fibrosis. *Int J Endocrinol.* 2010;2010:218691
25. Tangpricha V, Kelly A, Stephenson A, et al. An update on the screening, diagnosis, management, and treatment of vitamin D deficiency in individuals with cystic fibrosis: evidence-based recommendations from the Cystic Fibrosis Foundation. *J Clin Endocrinol Metab.* 2012; article first published online Mar 7
26. Levin AD, Wadhera V, Leach ST, et al. Vitamin D deficiency in children with inflammatory bowel disease. *Dig Dis Sci.* 2011;56:830-836
27. Pappa HM, Gordon CM, Saslowsky, et al. Vitamin D status in children and young adults with inflammatory bowel disease. *Pediatrics.* 2006;118:1950-1961
28. Pappa HM, Langereis EJ, Grand RJ, Gordon CM. Prevalence and risk factors for hypovitaminosis D in young patients with inflammatory bowel disease. *JPGN.* 2011;53:361-364
29. Pappa HM, Mitchell PD, Jiang H, et al. Treatment of vitamin D insufficiency in children and adolescents with inflammatory bowel disease: a randomized clinical trial comparing three regimens. *J Clin Endocrinol Metab.* 2012; article first published online Mar 28
30. Pascussi JM, Robert A, Nguyen, et al. Possible involvement of pregnane X receptor-enhanced CYP24 expression in drug-induced osteomalacia. *J Clin Invest.* 2005;115:177-186
31. Valsamis HA, Arora SK, Labban B, McFarlane SI. Antiepileptic drugs and bone metabolism. *Nutr Metab (Lond).* 2006;3:36
32. Wagner CL, Greer FR, Section on Breastfeeding and Committee on Nutrition. Prevention of rickets and vitamin D deficiency in infants, children, and adolescents. *Pediatrics.* 2008;122:1142-1152
33. Haagensen AL, Feldman HA, Ringelheim J, Gordon CM. Low prevalence of vitamin D deficiency among adolescents with anorexia nervosa. *Osteoporos Int.* 2008;19:289-294
34. DiVasta AD, Feldman HA, Brown JN, Giancaterino C, Holick MF, Gordon CM. Bioavailability of vitamin D in malnourished adolescents with anorexia nervosa. *J Clin Endocrinol Metab.* 2011;96:2575-2580
35. Bischoff-Ferrari HA, Dietrich T, Orav EJ, Dawson-Hughes B. Positive association between 25-hydroxyvitamin D levels and bone mineral density: a population-based study of younger and older adults. *Am J Med.* 2004;116:634-639
36. Lehtonen-Veromaa MK, Mottonen TT, Nuotio IO, Irjala KM, Leino AE, Viikari JS. Vitamin D and attainment of peak bone mass among peripubertal Finnish girls: a 3-y prospective study. *Am J Clin Nutr.* 2002;76:1446-1453
37. El-Hajj Fuleihan G, Nabulsi M, Tamim H, et al. Effect of vitamin D replacement on musculoskeletal parameters in school children: a randomized controlled trial. *J Clin Endocrinol Metab.* 2006;91:405-412
38. Winzenberg T, Powell S, Shaw KA, Jones G. Effects of vitamin D supplementation on bone density in healthy children: systematic review and meta-analysis. *BMJ.* 2011;342:c7254
39. Malabanan A, Veronikis IE, Holick MF. Redefining vitamin D insufficiency. *Lancet.* 1998;351: 805-806
40. Lips P. Vitamin D deficiency and secondary hyperparathyroidism in the elderly: consequences for bone loss and fractures and therapeutic implications. *Endocr Rev.* 2001;22:477-501
41. Abrams SA, Griffin IJ, Hawthorne KM, Gunn SK, Gundberg CM, Carpenter TO. Relationships among vitamin D levels, parathyroid hormone, and calcium absorption in young adolescents. *J Clin Endocrinol Metab.* 2005;90:5576-5581
42. Weaver CM, McCabe LD, McCabe GP, et al. Vitamin D status and calcium metabolism in adolescent black and white girls on a range of controlled calcium intakes. *J Clin Endocrinol Metab.* 2008;93:3907-3914
43. Hill KM, McCabe GP, McCabe L, Gordon CM, Abrams SA, Weaver CM. An inflection point of serum 25-hydroxyvitamin D for maximal suppression of parathyroid hormone is not evident from multi-site pooled data in children and adolescents. *J Nutr.* 2010;140:1983-1988

44. Tenforde AS, Sayres LC, Sainani KL, Fredericson M. Evaluating the relationship of calcium and vitamin D in the prevention of stress fracture injuries in the young athlete: a review of the literature. *PM R*. 2010;2:945-949
45. Loud KJ, Gordon CM, Micheli LJ, Field AE. Correlates of stress fractures among preadolescent and adolescent girls. *Pediatrics*. 2005;115:e399-406
46. Sonneville KR, Gordon CM, Kocher MS, Pierce LM, Ramappa A, Field AE. Vitamin D, calcium, and dairy intakes and stress fractures among female adolescents. *Arch Pediatr Adolesc Med*. 2012; article first published online Mar 5
47. Montgomery CO, Young KL, Austen M, Jo CH, Blasier RD, Ilyas M. Increased risk of Blount disease in obese children and adolescents with vitamin D deficiency. *J Pediatr Orthop*. 2010;30: 879-882
48. Stoffman N, Gordon CM. Vitamin D and adolescents: what do we know? *Curr Opin Pediatr*. 2009;21:465-471
49. Carter GD, Berry JL, Gunter E, et al. Proficiency testing of 25-hydroxyvitamin D (25-OHD) assays. *J Steroid Biochem Mol Biol*. 2010;121:176-179
50. Gordon CM, Williams AL, Feldman HA, et al. Treatment of hypovitaminosis D in infants and toddlers. *J Clin Endocrinol Metab*. 2008;93:2716-2721
51. Maalouf J, Nabulsi M, Vieth R, et al. Short- and long-term safety of weekly high-dose vitamin D3 supplementation in school children. *J Clin Endocrinol Metab*. 2008;93:2693-2701
52. Holick MF, Biancuzzo RM, Chen TC, et al. Vitamin D2 is as effective as vitamin D3 in maintaining circulating concentrations of 25-hydroxyvitamin D. *J Clin Endocrinol Metab*. 2008;93:677-681
53. Armas LA, Hollis BW, Heaney RP. Vitamin D2 is much less effective than vitamin D3 in humans. *J Clin Endocrinol Metab*. 2004;89:5387-5391
54. Khazai NB, Judd SE, Jeng L, et al. Treatment and prevention of vitamin D insufficiency in cystic fibrosis patients: comparative efficacy of ergocalciferol, cholecalciferol, and UV light. *J Clin Endocrinol Metab*. 2009;94:2037-2043

Adolesc Med 023 (2012) 471–492

Improving the Diets and Eating Patterns of Children and Adolescents: How Can Nutrition Education Help?

Isobel R. Contento, PhD*

Mary Swartz Rose Professor of Nutrition and Education, and Coordinator, Program in Nutrition, Department of Health and Behavior Studies, Teachers College Columbia University, 525 W. 120th Street, New York NY 10027

Good nutrition is essential for growth and development in children and for good health in people of all ages. Many dietary components are involved in the relationship between nutrition and health.[1] In more affluent countries, excesses and imbalances of some food constituents in the diet have replaced nutrient deficiencies that were, at one time, commonplace. Overweight and obesity in youth have increased considerably during the past several decades. Although the obesity rate has remained steady in the past few years, it is still high, having tripled from 5% of children being obese (>95th percentile) and 15% overweight and obese (>85th percentile) in the mid-1970s to about 17% and 32% respectively today.[2] Conditions such as diabetes and hypertension, which are associated with obesity in adults, are increasingly seen in youth.[3,4] There is scientific consensus that many of these health conditions are related, to some degree, to people's food choices and eating patterns. Thus, diet quality and physical activity levels play major roles in individuals for achieving overall health, reducing risk of chronic disease, and maintaining a healthy weight. Unfortunately, the diets of youth and their physical activity patterns need improvement.

In response to these concerns, interest in nutrition education, along with promotion of physical activity, has increased dramatically among both health professionals and the public. The field has also expanded enormously in scope and scale. This article focuses on nutrition education intervention studies directed at promoting healthy eating among youth. It explores lessons learned from these

*Corresponding author.
E-mail address: irc6@tc.columbia.edu (I. R. Contento).

 ISSN 1934-4287

studies, describes some new approaches, provides a stepwise procedure that can be used to design effective nutrition education, and suggests implications for research and practice.

WHAT ARE CHILDREN AND YOUTH EATING?

Government data show that although 33% of school-aged children and youth ate fruit or drank fruit juice a minimum of 2 times a day, and 14% ate vegetables 3 times a day,[5] only about 20% met the recommendations for 1½ cups of fruit per day and 4% for 2 to 2½ cups of total vegetables, including potatoes.[5,6] Of the vegetables, only 0.2% met the recommendations for dark green vegetables and 1.2 % for orange vegetables, eating about 0.1 servings each.[6,7] Most met the recommendations for starchy (eg, corn, potatoes, and peas) and other vegetables (eg, lettuce, onions). Youth generally met the recommendations for total grains (about 5-7 ounces, depending on age and sex), but 99% did not meet the recommendation that half of these, or about 3 ounces, should be whole grains, eating instead only a ½ ounce. About 15% drank 3 or more cups of milk a day as recommended. About 50% of boys and 40% of girls met the recommendations for meat and beans.[6] Children 2 to 19 years ate 21 teaspoons of added sugar a day and 63 grams of discretionary fats and oils. About 30% of teens drank regular soft drinks at least once per day. Teens are also eating too much saturated fat and salt.[8] The maximum discretionary calorie allowance (for solid fats and added sugars) is 300 to 400 calories a day for youth this age. In general, 90% to 99% of youth exceeded this allowance.[6] The diets of children and youth are in need of help, and nutrition education can play a role.

HOW EFFECTIVE IS NUTRITION EDUCATION IN IMPROVING DIETS OF CHILDREN AND YOUTH?

Healthy eating is the collective responsibility of many different entities in society, ranging from an individual, to families, schools, and communities, to government, industry, and the media. Schools, however, remain an important venue for nutrition education for youth because more than 95% of US children 5 to 17 years of age attend school. Consequently, numerous school-based nutrition education interventions have been conducted over the years.

Many people view nutrition education as merely the dissemination of food and nutrition information. A more recent consensus defines nutrition education as "any combination of educational strategies, accompanied by environmental supports, designed to facilitate the voluntary adoption of eating and other food- and nutrition-related behaviors conducive to health and well-being; it is delivered through multiple venues and involves activities at the individual, community, and policy levels."[9-11]

A comprehensive review, commissioned by United States Department of Agriculture (USDA), examined 74 studies with school-aged children that were conducted between 1981 and 1999.[9,12] Although some of the studies involved only a few schools, sample sizes were often large, involving dozens of schools and hundreds, if not thousands, of children in many cases. Studies were selected for review if they had control groups where classes or schools were randomly assigned to intervention or control conditions. The review concluded that nutrition education could be a significant factor in improving dietary practices when behavioral change was set as the goal and the educational strategies used were designed with that as a purpose. For example, it found that those programs that focused on specific behaviors resulted in more behavioral changes than general nutrition education interventions. Studies did not achieve across-the-board success on all study-specified criteria and components, and sometimes showed results with one gender but not the other. However, taken in the aggregate, nutrition education could contribute to improving dietary behaviors.

Several more recent reviews and meta-analyses have also found that nutrition education can be moderately effective in improving the diets of youth and reducing risk of chronic disease and obesity. For example, recent systematic reviews and meta-analyses of interventions to promote the intake of more fruits and vegetables that examined 7 to 14 studies each consistently found that interventions resulted in increases of 0.2 to 0.7 servings, with a mean of about 0.4 servings.[13-16] There are many systematic reviews and meta-analyses of interventions to reduce childhood obesity through a focus on promoting dietary and healthy lifestyle behaviors that lead to energy balance.[17,18] These have found that interventions taken as a group are statistically significantly effective, although there was considerable variation in outcomes, with improvements in some behaviors but not others, or with one subgroup but not another.[19,20] A Cochrane database systematic review and meta-analysis of 55 studies involving some 28,000 children also found that, taken as a group, the interventions were effective in reducing obesity risk through behavioral and environmental and policy changes.[21] These studies, taken together, suggest that nutrition education can contribute to significant improvements in diets of youth, though the changes are often modest and not consistent across all subgroups studies.

WHAT ELEMENTS CONTRIBUTE TO EFFECTIVENESS?

What are some lessons learned from these studies about elements that contribute to effectiveness of nutrition education? The main purpose of the extensive review commissioned by the USDA described earlier was to identify specific intervention elements that can contribute to the effectiveness of nutrition education.[9,12] Those identified are listed next. A recent review confirmed this list of elements of effectiveness.[22]

- Nutrition education is more likely to be effective when it is behavior- or action-focused. Behavior- or action-focused means that the focus of the educational and environmental support strategies is on food and nutrition-related behaviors, actions, and practices of interest or concern. Studies focusing on specific behaviors or actions are more effective than those focusing on general nutrition information or knowledge. The behaviors are identified from the needs, perceptions, motivations, desires, and assets of the target audience as well as from national nutrition and health goals and science-based research findings.

- Nutrition education interventions are more likely to be effective when they use educational strategies that are based on appropriate theory and research evidence and are directly relevant to the behavior or action focus. This means that nutrition education programs are more likely to be effective if they use a variety of contemporary theories and models of individual, social, and environmental change, usually in combination, to design the intervention. These theories and models help us understand how to systematically enhance awareness and motivation among children and youth, and they provide practice in skills to facilitate the ability to make the desired behavioral changes. They also emphasize the importance of environmental supports for taking action.
- Incorporation of student self-assessments with personalized feedback can be effective, particularly for older students. Most individuals have an optimistic bias, believing they are eating better than they actually are. When youth conduct self-assessments of their actual behaviors and then use them to set goals to make changes, they are more likely to follow through on their goals.
- Interventions need to devote adequate duration and intensity for nutrition education to be effective. Programs with longer durations, more contact hours, and more components tend to be more effective. On average, schools provide only 3 to 6 hours of nutrition education per year.[23] Yet studies suggest that such a small amount of time is expected to bring about only "small" effects in program specific knowledge (with 10-15 hours for general knowledge) and that 30 to 50 hours may be needed to bring about medium changes in attitudes and actual behavior.[24] Cumulative effects occur. To achieve needed hours for behavior change, children need to be exposed to nutrition education that is comprehensive, coherent, and delivered sequentially through all the grades. Additional channels, such as school-wide media campaign and interactive computer technologies, should also be used to increase intensity and duration of education.
- Family involvement enhances the effectiveness of school based-programs, particularly for younger children. Finding ways to engage families is a challenge. But direct methods, such as family workshops, family nights, and projects that children and families do together, are more effective than indirect methods, such as newsletters sent home through students.[25]
- Effective nutrition education includes intervening in the school food environment. This means encouraging healthful school meals and school-wide food and beverage availability to increase familiarity with healthful foods, see healthful food practices modeled, and reinforce classroom nutrition education.[26]
- Use of multiple components enhances effectiveness of nutrition education. In addition to classroom curriculum, healthy school meals, family involvement,

extra-curriculum environmental support strategies, such as supportive school-wide and classroom food and wellness policies, and special events and promotions should be used so that key messages are reinforced in multiple contexts.

- Interventions with links to the wider community can support and enhance school-based nutrition education. Engaging the larger community in the effort to improve the eating habits of youth, though challenging, can increase accessibility and acceptability of healthy foods and opportunities for being physically active.[27,28]

The recent review of studies[22] added:

- Use of innovative multimedia technology tools such as multimedia games, video, and Web-based activities may enhance children's interest and engagement in nutrition education. With the increasing familiarity and preference for new technologies by students and their availability in schools, interventions can incorporate these technologies in nutrition education.

Similar but more general features or elements have been recommended by a comprehensive meta-analysis,[19] as follows:

- Classroom (or after-school) instruction on improving dietary intake or increasing physical activity (PA)
- Parent involvement
- Participatory/hands-on, skill building student activities, the provision of print materials, student competitions
- Teacher training for program implementation
- Improvements to the nutritional environment (school cafeteria offerings, etc.)
- Implementation of PA programs in addition to routine physical education (PE); modifications to duration, frequency, or intensity of existing PE; use of noncompetitive PA
- Training in behavioral techniques (including self monitoring, goal setting, etc.) or coping skills (decreasing irrational thoughts, improving self-talk, etc.)
- Program tailoring for cultural relevance
- School policies and programs that weave nutrition, physical activity, or TV reduction lessons into the standard curriculum so that key messages are reinforced in multiple contexts

The Cochrane review[21] synthesis of findings from 55 studies indicates the following to be promising strategies and policies for improving energy-balance related behaviors and reducing obesity risk:

- School curriculum that includes healthy eating, physical activity, and body image
- Increased sessions for physical activity and the development of fundamental movement skills throughout the school week

- Improvements in nutritional quality of the food supply in schools
- Environments and cultural practices that support children eating healthier foods and being active throughout each day
- Support for teachers and other staff to implement health promotion strategies and activities (eg, professional development, capacity building activities)
- Parent support and home activities that encourage children to be more active, eat more nutritious foods, and spend less time in screen-based activities.

A synthesis of promising elements from these reviews and meta-analyses is provided in Table 1.

Table 1
Elements Contributing to Effectiveness of School-based Nutrition Education

Behavior- or action-focused	Nutrition education is more likely to be effective when it is behavior- or action-focused rather than knowledge-only focused.
Use of theory/evidence	Nutrition education interventions are more likely to be effective when they use educational strategies that are based on appropriate theory and research evidence. These include strategies for enhancing motivation and facilitating skill acquisition that are directly relevant to the behavior or action focus.
Self-assessments	Incorporation of student self-assessments with personalized feedback can be effective, particularly for older students.
Duration and intensity	Interventions need to devote adequate duration and intensity for nutrition education to be effective. This can be accomplished by using multiple venues so that messages in the classroom are reinforced and extended.
Family involvement	Parent support and home activities that encourage children to eat more nutritious foods and to be more active enhance the effectiveness of school based-programs, particularly for younger children.
Tailoring for cultural relevance	Making curricula and programs culturally relevant enhances engagement of students and is likely to enhance effectiveness.
Innovative multimedia technology	Use of innovative multimedia technology tools such as multimedia games, video, and Web-based activities may enhance children' interest and engagement in nutrition education.
Teacher professional development	Teacher professional development (PD) and capacity-building activities are essential to provide support for teachers and other staff to implement health promotion strategies and activities. Ongoing support is more effective than one-time-only PD.
School food environment	Effective nutrition education includes intervening throughout the school food and beverage environment (school-wide, classrooms, parent activities) to make them more healthful.
Multiple components	Use of multiple components enhances effectiveness of nutrition education. These include family component, school food and wellness policies, or school-wide media promotions.
Wider community	Interventions with links to the wider community can support and enhance school-based nutrition education.

USING THEORY AND RESEARCH TO INCREASE NUTRITION EDUCATION EFFECTIVENESS

An important finding from all reviews of studies is that nutrition education is more likely to be effective if it is not only behavior- or action-focused, but also based on use of appropriate contemporary theories or models of behavioral and environmental change. By theory or model, we mean a conceptual map, derived from evidence, to help us understand how various influences on food-related behavior are related to, or predict, behavior or behavior change. Contemporary theories or models propose that effective behavior change involves enhancing awareness and motivation, facilitating the ability to take action, and fostering health-promoting environments.[10]

- **Enhancing awareness and motivation.** To enhance awareness and motivation, attitude change models, theory of planned behavior, and related theories can be used effectively, whether through classroom curricula or school-wide promotions. The central concept of these models is that motivation is enhanced when individuals recognize the positive outcomes (benefits) to be experienced by taking action and come to value these outcomes. These benefits can be cognitive or affective. One theory used in interventions with youth is *the theory of planned behavior*,[29] where attitudes (cognitive attitudes based on beliefs or benefits and affective attitudes based on anticipated taste or emotion) and social norms (perceived group pressure) influence behavioral intention, which in turn influences behavior. Behavioral intent and behavior are also influenced by the degree of control over circumstances youth feel they have and whether they can perform the behavior, which is called *perceived behavioral control*. Because food can be laden with emotional meanings based on prior experience or taste, particularly for children, emotional or affective attitudes can be a major influence on eating behavior. Nutrition education programs can use these theories to design interventions to influence beliefs, attitudes, social norms, and perceived control or barriers.
- **Facilitating the ability to take action.** Variations or combinations of several theories can be used to provide strategies for bringing about behavioral change or "how to take action." Social cognitive theory (SCT) is the most widely used theory in nutrition education and proposes that personal, behavioral, and environmental factors work in a dynamic and reciprocal fashion to influence behavior.[30,31] The sense of ability to exert personal influence over one's environment as well as over one's behaviors is described as personal agency.[31] This is enhanced by: beliefs that the outcome of taking action will be beneficial (outcome expectations); proactive commitment to take action (goal intention); self-efficacy (individuals' confidence in their ability to organize and execute particular behaviors); and self-regulation of behavior through self-assessment and goal-setting processes. Self-determination theory (SDT) has been used in some studies as well. It postulates that individuals have innate psychological needs for autonomy, competency, and relatedness,

which, when satisfied, enhance their autonomous motivation and well-being.[32] Autonomy refers to the need to experience one's actions as results of volitional choice; competence refers to the generalized need to experience oneself as competent in dealing with one's life and with the environment; and relatedness refers to the need to experience satisfaction in involvement with the social world. These theories are used to design interventions that focus on self-regulation processes of behavior change: self-assessment, goal-setting, acquiring the knowledge and skills to achieve goals, and self-monitoring one's progress toward those goals.

The stages of change framework suggests that people who intentionally change habitual behaviors do not do so all at once, but through a series of stages.[33] At each stage, individuals use different psychological processes, and thus require different kinds of motivational and informational approaches and skills to move to the next stage.

- **Fostering health-promoting environments.** A social ecological model has become increasingly used in nutrition education for health promotion. In this model, programs are directed at changing not only personal lifestyle factors, but also the interpersonal, organizational, community, and policy and systems factors that support and maintain unhealthy behaviors.[1,26,34,35] The social ecological model is shown in Figure 1. Evidence suggests that such comprehensive, multicomponent interventions directed at multiple levels of influence are more likely to be effective in providing "environmental support for action".[27,28,36,37] Developing and implementing such programs requires that nutrition professionals work in collaboration with school decision-makers and policy-makers, such as school administrators, teachers, and food service providers, to create a healthy school environment and health-enhancing policies.

ARE NUTRITION EDUCATION INTERVENTIONS INCORPORATING EVIDENCE-BASED BEST PRACTICES?

School-based interventions have increased in number and sophistication in the past decade, generating many interesting findings. Some of them focus on increasing fruits and vegetables only, whereas others focus on a set of behaviors related to maintaining energy balance and reducing the risk of chronic disease. These behaviors include the intake of sweetened drinks, high-energy processed snacks, and high-fat fast food, in addition to fruits and vegetables. A review of peer-reviewed studies published between 2000 and 2008 was conducted to specifically assess the extent to which the interventions used the elements of effectiveness that are outlined previously and shown in Table 2.[28] The review found that 100% of 26 studies reviewed were *behaviorally focused* and 96% measured behavior change. In this review, behaviorally focused interventions were defined as programs that provided a theoretical framework or *appeared* to address personal factors, environmental factors, and the behavioral change process based

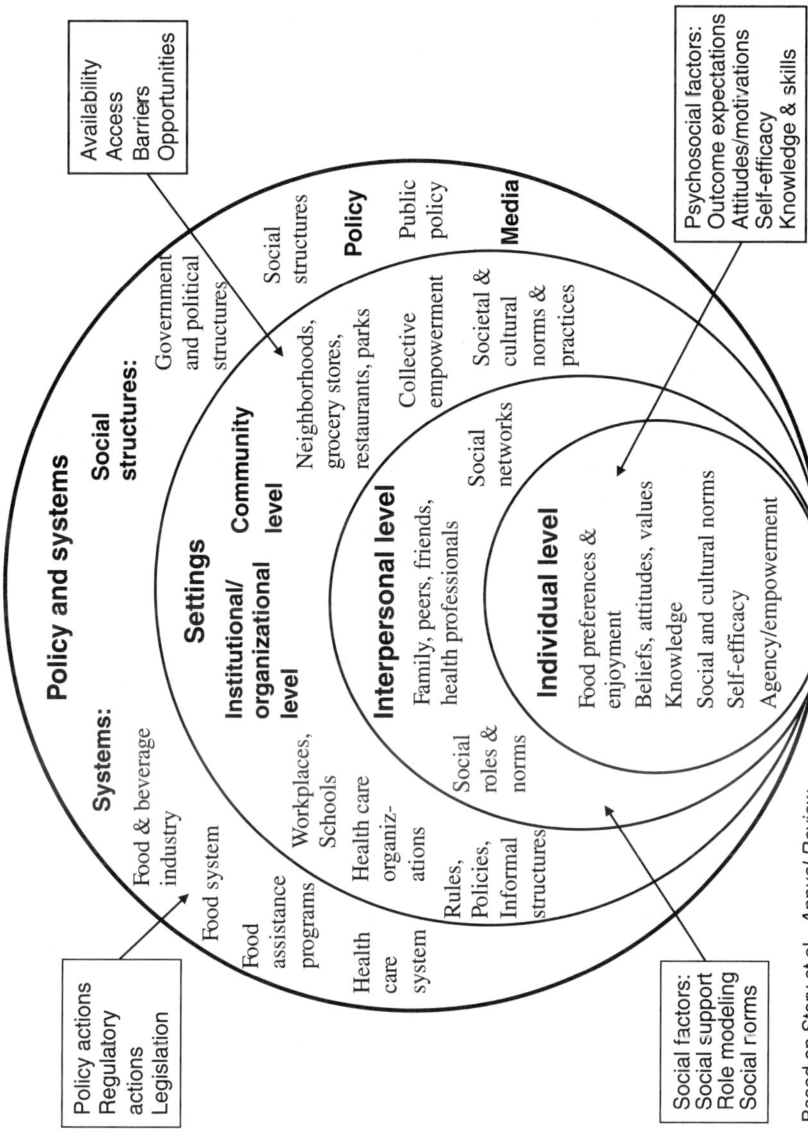

Based on Story et al., *Annual Review of Public Health 2008*

Fig 1. Social Ecological Model

on an examination of the nature of the intervention. *Use of self-assessments* was assessed only for the 9 middle and high school interventions, and only 33% used them. *Duration and intensity* of at least 6 months was achieved in 42% of interventions, and *family involvement* was included in 62%. *Innovative or multimedia technology* was used in 35% of interventions, and *teacher professional development* in 42%. Changes in *school meals* were incorporated into 31% to 38% of interventions, and changes in other aspects of the school food environment in 38%. Most interventions involved *multiple components* (88%), but only 15%

involved *the wider community*. These results are similar to those found in a review that examined 65 school-based health promotion interventions by levels of the social ecological model[35] and are thus encouraging.

Innovative Approaches

Studies that illustrate some innovative approaches are described briefly and shown in Table 2.

Use of Newer Technologies Video games designed to promote behavior change are a promising venue and have been evaluated in several studies. These are very expensive to produce but are likely to be engaging for students.

"Escape from Diab" (Diab) and "Nanoswarm: Invasion from Inner Space" (Nano) are 2 computer-based "serious" video games, designed to be played in tandem, that were developed to increase consumption of fruit, vegetables, and water and increase moderate to vigorous physical activity. The games are theory based.[38] The effectiveness of these games was investigated in a 2-group randomized controlled trial involving a convenience sample of 133 children aged 10 to 12 years.[39] The treatment group played Diab and Nano in sequence. The control group played diet and physical activity knowledge-based games available on popular Web sites. Each game had 9 sessions and a minimum of approximately 40 minutes of game-play per session. Children playing these video games increased fruit and vegetable consumption by about 0.67 servings per day ($p<0.018$), but not water or moderate-to-vigorous physical activity. There were no significant differences in body composition probably because average body mass index (BMI) was at the 78th percentile.

Garden-Enhanced and Garden-Based Strategies The use of school gardens for educational purposes has received increasing attention.[40] The few formal studies conducted show some promise in increasing preference for, and consumption of, fruits and vegetables.[41] One study examined the outcomes of a 12-week garden-based curriculum on fruit and vegetable intake in 99 sixth grade students in 3 schools. A control school and one intervention school, randomly assigned, received nutrition and horticulture curriculum, and a matched school had a garden.[42] At the second intervention school students also participated in hands-on, garden-based activities and in food experiences with the products of the garden. Based on three 24-hour food-recall workbooks, those who participated in the garden-based intervention significantly increased their servings of fruits and vegetables (from 2 to 4.5 servings).

School Nutrition Policy The School Nutrition Policy Initiative was a 2-year cluster randomized intervention-control study involving 10 schools, and 1349 students in 4th through 6th grades.[43] The Initiative consisted of the following components: school-wide self-assessment of the food environment, nutrition education,

Table 2
Selected studies with innovative approaches in nutrition education

Study	Study Sample	Study Design/ Intervention	Theory/Constructs	Measures	Main Findings
Baranowski et al, 2010, 2011[38,39] *Diab* and *Nano* video games	Ages 10-13 years n = 133 Multiethnic	Randomized controlled trial of convenience sample. Purpose: to reduce risk of obesity and diabetes though diet and physical activity. Two computer-based video games "Escape from Diab" and "Nanoswarm" played in sequence; nine 40-minute sessions each game; total 6 hours/game.	SCT, SDT, BIT. Goal setting, problem-solving.	BMI, triceps, waist circumference Behaviors: fruit, vegetable, and water from 3 nonconsecutive 24hr recalls; 5 consecutive days of physical activity using accelerometers.	Children playing these video games increased fruit and vegetable consumption by 0.67 servings per day ($p<0.018$), but not water, moderate-to-vigorous physical activity, or body composition.
McAleese & Rankin, 2007[42] Garden-based	Ages 10-13 years Grade 6 n = 99 Multiethnic 3 schools	Nonequivalent control group design. A control school and 1 experimental school were randomly assigned, and a second matched experimental school was assigned based on garden availability. 12-week curriculum that combined nutrition and horticulture. Curriculum plus garden-based students also tended garden with a large variety of vegetables and had workshops about, and food experiences with, vegetables grown.	Theory not stated.	Analysis of food and nutrient intakes based on three 24-hour food-recall workbooks that included portion size illustrations.	Students participating in the nutrition education curriculum along with garden-based activities increased their fruit and vegetable servings (from 2 to 4.5; $p<0.001$), intakes of vitamins A and C, and fiber more than students in control school and students receiving curriculum without garden activities.

Table 2
Selected studies with innovative approaches in nutrition education

Study	Study Sample	Study Design/ Intervention	Theory/Constructs	Measures	Main Findings
Foster et al, 2008[43] *School Nutrition Policy Initiative*	Ages 11-13 years n = 1349 Multiethnic 10 schools 2 years	Cluster randomized controlled trial. Intervention: 5 components: (1) school self-assessment, (2) nutrition education (50 hours), (3) nutrition policy (changes in school meals and policy on a la carte and vending machines), (4) social marketing (5) parent outreach.	SCT	The incidence and prevalence of overweight and obesity Behaviors: 152-item FFQ (Youth/Adolescent Questionnaire), hours of activity and inactivity (24-item Youth/Adolescent Activity Questionnaire).	At 2 years, incidence of overweight in intervention was 7.5% vs. 14.9% in control; prevalence decreased 10.3% in intervention schools, increased 25.9% in controls. No impact for obesity. Similar decreases in self-reported intakes of energy, fat, FV, and PA in both intervention and control schools. 9% decrease in inactivity, 3% increase in controls.
HEALTHY writing group 2009, 2010[44, 45] Multicomponent	Ages 10-13 years Grades 6 to 8 n = 4603 Multiethnic 42 schools 2 years	Cluster randomized controlled trial. Intervention: 4 components: (1) nutritional quality of foods throughout the school; (2) PA/physical education; (3) classroom curriculum.	SCT: focus: self-awareness, knowledge, decision-making skills, peer involvement, self-monitoring.	Prevalence of overweight and obesity combined, waist circumference, fasting glucose and insulin, 100-item FFQ (Block Kids) analyzed for foods and nutrients.	No significant decreases in prevalence but significant decreases in obesity, waist circumference, fasting insulin. Increases in fruit and water intakes but no changes in energy, vegetables, grains, sweetened beverages, or milk.

Hoelscher et al, 2010[28] *CATCH* Community involvement[27]	Mean age: 10 years Grade 4 to 6 Multiethnic n = 1107 30 schools 2 years	Matched pairs. Basic Program (BP): (1) classroom curricula, (2) physical education program, (3) food service, (4) family involvement (5) teacher-led activity breaks, (6) social marketing. Basic Program plus Community (BPC): in addition, partnerships between school and external community organizations.	SCT, social ecological model	Prevalence of overweight and obesity combined, dietary intakes from food and practices frequency questionnaire (SPAN), also used to calculate healthy and unhealthy food indices.	BP resulted in decreased consumption of sweetened beverages and unhealthy foods. BPC additional increases in percent eating breakfast and numbers of fruits and vegetables, a decrease in the unhealthy foods.
Contento et al, 2010 *Choice, Control & Change* Science education-based[46]	Ages 11-13 years Grade 7 Predominantly Hispanic and black n = 1136 10 schools 8 weeks	Cluster randomized controlled trial. 19-lesson curriculum, 45-min lessons, 6-8 weeks. Used science inquiry-based methods to enhance motivation, and behavioral theory procedures for self-regulation skills (goal-setting, self-monitoring).	SCT, SDT	Intake of targeted foods from validated food frequency questionnaire; psychosocial variables: outcome expectations, intention, self-efficacy, agency/autonomous motivation.	Significant decreases in sweetened drinks and packaged snacks; smaller sizes of fast food; no increases in intakes of water, fruits, and vegetables. Increases in positive outcome expectations, self-efficacy, intentions, competence, and autonomy.

BIT = behavioral inoculation theory; FV= fruit and vegetable intake; FFQ = food frequency questionnaire; PA = physical activity; SCT = social cognitive theory; SDT = self-determination theory.

nutrition policy, social marketing, and parent outreach. The focus was on policy activities. All of the foods served had to meet standards from the Dietary Guidelines for Americans including those in vending machines, school stores, and those sold in cafeterias separate from the official school meals. Social marketing provided incentives to purchase healthy snack and beverage items. Parent outreach discouraged unhealthy snack purchases on the way to school, unhealthy foods at parent fundraisers, and sending sweets into the classroom. The intervention resulted in a 50% reduction in the incidence of overweight. Students in both groups reported similar decreases in energy intake, fat, and fruits and vegetables, as well as a decrease in physical activity. However there was a significant difference in the decrease in sedentary activity, with the intervention group decreasing more. It thus had mixed results on weight-related parameters, healthy eating, and physical activity.

Multicomponent Intervention There is an increasing number of school-based interventions that use multiple components to achieve health goals. The HEALTHY study addressed risk factors for diabetes.[44] Using a cluster design, 42 schools were randomly assigned to intervention or assessment only (control) conditions. The intervention used 4 integrated components: changes in school meals and foods served throughout the school environment, physical activity through physical education classes, a classroom curriculum (FLASH) emphasizing behavioral knowledge and skills, and communications and social marketing. The results were mixed. The intervention schools did not have greater decreases in the combined prevalence of overweight and obesity than those in the control schools, but the odds of being obese and having a high waist circumference were significantly reduced in the intervention schools. There were no differences in serum glucose or insulin levels. There were increases in fruit and water intake, but no change in grains, vegetables, legumes, sweetened beverages, or milk.[45]

Involvement of the Community The additional role of the community in a multicomponent intervention was investigated in a study of CATCH (Coordinated Approach To Child Health), where 15 schools received the Basic Program (BP) (K-5 classroom curricula, physical education program, child food services component, and family involvement) and 15 matching schools received the Basic Program plus Community (BPC), involving partnerships between the school and external community organizations to extend school programs to the surrounding community.[28] The BP resulted in decreased consumption of sweetened beverages and unhealthy foods and increased physical activity. Adding the community component (BPC) resulted in significant additional increases in percentage eating breakfast and numbers of fruits and vegetables, a decrease in the unhealthy foods, a decrease in sedentary activity, and a decrease in prevalence of overweight and obesity combined (which was not significant for the BP). This study demonstrates the usefulness of adding additional levels of influence as suggested by the social ecological model.

THE "DESIGN" STEPWISE PROCEDURE FOR DEVELOPING THEORY-BASED NUTRITION EDUCATION PROGRAMS

Designing theory-based programs is made easier by following a procedure, such as the one provided by Contento,[10] the DESIGN Stepwise Procedure. Its key feature is to provide a method for effectively translating theory-based mediators of change into educational plans that are used to teach group sessions and provide environmental support or policy change activities. The DESIGN Stepwise Procedure is flexible and can be used for one session in a pediatric outpatient setting, a school-based curriculum, or an intervention with several components, such as classroom lessons, family newsletters, social media, and posters. It is based on a logic model in which nutrition educators plan the inputs, outputs, and outcomes of an intervention. *Inputs* are the people and resources needed as well as the needs analysis or assessment process. *Outputs* are the nutrition education activities. *Outcomes* are the effects of the nutrition program on the behaviors or practices that are the focus of the program. The DESIGN Procedure involves 6 steps as shown in Table 3. *Choice, Control & Change (C3)*, a middle school curriculum, is used to illustrate the DESIGN Procedure.[46,47]

Decide Issue and Behaviors (Step 1)

The first 2 steps analyze *inputs.* The first step involves deciding the health issue of concern for the intended audience. Then, using national nutrition and health goals, science-based research findings, and the current eating practices of the

Table 3
The DESIGN Stepwise Procedure for developing behaviorally focused, theory-informed school-based nutrition education for youth

Inputs	**D**ecide Issue and Behavior(s)	Step 1: Decide on health condition of intended audience to be addressed and decide behaviors that contribute to it
	Explore Mediators/Determinants	Step 2: Explore determinants or motivators of behavior and mediators or facilitators of behavior change
Outputs	**S**elect Theory, Philosophy, and Components	Step 3: Select a theoretical framework or model, state philosophy, and determine components of program
	Indicate Objectives	Step 4: Indicate educational objectives for the mediators / determinants of change in the theory model; and environmental /policy component objectives
	Generate Plans	Step 5: Generate educational strategies and sequence into an educational plan for sessions and develop a plan for environmental /policy components
Outcomes	**N**ail Down Evaluation	Step 6: Plan the evaluation for health and/or behavioral outcomes, mediators of behavior change, and environmental /policy change

audience, program planners decide on the target behaviors that improve the health issue of concern.

For *C3*, the health issue of concern was the risk for obesity with its related health risks, which was identified from the literature[2] and surveys. The energy-balance related behaviors that would reduce obesity risk according to the literature and assessment of the students were: increasing intakes of fruits and vegetables; decreasing intakes of sweetened beverages, energy-dense processed snacks, and fast foods; increasing physical activity; and decreasing sedentary behaviors.[5,6,48] Because *C3* was a 19-lesson curriculum, all of these behaviors were targeted. For programs with fewer sessions, the program should target fewer behaviors.

Explore Mediators or Determinants (Step 2)

Next, planners explore mediators in all 3 aspects of nutrition education: enhance motivation (information for "why to" take action); facilitate ability to take action (knowledge and skills for "how to" take action), and promote environmental supports (including changing policies) to determine which mediators could potentially help the audience makes changes on the targeted behavior(s).

In the case of the *C3* audience—inner city middle school youth—the potential mediators of *behavior change* were beliefs or outcome expectations about the benefits of these behavior changes on their health (drawing on their experiences with the high chronic disease prevalence among members of their families and communities) and an increase in their self-efficacy. The barriers were primarily taste and habit. These were based on pilot studies and the literature.[49]

Select Theory, Philosophy, and Components (Step 3)

This step and the next 2 are the *outputs*, or activities, of the program. Based on the potential mediators, planners now select a theoretical framework, state the educational philosophy of the program, and determine its components.

For *C3*, a theory model of behavior change was created based on social cognitive theory and self-determination theory variables to enhance personal agency of youth to make healthy food and activity choices.[47] The model included the following components of SCT: *outcome expectations* based on a scientific rationale for taking action and on an analysis of personal behavior and environment as factors that are health risks; *self-efficacy/perceived barriers* and *behavioral intentions*; *behavioral capabilities* (knowledge and skills related to achieving behavioral goals); and *self-regulation processes* (goal setting, action plans, and self-monitoring). The following components of SDT were included in the model: *autonomy* and *competence*. The philosophy of *C3* was to combine inquiry-based learning processes from science education, and behavior change and skill-building processes from behavioral theory to empower youth to navigate the obesogenic food and activity environments of their low-income urban neighborhoods. *C3* had only one component, a curriculum, to be taught in science education classes.

Indicate Objectives (Step 4)

In this step, program planners indicate educational objectives for the mediators in the theory model, and also indicate specific environmental support objectives. They create these objectives in conjunction with the next step of generating educational plans.

Generate Educational and Environmental Support Plans (Step 5)

This step is the core of program design. It involves developing activities to address the mediators in the theory model and carefully organizing and sequencing them into educational plan(s), one plan for each session. It is best to have activities in every session that enhance motivation ("why to" activities) and that facilitate behavior change ("how to" activities). Also generate a plan to address the environmental support objectives.

In *C3*, for the potential mediator *outcome expectations* ("why to" information) students explore the scientific evidence to enable them to understand why healthful eating and ample physical activity are important. They learn about their biological predispositions to liking the tastes of sugar, salt, and fat and examine their obesogenic neighborhoods to appreciate the barriers to healthful behaviors. Students also collect and analyze their own food and activity data. They learn *self-regulation skills* and gain *self-efficacy* by comparing their data to the *C3* behavioral goals, creating action plans for change, learning behavior-relevant food and nutrition information, and monitoring their change process ("how to" information and skills). Each lesson in *C3* addresses "why to" and "how to" take action through a sequential series of activities.

Nail Down Evaluation (Step 6)

This final step is the *outcomes* of the program on the health issue of concern, targeted behavior(s), theory-based mediators, and the environmental support component. Evaluating all of the outcomes is important in both research and practice, to judge whether a program was effective and also to identify which components were effective and why. Even though evaluation is the final step, it needs to be planned in conjunction with the first 5 steps.

For *C3*, an instrument called the EatWalk survey was developed that included a food frequency questionnaire that asked about the specific behaviors targeted by the curriculum and the psychosocial mediators of behavior change. The instrument was assessed for validity and reliability. The curriculum was then evaluated using a cluster-randomized, intervention-control, pre- and post-test study design involving 10 schools (41 classrooms).

If a nutrition education program involves more than one component, then the DESIGN Procedure needs to be conducted for each component. For example, if *C3* had an additional parent or family component, then while the health issue would be the same—obesity with its associated health risks—an assessment would have to be made of parental behaviors in relation to their child, the motivators for parents to change their behaviors where indicated, and parenting skills they might need. If *C3* had an environmental support component, then an assessment needs to be conducted to identify the necessary changes in the school's food and activity environment and organizational food and wellness policy. Specific objectives need to be stated and activities designed to address those objectives. All the activities need to be conducted with school partners.

This systematic procedure can be done quickly for a single session or thoroughly for larger programs, but in all cases, all DESIGN procedure steps should be considered to ground nutrition education in research and theory, enhancing the likelihood of its effectiveness.

CONCLUSIONS

This article has found that the field of nutrition education has made considerable progress in the past decade. Nutrition education is about helping people eat better, not just providing nutrition information. Consequently, nutrition education needs to be more behaviorally focused and theory-based, directed at enhancing awareness and motivation, facilitating knowledge and skills in healthful eating, and providing environmental supports for action. Although nutrition education interventions in school-based settings have not resulted in substantial across-the-board improvements in all behaviors, taken as a whole they seem to make a significant contribution to behavior changes that address important health priorities. Several elements or features have been identified that may improve the effectiveness of nutrition education. Many new approaches are being tried.

The recommendations on the elements of effectiveness emerging from several recent comprehensive reviews are consistent with each other and are practical and feasible. Full implementation of these in practice would go a long way to addressing current nutrition-related health priorities for youth. Of these, family involvement and the use of multiple components are now more widespread, but other elements have lower rates of incorporation, such as appropriate duration and intensity of intervention, use of innovative technology, improvement in the healthfulness of school meals, changes in the school food environment, and engagement of the wider community. This probably reflects the realities of the school environment, where there are many competing imperatives. These changes require collaborations among many stakeholders and need to be supported. Health professionals can play an important role by helping schools connect with organizations and services that can support school's health promotion efforts.

Although we know more about enhancing effectiveness in broad outline, knowing what to do specifically to ensure that nutrition education is effective remains a challenge. More research is needed for designing each step of the intervention process.[50] Using the Stepwise DESIGN Procedure steps as a framework, after the selection of the key health issues for the school-aged population, research is still needed to identify the key *behaviors or patterns of behavior* that causally contribute to the health issue for the given group. For example, although a certain behavior such as sweetened beverages may be a contributor to overweight and chronic disease risk in some research studies with adolescents, this behavior may not be the most important for younger children or it may be important for boys but not girls. Thus, the specific problem behavior(s) must be validated for the particular group for a *decision* to be made as to which behaviors to target. Research is also needed to validate which of the many potential personal, social, or environmental variables are actually relevant mediators or determinants of change for the given group and to create a *conceptual* or *theory model* that clearly specifies how these influences interrelate and are related to the targeted behavior(s). Ideally this should include an estimation of effect sizes for the associations between the variables and the behavior. To do this, validated instruments must be available to measure these mediating variables. This is an area of considerable difficulty as the psychometric properties of the instruments must be examined, and large samples and longitudinal designs may be necessary.

With a clearly specified theory model, program planners must now generate educational plans for the intervention sessions consisting of strategies and activities that are known to be effective ways to operationalize or convert the mediating variables from behavioral theory into educational terms. Most often strategies and activities are created based on general educational principles and experience. Such activities should be hands-on, involve group activity, include food experiences, and so forth. But research is needed to clearly specify the nature and spacing of activities that are most likely to contribute to effectiveness. Also, research is needed to establish specific environmental and policy strategies that are effective. Finally, in terms of planning the evaluation, research is needed on the most appropriate measures for the health outcomes for a given group and on developing validated instruments for each of the behaviors and for the mediating variables as well as for the environmental influences. Thus although immediate and full implementation of the elements recommended from the existing literature will likely improve the health of youth, research that results in refinements of these elements would be expected to enhance intervention effectiveness more consistently and with stronger outcomes and thus to help achieve national health goals.

References

1. Dietary Guidelines for Americans. US Department of Health and Human Services and US Department of Agriculture. *US Government Printing Office*, Mail Stop SSOP, Washington DC 20402-0001, 2010
2. Ogden CL, Carroll MD, Kit GK, Flegal KM. Prevalence of obesity and trends in body mass index among US children and adolescents, 1999-2010. *JAMA*. 2012;307(5):483-490
3. Jago R, Harrell JS, McMurray RG, Edelstein S, El Ghormli L, Bassin S. Prevalence of abnormal lipid and blood pressure values among an ethnically diverse population of eighth-grade adolescents and screening implications. *Pediatrics.* 2006;117(6):2065-2073
4. Nelson RA, Bremer AA. Insulin resistance and metabolic syndrome in the pediatric population. *Metab Syndr Relat Disord.* 2010;8(1):1-14
5. Centers for Disease Control and Prevention. Youth Risk Behavior Surveillance – United States 2009. Surveillance Summaries. June 4, 2010. *Morbidity and Mortality Weekly.* 2010;59 (No. SS5)
6. Krebs-Smith SM, Guenther PM, Subar AF, Kirkpatrick SI, Dodd KW. Americans do not meet federal dietary recommendations. *J Nutr.* 2010;140:1832-1838
7. Guenther PM, Dodd KW, Reedy J, Krebs-Smith SM. Most Americans eat much less than recommended amounts of fruits and vegetables. *J Am Diet Assoc.* 2006;106:1371-1379
8. NHANES 2005-08. Two-day averages for individuals age 2 and older who are not pregnant or lactating. Available at: http://www.ers.usda.gov/Briefing/DietQuality/Data/. Accessed March 3, 2012
9. Contento IR, Balch GI, Bronner YL, Lytle LA, Maloney SK, Olson CM, Swadener SS. The effectiveness of nutrition education and implications for nutrition education policy, programs and research. A review of research. *J Nutr Educ.* 1995;27:279-418
10. Contento IR. *Nutrition Education: Linking Research, Theory, and Practice.* Sudbury, MA: Jones and Bartlett Publishers; 2011
11. Society for Nutrition Education and Behavior Home page. Available at: www.sne.org. Accessed March 3, 2012
12. Contento IR, Randell JS, Basch CE. Review and analysis of evaluation measures used in nutrition education intervention research. *J Nutr Educ.* 2002;34: 2-25
13. Stables GJ, Young EM, Howerton MW, Yaroch AL, Kuester S, Solera MK, Cobb K, Nebeling L. Small school-based effectiveness trials increase vegetable and fruit consumption among youth. *J Am Diet Assoc.* 2005;105(2):252-256
14. Knai C, Pomerleau J, Lock K, McKee M. Getting children to eat more fruit and vegetables: a systematic review. *Prev Med.* 2006;42:85-95
15. Howerton MW, Bell BS, Dodd KW, Berrigan D, Stolzenberg-Solomon R, Nebeling L. School-based nutrition programs produced a moderate increase in F&V consumption: meta and pooling analyses from 7 studies. *J Nutr Educ Behav.* 2007;39:186-196
16. Thomson CA, Ravia J. A systematic review of behavioral interventions to promote intake of F&V. *J Am Diet Assoc.* 2011;111:1523-1535
17. Doak CM, Visscher TL, Renders CM, Seidell JC. The prevention of overweight and obesity in children and adolescents: a review of interventions and programmes. *Obes Rev.* 2006;7:111-136
18. Zenzen W, Kridli S. Integrative review of school-based childhood obesity prevention programs. *J Pediatr Health Care.* 2009;23(4):242-258
19. Katz DL, O'Connell M, Njike VY, Yeh MC, Nawaz H. Strategies for the prevention and control of obesity in the school setting: systematic review and meta-analysis. *Int J Obes (Lond).* 2008;32(12):1780-1789
20. Gonzalez-Suarez C, Worley A, Grimmer-Somers K, Dones V. School-based interventions on childhood obesity: a meta-analysis. *Am J Prev Med.* 2009;37(5):418-427
21. Waters E, de Silva-Sanigorski A, Hall BJ, Brown T, Campbell KJ, Gao Y, Armstrong R, Prosser L, Summerbell CD. Interventions for preventing obesity in children. *Cochrane Database Syst Rev.* 2011;12:CD001871
22. Roseman MG, Ridell MC, Haynes JN. A content analysis of kindergarten-12th grade school-based nutrition interventions: taking advantage of past learning. *J Nutr Educ Behav.* 2011;43:2-18

23. Kann L, Telljohann SK, Wooley SF. Health education: results from the School Health Policies and Programs Study 2006. *J Sch Health.* 2007;77:408-434
24. Connell DB, Turner RR, Mason EF. Summary of findings of the School Health Education Evaluation: health promotion effectiveness, implementation, and costs. *J Sch Health.* 1985;55: 316-321
25. Hingle MD, O'Connor TM, Dave JM, Baranowski T. Parental involvement in interventions to improve child dietary intake: a systematic review. *Prev Med.* 2010;51(2):103-111
26. Story M, Kaphingst KM, Robinson-O'Brien R, Glanz K. Creating healthy food and eating environments: policy and environmental approaches. *Annu Rev Public Health.* 2008;29:253-272
27. Economos CD, Hyatt RR, Goldberg JP, Must A, Naumova EN, Collins JJ, Nelson ME. A community intervention reduces BMI z –score in children: Shape Up Somerville first year results. *Obesity.* 2007;15:1325-1336
28. Hoelscher DM, Springer AE, Ranjit N, Perry CL, Evans AE, Stigler M, Kelder SH. Reductions in child obesity among disadvantaged school children with community involvement: the Travis County CATCH Trial. *Obesity (Silver Spring).* 2010;18(Suppl 1):S36-S44
29. Ajzen I. The theory of planned behavior. *Organ Behav Hum Decis Process.* 1991;50:179-211
30. Bandura A. *Social Foundations of Thought and Action: Social Cognitive Theory.* Englewood Cliffs, NJ: Prentice-Hall; 1986
31. Bandura A. Social cognitive theory: an agentic perspective. *Annu Rev Psychol.* 2001;52:1-26
32. Ryan RM, Deci EL. Self-determination theory and the facilitation of intrinsic motivation, social development, and well-being. *Am Psychol.* 2000;55:68-78
33. Prochaska JO, Velicer WF, Rossi JS, Goldstein MG, Marcus BH, Rakowski W, et al. Stages of change and decisional balance for 12 problem behaviors. *Health Educ Q.* 1994;13:39-46
34. McLeroy KR, Bibeau D, Steckler A, Glanz K. An ecological perspective on health promotion programs. *Health Educ Q.* 1988;15:351-377
35. Golden SD, Earp JAL. Social ecological approaches to individuals and their contexts: twenty years of *Health Education & Behavior* health promotion interventions. *Health Educ Behav.* 2012;39(3): 64-372; article first published online Jan 20, 2012
36. Birnbaum AS, Lytle LA, Story M, Perry CL, Murray DM. Are differences in exposure to a multicomponent school-based intervention associated with varying dietary outcomes in adolescents? *Health Educ Behav.* 2002;29:427-443
37. Cullen KW, Baranowski T, Baranowski J, et al. Influence of school organizational characteristics on the outcomes of a school health promotion program. *J Sch Health.* 1999;69:376-380
38. Thompson D, Baranowski T, Buday R, Baranowski J, Thompson V, Jago R, Griffith MJ. Serious video games for health: how behavioral science guided the development of a serious video game. *Simulation & Gaming.* 2010;41(4):587-606
39. Baranowski T, Baranowski J, Thompson D, Buday R, Griffith MJ, Ngyen N, Watson KB. Video game play, child diet, and physical activity behavior change: a randomized clinical trial. *Am J Prev Med.* 2011;40(1):33-38
40. Ozer EJ. The effects of school gardens on students and schools: conceptualization and considerations for maximizing healthy development. *Health Educ Behav.* 2007;34:846-863
41. Robinson-O'Brien R, Story M, Heim S. Impact of garden-based youth nutrition intervention programs: a review. *J Am Diet Assoc.* 2009;109(2):273-280
42. McAleese JD, Rankin LL. Garden-based nutrition education affects fruit and vegetable consumption in sixth-grade adolescents. *J Am Diet Assoc.* 2007;107:662-665
43. Foster GD, Sherman S, Borradaile KE, Grundy KM, Vander Veur SS, Nachmani J, Karpyn A, Kumanyika S, Shults J. A policy-based school intervention to prevent overweight and obesity. *Pediatrics.* 2008;121(4):e794-802
44. Foster GD, Linder B, Baranowski T, and the HEALTHY Study Group. A school-based intervention for diabetes risk reduction. *N Engl J Med.* 2010;363(5):443-453
45. Siega-Ritz AM, El Ghormli L, Mobley C, Gillis B, Stadler D, Hartstein J, Volpe SL, Bridgman J; HEALTHY Study Group. The effects of the HEALTHY study intervention on middle school student dietary intakes. *Int J Behav Nutr Phys Activity.* 2011;8:7

46. Koch PA, Contento IR, Calabrese-Barton, A. *Choice, Control & Change: Using Science to Make Food and Activity Decisions. Linking Food and the Environment Curriculum Series.* South Burlington, VT: National Gardening Association; 2010
47. Contento IR, Koch PA, Lee H, Calabrese-Barton A. Adolescents demonstrate improvement in obesity risk behaviors after completion of Choice, Control & Change (C3), a curriculum addressing personal agency and autonomous motivation. *J Am Diet Assoc.* 2010;110:1830-1839
48. Barlow SE. Expert committee recommendations regarding the prevention, assessment, and treatment of child and adolescent overweight and obesity: summary report. *Pediatrics.* 2007;120(Suppl 4):S164-S192
49. Cerin E, Barnett A, Baranowski T. Testing theories of dietary behavior change in youth using the mediating variable model with intervention programs. *J Nutr Educ Beh.* 2009;41:309-318
50. Baranowski T, Cerin E, Baranowski J. Steps in the design, development and formative evaluation of obesity-prevention-related behavior change trails. *Int J Beh Nutr Phys Activity.* 2009;6:6

Adolesc Med 023 (2012) 493–510

Promoting Youth Physical Activity through Physical Education and After-School Programs

James F. Sallis, PhD[a*], Jordan A. Carlson, MA[b], Alexandra M. Mignano, BA[c]

[a]*Distinguished Professor of Family and Preventive Medicine, University of California, San Diego, 3900 Fifth Avenue, Suite 310, San Diego, CA 92103*
[b]*Doctoral Student in Public Health, University of California, San Diego and San Diego State University, San Diego, 3900 Fifth Avenue, Suite 310, San Diego, CA 92103*
[c]*Department of Family and Preventive Medicine, University of California, San Diego, 3900 Fifth Avenue, Suite 310, San Diego, CA 92103*

HEALTH BENEFITS OF PHYSICAL ACTIVITY IN ADOLESCENTS

Adolescents who engage in regular physical activity are likely to have better cardiovascular health and musculoskeletal fitness compared with those who are inactive.[1] Regular physical activity can also facilitate weight control, prevent or treat symptoms of depression and anxiety, and decrease the likelihood of developing risk factors for chronic diseases in adulthood.[1]

PREVALENCE AND TRENDS OF PHYSICAL ACTIVITY IN ADOLESCENTS

The Centers for Disease Control and Prevention (CDC) and US Department of Health and Human Services (DHHS), among others, recommend adolescents engage in 60 minutes of moderate to vigorous physical activity (MVPA) every day for optimal health and disease prevention.[1] The physical activity guidelines do not address total sedentary time but recommend no more than 2 hours per day of television viewing.

*Corresponding author.
E-mail address: jsallis@ucsd.edu (J. F. Sallis).

 ISSN 1934-4287

National self-report data from the Youth Risk Behavior Surveillance System (YRBS) indicate that only 26% of adolescents engage in moderate physical activity for 30 or more minutes per day on at least 5 days per week, and 64% engage in vigorous physical activity 20 or more minutes per day on at least 3 days per week.[2] Trends over the past decade show that adolescent physical activity has not increased.

Objective data from accelerometers (motion sensors worn on the waist) document even lower activity levels. Adolescents engage in an average of 31 minutes per day of MVPA, and only 8% of adolescents meet the recommended 60 minutes per day.[3] Average sedentary time for adolescents is 7.5 to 8 hours per day.[4] Older adolescents and girls engage in less physical activity and more sedentary time than their counterparts, and adolescents have among the lowest rates of physical activity and highest rates of sedentary time of any age group.[3-5]

Contrary to self-report data, objective measures show white non-Hispanic adolescents engage in less physical activity as compared to black and Mexican American adolescents.[3] Mexican American adolescents engage in lower amounts of sedentary time as compared to non-Hispanic whites and blacks.[4]

PHYSICAL ACTIVITY LOCATIONS AND TIME

Understanding when and where youth are active can help design programs and policies that maximize the opportunity for youth to meet physical activity recommendations. The most commonly used sites for physical activity among adolescents include fields/courts (43%), swimming pools (38%), indoor recreation facilities (37%), and parks (31%).[6] Adolescents with limited access to public and private recreation sites are less physically active.[7] Adolescents do most of their MVPA during the hours immediately after school.[8,9] In one study, adolescents were more than twice as active after school than during school.[8] Some interventions produced the largest increases in physical activity immediately after school hours, suggesting this may be a particularly promising time to target interventions.[10]

ECOLOGICAL MODELS TO GUIDE INTERVENTIONS

Recommendations for youth physical activity promotion and childhood obesity prevention interventions, such as those from the Institute of Medicine,[11] Centers for Disease Control and Prevention,[1] Healthy People 2020,[12] and the US National Physical Activity Plan,[13] are based on ecological models of behavior change. A guiding principle of ecological models is there are multiple levels of influence on physical activity, including individual (ie, biological, psychological), social/cultural (social support, crime), built environment (parks), and policy factors (physical education in school).[14] Because there is evidence that variables at all these levels are related to physical activity,[15] another principle is that the most effective interventions operate at all these levels. Thus, interventions are needed that target changes in children, families, environments, and policies.

There are opportunities for youth to be active in several places or settings, so interventions need to be developed for the main settings where children spend their lives, such as homes, schools, neighborhoods, parks and recreation facilities, and community organizations. Multilevel intervention approaches can be devised for each setting. One example is the program Safe Routes to Schools, which aims to slow down traffic near schools, improve street crossings, organize walking school buses, and encourage walking to school.[16] Some interventions can be designed to increase walking and bicycling for transportation by ensuring neighborhoods are designed to have stores and schools near homes and well-maintained sidewalks and bike paths. Other interventions can increase active recreation by ensuring neighborhoods have safe parks, sports, or other activity programs open to all and parental education to take advantage of opportunities. The US Institute of Medicine[17] and the National Physical Activity Plan[13] recommend a wide range of strategies for increasing youth physical activity, but we focus on interventions implemented by or in partnership with schools.

PURPOSE

The purpose of this article is to review evidence about the numerous options for interventions in and around schools as well as after-school programs sponsored by schools or community groups. Consistent with ecological models, we cover interventions at multiple levels of influence, though few studies have evaluated multilevel approaches. We emphasize policy, environmental, and multilevel approaches that can affect large proportions of adolescents for months or years, because ongoing intervention support is needed for long-term change. Even though adolescent medicine specialists cannot directly implement these programs, physicians can be effective educators and advocates to school officials and community groups about the need for evidence-based approaches to improving physical activity among all young people.

PHYSICAL EDUCATION AND AFTER-SCHOOL PHYSICAL ACTIVITY RECOMMENDATIONS

Health organizations recommend 225 minutes per week of physical education (PE) in middle and high schools, and many recommend 50% of PE time be spent in MVPA.[17-23] The National AfterSchool Association and National Institute on Out-of-School Time recommend at least 20%, or 30 minutes, of after-school program time be dedicated to physical activity and that children be active at least 50% of this time.[24,25]

POLICIES AND PRACTICES RELATED TO TIME IN PE

Currently, 41 states require PE in middle school and 48 require PE in high school. However, only 1 state requires the recommended 225 minutes per week of PE in middle schools, and no states require 225 minutes per week in high school.[26] Examination of district-level policies shows that only 2% of school districts nationwide require 225 minutes per week of PE in middle and high schools.[27] The number of youth receiving PE declines as children move from primary to secondary schools.[28,29] Adolescent reports from the YRBS suggest that the percent of adolescents who receive any PE on a daily basis has remained low, at 30%, over the past decade.[2]

Few studies have investigated whether schools that require the recommended 225 minutes of PE per week provide more PE. Only 1 study has investigated this in secondary schools. PE increased from 2 to 3.7 sessions per week in the 16 schools studied after the Texas Legislature passed a bill requiring 135 minutes of PE per week.[30] In a national study, elementary schools in states that had a policy requiring the recommended minutes of PE (150 minutes per week for elementary schools) were almost 3 times as likely to report meeting the standard; schools in districts that had a policy requiring the recommended minutes of PE were almost 2.5 times as likely to report meeting the standard.[31]

POLICIES AND PRACTICES RELATED TO PHYSICAL ACTIVITY IN PE

Historically, the focus of PE has been primarily teaching skills,[32] although more recent efforts have been made by the field of public health to harness the health-promoting effects of PE.[33] The health benefits of PE are related to the amount time spent being physically active, so the primary goal of PE should be to provide students with a large proportion of the daily recommended amount of physical activity. Other important health-related goals of PE include skills development (ie, cognitive, social, and physical) and promotion of physical activity beyond the school day.[33]

A review of MVPA in PE found that middle school students spend 27% to 47% of PE class time in MVPA, depending on the type of measurement. Accelerometer studies suggest lower amounts of MVPA than do studies using direct observations or heart rate monitoring.[34] Although all measurement methods indicate that few schools are meeting the guideline of 50% of PE time in MVPA.

Several evidence-based strategies to increase physical activity in PE have been recommended by health organizations, particularly enhanced curricula.[35] Enhanced curricula replaces less physically active games with those that are more active, uses modified game rules that increase adolescents' physical activity, maximizes equipment use to prevent inactivity and build sports skills, and incorporates physical activity into otherwise sedentary activities like roll call and skill demonstrations.[35-37]

Several enhanced PE curricula have been developed and tested, and most have been successful in increasing MVPA in PE (Fig 1). The Middle School Physical Activity and Nutrition (M-SPAN) PE intervention led to increases in MVPA

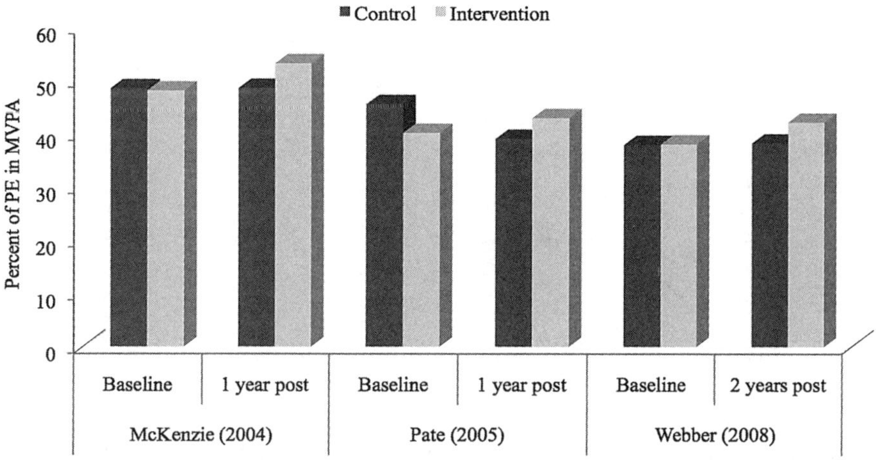

Fig 1. Increases in physical activity in PE for enhanced PE interventions
Note: McKenzie (2004)[38] included boys and girls who were in 6th to 8th grades at baseline and follow up and used SOFIT to assess MVPA. Pate (2005)[39] included girls who were in 8th grade at baseline and used the 3-day Physical Activity Recall (PAR) to assess vigorous physical activity. Webber (2008)[10] included girls who were in 6th grade at baseline and used SOFIT to assess MVPA.

from 49% at baseline to 53% at 1-year follow up (3 minute increase per session) as compared to no increase in the control group.[38] The Trial of Activity in Adolescent Girls (TAAG) enhanced PE intervention in middle school girls and resulted in 42% of class time spent in MVPA versus 38% in controls.[10] Enhanced PE has been investigated in high schools but only in girls. The Lifestyle Education for Activity Program (LEAP) was successful in increasing the percent of girls engaging in 30 or more minutes of self-reported vigorous physical activity during PE to 45% as compared to 36% in the control group after accounting for baseline differences.[39]

Other factors related to PE quality include class size, teacher credentials and training, and socioeconomic status (SES) of the school. Class size was the main barrier to quality PE mentioned by PE specialists in 1 study.[40] Larger class sizes typically have a lower percent of MVPA in PE time,[41] with classes of more than 45 students engaging in half the amount of MVPA during PE as compared to classes with fewer than 25 students.[42] Lower income schools typically have less MVPA in PE as compared to higher income schools.[42] Two enhanced PE interventions found that trained PE specialists provided more minutes of MVPA during each PE class as compared to classroom teachers, but both interventions increased the amount of MVPA provided by classroom teachers through training and ongoing support.[41,43]

Currently, only 5 states (10%) have adopted a policy requiring at least 50% of PE time to be spent physically active, which is an important marker of PE quality (Fig 2).[44] Each of these policies has been adopted within the past 6 years, sug-

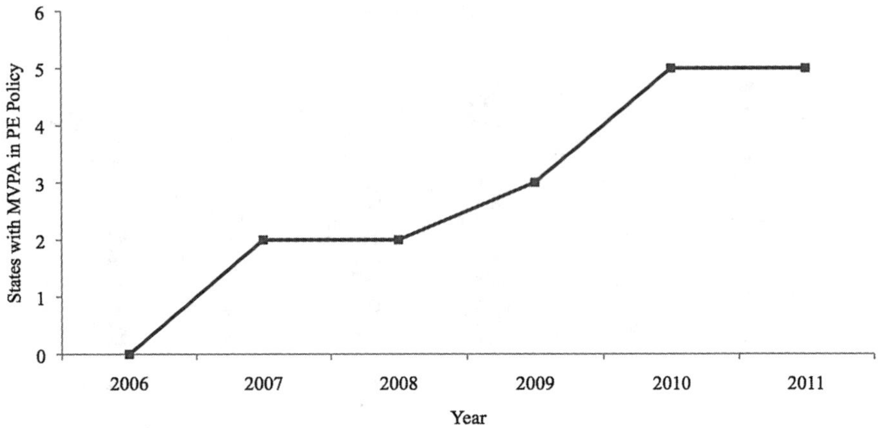

Fig 2. Cumulative number of states by year with policies specifying 50% of PE be spent in moderate-to-vigorous physical activity (MVPA)
Note: Data from Carlson (2012)[44].

gesting a trend of improved legislation surrounding PE, but their impact on PE quality has not been evaluated.

AFTER-SCHOOL PROGRAMS

In the United States, 8.4 million youth participate in after-school programming, and more than 18 million would be interested in after-school programming if it were available.[45] After-school programs are difficult to define because they vary by sponsoring organization, goals (academic, physical activity, or both), setting (school, other), facilities available, leader qualifications, frequency, and duration. After-school programs can include activities such as youth sports, academic enrichment, religion, and arts.[46] Unfortunately these programs are not coordinated at either the state or national level. More research is needed to develop and evaluate program curricula that comply with standards and provide opportunities for physical activity.

After-school programs are an attractive setting for physical activity interventions. The goals are different from PE in that after-school physical activity programs are typically for recreation, not instruction. Programs provide a safe and supervised place for enjoyable physical activity. Two reviews of physical activity interventions in after-school programs have been published,[47,48] both finding a positive pooled effect on physical activity (Fig 3). The amount of physical activity provided in these interventions varied considerably and depended on the frequency of the program.[49-54] Beyond increasing physical activity, there is evidence of modest intervention effects on cardiovascular fitness, body mass index (BMI), and blood lipids.[47] Several of the interventions were found to be effective with girls, blacks, low-income, and overweight students. Enjoyment was reported

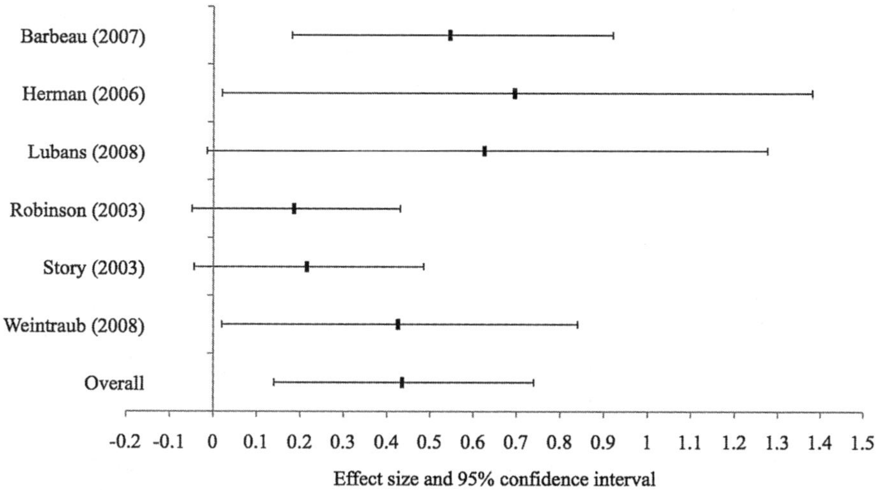

Fig 3. Effect sizes with 95% confidence intervals for the effect of after-school programs on physical activity

Note: Data from Beets (2009) review study;[47] Barbeau (2012),[49] Herman (2006),[50] Lubans (2008),[51] Robinson (2003),[52] Story (2003),[53] and Weintraub (2008)[54] were original studies referenced in the Beets review study.

to be high and attendance was high, but a common barrier to participating in after-school programs was lack of transportation to the after-school setting, or to home after the program. A controlled study in 32 YMCAs in 4 communities found physical activity increased 10.5 minutes per day more often at intervention sites than at control sites.[55] Thus, after-school programs provide a promising platform for interventions, though the characteristics of the most effective interventions have not been identified. Another challenge is to increase access to quality after-school programs.

Most of the studies evaluated interventions designed by researchers to provide substantial amounts of physical activity, but it is useful to document what is occurring in nonresearch programs. One study reported a middle school program provided only about one-third of the recommended 60 minutes of MVPA per day.[56] A study of 25 community-based programs also found modest levels of physical activity, with the average 2-hour program providing about 27 minutes of MVPA.[57] A fruitful approach to research on after-school programs is to evaluate strategies designed to improve physical activity in existing programs and implementation of guidelines,[25] then evaluate concerted efforts to disseminate effective strategies, especially in large organizations, such as Boys and Girls Clubs, that could affect many children. A recent study evaluated statewide dissemination of an after-school program shown to increase physical activity in Hawaii.[58] The program, along with a nutrition component, was implemented in more than 90% of state-mandated elementary after-school programs and maintained over 4 years. Percent MVPA during the program activities, assessed by direct observation, more than doubled from 14% to 32% over the 4 years. Keys to success seemed to be training staff to use an evidence-based program, close communication with program staff, ongoing evaluation informing program improvements, and annual booster training for new staff.

SPORTS

About 44 million youth participate in organized sports in the United States, and roughly 70% of the participants are adolescents.[59] A major finding with organized youth sports is that, with increasing age, there is more emphasis placed on competition and skill. An estimated 45% of youth drop out of sports, and the primary reason for dropout is lack of fun, which is often related to skill level.[60]

Youth who participate in organized sports have been found to expend more energy per day compared to nonparticipants.[61] However, activity levels during sports can be low. In 1 study, only 24% of softball/baseball and soccer players met the physical activity guidelines of 60 minutes during practice (Fig 4). Softball/baseball players, girls, and older youth accumulated significantly less MVPA,

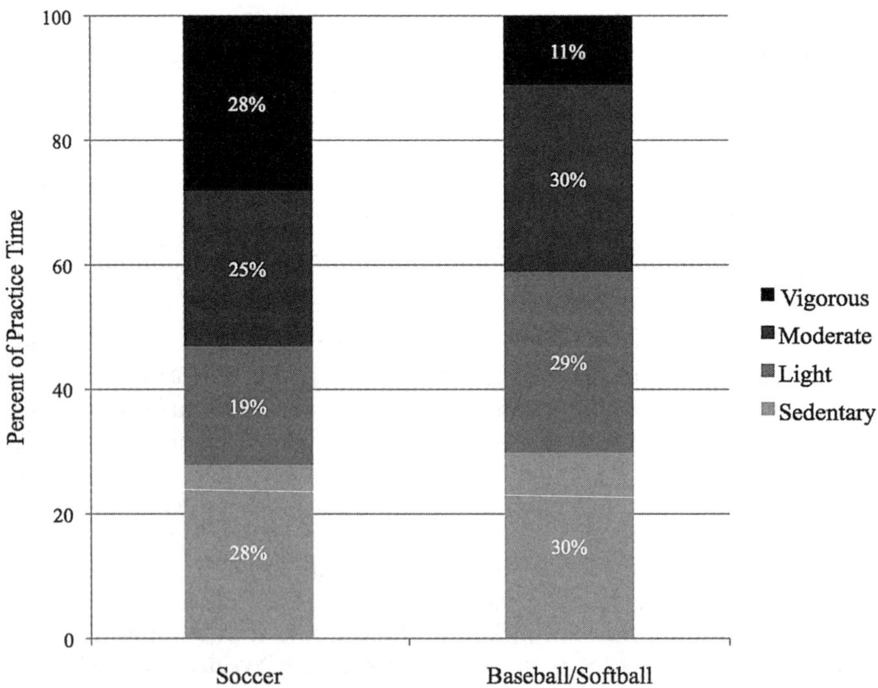

Fig 4. Percent of youth sports practice time spent in sedentary, light, moderate and vigorous physical activity
Note: Data from Leek (2010)[62].

compared to soccer players, boys, and younger children.[62] These findings are consistent with other research that found middle school sports participants were sedentary for 53% of practice time.[63] Thus, it is recommended that sports participants also engage in physical activity outside of sports to meet the recommended 60 minutes per day of MVPA. No studies could be located that evaluated programs to increase physical activity among youth sports participants.

In contrast to varsity level sports, intramural sports provide greater access to youth because leagues are less expensive, invite all skill levels, and both boys and girls can participate. Physical activity levels were higher in intramural sports compared to varsity sports in 1 study.[63] Another study predicted that offering intramural sports in middle schools could lead to an increase in the number of adolescents participating in sports, from 36% to 72%.[64] Future research should focus on evaluating school sport policies that can lead to more prolonged physical activity in school sports, improved access by disadvantaged youth, and ensuring that programs are available to participants of all skill levels throughout adolescence.

ACTIVE COMMUTING TO SCHOOL

Active commuting to school (ACS) is an effective means to increase adolescents' total daily physical activity.[65,66] Unfortunately, the number of youth who walk or bike to school in the United States has been decreasing, from 40.7% in 1969 to about 15% currently.[67-69] Adolescents who are economically disadvantaged or of racial/ethnic minority are more likely to engage in ACS compared to their counterparts. ACS peaks during middle school years and declines among adolescents who reach the legal age to obtain a driver's license.[65,68] Distance to school is the strongest predictor of ACS,[65] which may explain approximately half of the decline in ACS, as distance to school has increased over the past several decades because of low-density residential-only development patterns.[68] School size has continued to expand, and some state policies favor constructing new schools away from the city center.[70] Neighborhood walkability, measured by characteristics such as mixed land use and connected street patterns, as well as presence of sidewalks and parent concerns about traffic safety and crime, also influence ACS.[65,71]

The federally funded Safe Routes to School (SRTS) initiative began in 1997 to promote walking and biking to school by funding educational and construction projects to address barriers to ACS. Most SRTS programs include construction projects such as installing sidewalks, improving street crossings, and slowing traffic near schools. These are often complemented with funding for crossing guards, promotional materials, enforcement of speed limits around schools, and the organization of walking school buses.[16] By 2011, $584 million had been funded to more than 10,000 schools nationwide.[16] However, few studies evaluating the effectiveness of these interventions have been conducted, and results are encouraging. An early study surveyed parents of 10 California elementary schools with

SRTS projects and showed that 11% of parents reported their child walked/biked to school more after the intervention, with 72% reporting no difference.[72] A recent report on 569 federally funded SRTS projects in 5 states affecting 1410 schools found the most common improvements were for sidewalks, street crossings, and signage. The pre-post evaluation showed an increase in walking and cycling from about 12% to 16% of students, which was highly significant.[73]

SRTS programs are promising, but limited evaluations and methodological shortcomings such as lack of control conditions and unknown measurement accuracy make it difficult to draw conclusions about the effect of these programs. Future research should investigate ACS interventions among middle and high school-aged youth and vulnerable populations like minorities and economically disadvantaged youth.

JOINT USE AGREEMENTS

Joint use agreements can be made between schools and parks departments or independent activity providers to allow use of school facilities for recreational use by students or the community at large. The agreements specify which party is responsible for security and maintenance of school facilities and who is eligible to use them. Many districts and schools have policies that prohibit use of school facilities for recreational purposes. A major appeal of joint use agreements is that they can provide recreational facilities in neighborhoods that otherwise lack them. It is well documented that low-income, mostly Latino, and mostly black neighborhoods are less likely to have public parks and private facilities like health clubs and dance studios.[7,74] Commonly cited barriers to joint use agreements include legal/security (liability, vandalism), resources (maintenance costs, activity costs), and social support (from school officials and community groups).[75] However, legal research shows actual risk from joint use is minimal, and 42 states have laws that provide some liability protection for use of schools for recreation and sports purposes.[76]

No studies evaluating the impact of joint use agreements per se could be located, but a few studies evaluated related interventions or provide relevant data. For example, in a 3-city study, 25% to 30% of children and adolescents used school recreation facilities outside of school hours for physical activity.[6] This suggests school facilities are widely used, but there is room to increase facility availability. The Learning Landscapes program in Denver, Colorado, redesigned schoolyards in low-income neighborhoods, transforming them, with extensive input from local residents, into community parks. Renovations included new playground equipment, asphalt play areas painted with game designs, and open spaces. The program was evaluated by observing youth's physical activity on 6 renovated and 3 unrenovated school grounds (Fig 5). They found significantly higher numbers of youth and 24% and 35% overall higher energy expenditure on renovated grounds.[77] There is the potential for supervised programs to provide even more

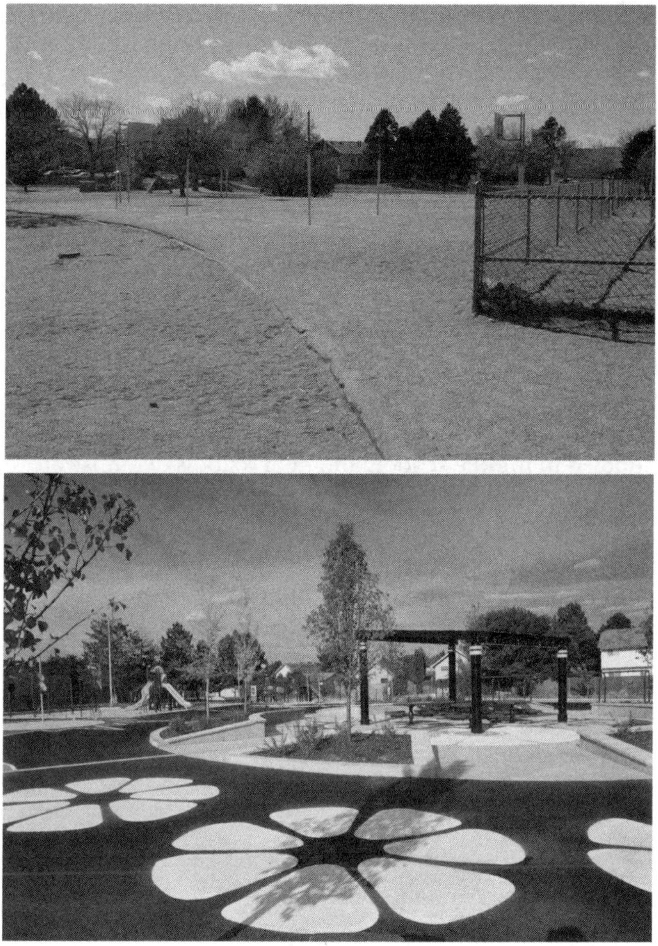

Fig 5. Example of before and after schoolyard renovation
Note: Photos taken by Learning Landscapes[77].

physical activity. The most common model for joint use agreements is to open existing facilities for supervised programs, but no evaluation of this approach could be found. Nevertheless, there are efforts being made to promote joint use agreements, and resources are available (Table 2).

SUMMARY AND CONCLUSIONS

Physical activity provides a wide range of physical and mental health benefits to adolescents, but most adolescents are not meeting the guidelines of at least 60 minutes per day of MVPA.[1,3] Authoritative US health organizations, including the CDC, IOM, American Heart Association, and the National Physical Activity Plan, recommend a range of interventions to increase youth physical activity that can be implemented in, around, and in collaboration with schools (see Table 1).[13,17,20,22] There is a consensus that interventions should involve educational, environmental, and policy changes, so they can affect the greatest number of youth throughout the year and over multiple years. However, recommended interventions are usually not implemented, and opportunities for increasing physical activity in adolescents are far from being used optimally.

Fortunately, there are evidence-based interventions shown to be effective in increasing youth physical activity that can be adopted and implemented, as recommended by national organizations. The public health effect of these interventions depends on (a) the duration, frequency, and intensity of physical activity delivered by the program, and (b) the number of youth served or affected by the program. School physical education probably has the greatest reach, though the percent of participating youth declines dramatically in high school.[28,29] Several studies conducted in middle schools and high schools demonstrate that it is feasible to improve the quantity and quality of school PE through policies, teacher training, use of activity-focused "enhanced" curricula, and smaller class sizes.[10,38,39] States are increasingly adopting policies to improve PE, but those policies need better accountability and monitoring, as well as adequate fund-

Table 1
School physical activity recommendations from health organizations

	AAP	AHA	CDC	IOM	National PA Plan
Provide at least 225 minutes of PE weekly	✗	✗	✗	✗	✗
Provide physical activity for at least 50% of PE time		✗	✗	✗	✗
Use planned PE curriculum that enhances physical activity		✗	✗		✗
Provide physical activity opportunities outside of PE and recess	✗	✗	✗	✗	
Encourage and support students to walk or bike to school		✗		✗	✗
Dedicate/identify funding for school physical activity	✗				✗
Monitor physical activity and set up accountability systems		✗	✗	✗	✗
Evaluate policies related to physical activity			✗	✗	
Require qualifications of those who teach PE and supervise recess	✗	✗	✗		✗
Include physical activity in professional development of teachers			✗		✗
Identify and partner with community resources	✗	✗	✗		

Note: AAP = American Academy of Pediatrics;[18,19] AHA = American Heart Association;[22] CDC = Centers for Disease Control and Prevention;[20] IOM = Institute of Medicine of the National Academies;[17] National PA (Physical Activity) Plan[13]

ing.[44] Most youth physical activity occurs in the after-school hours,[8,9] and there are specific after-school programs that could be delivered to the millions of adolescent participants in after-school programs, often on a daily basis.[47] Critical elements of these programs are staff training, an activity-focused curriculum, and ongoing communication to solve implementation problems.[58] Youth sports are a good source of physical activity, but participation declines among adolescents as sports become more competitive and elite-oriented.[60] Furthermore, participation in sports should be supplemented with other sources of physical activity for youth to meet physical activity guidelines.[62]

Active transportation to school has declined dramatically in recent decades,[68] and because of suburban development trends, fewer youth live close enough to walk or bicycle to school. This problem has been addressed by major federal funding for SRTS, and there is evidence that such programs can be effective.[16,73] Because many schools have received funds for SRTS programs, there are abundant opportunities for research and evaluation. The final intervention topic reviewed was joint use agreements between schools and physical activity providers. There are no direct evaluations of joint use agreements, but schoolyard renovations have been found to lead to substantial increases in physical activity.[77]

All of the interventions highlighted here have the potential for long-term effects on millions of adolescents. Though it may seem like adolescent medicine physicians are not able to implement these nonclinical interventions, they can make critical contributions. Physicians are held in high regard by decision makers in the education, transportation, and youth sports agencies that set policies. These decision makers may not be considering the effects of their decisions on youth physical activity and health. Thus, they could benefit from education, and adolescent medicine physicians who confront the health consequences of inactive youth are credible and compelling educators. There are increasing efforts of physician-based organizations to become involved in advocacy for physical activity promotion and obesity prevention. It is clear that the problems of physical inactivity, obesity, and related health conditions cannot be solved solely by clinical interventions. The National Initiative for Children's Healthcare Quality developed the Childhood Obesity Activity Network that includes an online training program for physicians to support their advocacy for obesity prevention policies (www.nichq.org).[78] Policy advocacy does not have to be time-consuming, but it can be fulfilling and have a positive effect. Physicians can use their time efficiently by working with credible advocacy organizations, such as those listed in Table 2.

Table 2
Resources for school physical activity advocacy

Physical Education
National Association for Sport and Physical Education *http://www.aahperd.org/naspe/* US Department of Health and Human Services *http://www.cdc.gov/HealthyYouth/physicalactivity/pdf/quality_pe.pdf*
After-School Programs
National After School Association *http://www.naaweb.org/* National Institute on Out-of-School Time *http://www.niost.org/*
Sports
National Alliance for Youth Sports *http://www.nays.org/* National Council on Youth Sports *http://www.ncys.org/*
Active Commuting to School
International Walk to School *http://www.walktoschool.org/* National Center for Safe Routes to School *http://www.saferoutesinfo.org/* Safe Routes to School National Partnership *http://www.saferoutespartnership.org*
Joint-Use Agreements
Joint Use.org *http://www.jointuse.org/* ChangeLab Solutions *http://changelabsolutions.org/publications/opening-school-grounds-community-after-hours*
Physician Advocacy
National Initiative for Children's Healthcare Quality, "Be My Voice" *http://www.nichq.org/advocacy/*

References

1. U.S. Department of Health and Human Services. 2008 physical activity guidelines for Americans. Available at: http://www.health.gov/paguidelines/pdf/paguide.pdf. Accessed February 3, 2012
2. Lowry R, Lee SM, Fulton JE, Kann L. Healthy People 2010 objectives for physical activity, physical education, and television viewing among adolescents: national trends from the Youth Risk Behavior Surveillance System 1999-2007. *J Phys Act Health*. 2009;6(Suppl 1):S36-S45
3. Troiano RP, Berrigan D, Dodd KW, Masse LC, Tilert T, McDowell M. Physical activity in the United States measured by accelerometer. *Med Sci Sports Exerc*. 2008;40(1):181-188

4. Mathews CE, Chen KY, Freedson PS, Buchowski MS, Beech BM, Pate RR, Troiano RP. Amount of time spent in sedentary behaviors in the United States, 2003-2004. *Am J Epidemiol.* 2008;167(7):875-881
5. Whitt-Glover MC, Taylor WC, Floyd MF, Yore MM, Yancey AK, Mathews CE. Disparities in physical activity and sedentary behaviors among U.S. children and adolescents: prevalence, correlates, and intervention implications. *J Public Health Policy.* 2009;30(Suppl 1):S309-S334
6. Grow HM, Saelens BE, Kerr J, Durant NH, Norman GJ, Sallis JF. Where are youth active? Roles of proximity, active transport, and built environment. *Med Sci Sports Exer.* 2008;40(12):2071-2079
7. Gordon-Larsen P, Nelson MC, Page P, Popkin BM. Inequality in the built environment underlies key health disparities in physical activity and obesity. *Pediatrics.* 2006;117(2):417-424
8. Jago R, Anderson CB, Baranowski T, Watson K. Adolescent patterns of physical activity: differences in gender, day and time of day. *Am J Prev Med.* 2005;28(5):447-452
9. Mota J, Silva P, Aires L, Santos MP, Oliveria J, Ribeiro JC. Differences in school-day patterns of daily physical activity in girls according to level of physical activity. *J Phys Act Health.* 2008;5(Suppl 1S):S90-S97
10. Webber LS, Catellier DJ, Lytle LA, Murray DM, Pratt CA, Young DR, Elder JP, Lohman TG, Stevens J, Jobe JB, Pate RR. Promoting physical activity in middle school girls: Trial of Activity for Adolescent Girls. *Am J Prev Med.* 2008;34(3):173-184
11. Institute of Medicine. *Health and Behavior: The Interplay of Biological, Behavioral, and Societal Influences.* Washington, DC: The National Academy Press; 2001
12. U.S. Department of Health and Human Services. Healthy People 2020. 2012. Available at: http://www.healthypeople.gov/2020/topicsobjectives2020/overview.aspx?topicid=33. Accessed March 16, 2012
13. U.S. National Physical Activity Plan. 2010. Available at: http://www.physicalactivityplan.org/. Accessed March 16, 2012
14. Sallis JF, Cervero RB, Ascher W, Henderson KA, Kraft MK, Kerr J. An ecological approach to creating active living communities. *Annu Rev Public Health.* 2006;27(4):297-322
15. Smith AL, Biddle SJH, eds. *Youth Physical Activity and Sedentary Behavior.* Champaign, IL: Human Kinetics; 2008
16. National Center for Safe Routes to School. Federal safe routes to school program progress report, 2011. Available at: http://www.saferoutesinfo.org/program-tools/federal-safe-routes-school-program-progress-report. Accessed March 15, 2012
17. Koplan J, Liverman CT, Kraak VI. *Preventing Childhood Obesity: Health in the Balance.* Washington, DC: National Academy Press; 2005
18. American Academy of Pediatrics. Active healthy living: prevention of childhood obesity through increased physical activity. *Pediatrics.* 2006;117(5):1834-1842
19. American Academy of Pediatrics. Prevention and Treatment of Childhood Overweight and Obesity Policy Opportunities tool. Available at: http://www2.aap.org/obesity/matrix_1.html. Accessed March 29, 2012
20. Centers for Disease Control and Prevention. School health guidelines to promote healthy eating and physical activity. *Morbidity & Mortality Weekly Report.* 2011;60(5):1-71
21. National Association for Sport and Physical Education. Physical education guidelines. 2012. Available at: http://www.aahperd.org/naspe/standards/nationalGuidelines/PEguidelines.cfm. Accessed February 6, 2012
22. Pate RR, Davis MG, Robinson TN, Stone EJ, McKenzie TL, Young JC. Promoting physical activity in children and youth: a leadership role for schools: a scientific statement from the American Heart Association Council on Nutrition, Physical Activity, and Metabolism (Physical Activity Committee) in collaboration with the Councils on Cardiovascular Disease in the Young and Cardiovascular Nursing. *Circulation.* 2006;114(11):1214-1224
23. The Community Guide Branch, Epidemiology Analysis Program Office (EAPO), Office of Surveillance, Epidemiology, and Laboratory Services (OSELS), Centers for Disease Control and Prevention. The Guide to Community Preventive Services. Available at: http://www.thecommunityguide.org/index.html. Accessed February 15, 2012

24. National Afterschool Association. Healthy eating and physical activity. Available at: http://www.naaweb.org/downloads/resources/HEPAStandards8-4-11final.pdf. Accessed March 15, 2012
25. Wiecha JL, Gannett L, Hall G, Roth BA. National Afterschool Association standards for healthy eating and physical activity in out-of-school time programs. 2011. Available at: www.niost.org. Accessed January 15, 2012
26. National Cancer Institute. Classification of laws associated with school students. Available at: http://class.cancer.gov/. Accessed February 15, 2012
27. Chriqui JF, Schneider L, Chaloupka FJ, Gourdet C, Bruursema A, Ide K, Pugach O. *School District Wellness Policies: Evaluating Progress and Potential for Improving Children's Health Three Years After the Federal Mandate.* Vol. 2. Chicago, IL: Bridging the Gap Program, Health Policy Center, Institute for Health Research and Policy, University of Illinois at Chicago; 2010
28. Lee SM, Burgeson CR, Fulton JE, Spain CG. Physical education and physical activity: results from the School Health Policies and Programs Study 2006. *J Sch Health.* 2007;77(8):435-463
29. Johnston LD, O' Malley PM, Terry-McElrath YM, Freedman-Doan P, Brenner JS. *School Policies and Practices To Improve Health and Prevent Obesity: National Secondary School Survey Results, School Years 2006–07 and 2007–08.* Vol. 1. Ann Arbor, MI: Bridging the Gap Program, Survey Research Center, Institute for Social Research; 2011. Available at: http://www.bridgingthegapresearch.org/research/secondary_school_survey. Accessed April 8, 2012
30. Barroso CS, Kelder SH, Springer AE, Smith CL, Ranjit N, Ledingham C, Hoelscher DM. Senate Bill 42: implementation and impact on physical activity in middle schools. *J Adolesc Health.* 2009;45:S82-S90
31. Slater SJ, Nicholson L, Chriqui J, Turner L, Chaloupka F. The impact of state laws and district policies on physical education and recess practices in a nationally representative sample of US public elementary schools. *Arch Pediatr Adolesc Med.* 2012;166(4):311-316; article first published online 2011 Dec 5
32. Pate RR, Hohn RC, eds. *Health And Fitness through Physical Education.* Champaign, IL: Human Kinetics Publishers; 1994
33. Sallis JF, McKenzie TL, Beets MW, Beighle A, Erwin H, Lee S. Physical education's role in public health: steps forward and backward over 20 years and hope for the future. *Res Q Exerc Sport.* 2012; 83(2):125-135
34. Fairclough S, Stratton G. Physical activity levels in middle and high school physical education: a review. *Pediatr Exerc Sci.* 2005;17(3):217-236
35. U.S. Department of Health and Human Services, Centers for Disease Control and Prevention, National Center for Chronic Disease Prevention and Health Promotion, Division of Adolescent and School Health. Strategies to improve the quality of physical education. 2010. Available at: http://www.cdc.gov/healthyyouth/physicalactivity/pdf/quality_pe.pdf. Accessed April 8, 2012
36. Partnership for Prevention. *School Based Physical Education: Working with Schools to Increase Physical Activity among Children and Adolescents in Physical Education Classes.* Washington, DC: Partnership for Prevention; 2008. Available at: http://www.prevent.org/The-Community-Health-Promotion-Handbook/School-Based-Physical-Education.aspx. Accessed April 8, 2012
37. San Diego State University, the Active Living Research Program, UCLA School of Public Health' s Center to Eliminate Health Disparities, The California Center for Public Health Advocacy. *Physical Education Matters: A Full Report.* Los Angeles, CA: The California Endowment; 2007. Available at: http://www.calendow.org/uploadedFiles/Publications/By_Topic/Disparities/Obesity_and_Diabetes/PE%20Matters%20Long%20VersionFINAL.pdf. Accessed January 15, 2012
38. McKenzie TL, Sallis JF, Prochaska JJ, Conway TL, Marshall SJ, Rosengard P. Evaluation of a two-year middle-school physical education intervention: M-SPAN. *Med Sci Sports Exerc.* 2004;36(8):1382-1388
39. Pate RR, Ward DS, Saunders RP, Felton G, Dishman RK, Dowda M. Promotion of physical activity among high-school girls: a randomized controlled trial. *Am J Public Health.* 2005;95:1582-1587
40. Barroso CS, McCullum-Gomez C, Hoelscher DM, Kelder SH, Murray NG. Self-reported barriers to quality physical education by physical education specialists in Texas. *J Sch Health.* 2005;75(8):313-319

41. McKenzie TL, Stone EJ, Feldman HA, Epping JN, Yang M, Strikmiller PK, Lytle LA, Parcel GS. Effects of the CATCH physical education intervention: teacher type and lesson location. *Am J Prev Med.* 2001;21(2):101-109
42. UCLA Center to Eliminate Health Disparities, Samuels & Associates, the Active Living Research Program. *Failing Fitness: Physical Activity and Physical Education in Schools.* Los Angeles, CA: The California Endowment; 2007. Available at: http://www.calendow.org/uploadedFiles/failing_fitness.pdf. Accessed April 8, 2012
43. Sallis JF, McKenzie TL, Alcaraz JE, Kolody B, Faucette N, Hovell MF. The effects of a 2-year physical education program (SPARK) on physical activity and fitness in elementary school students. *Am J Public Health.* 1997;87(8):1328-1334
44. Carlson JA, Sallis JF, Chriqui JF, Schneider L, McDermid LC, Agron P. State policies about physical activity minutes in physical education or during the school day. *J Sch Health.* In press
45. Afterschool Alliance. America After 3 PM, 2009. Available at: http://www.afterschoolalliance.org/AA3_Full_ Report.pdf. Accessed March 13, 2012
46. Carver PR, Iruka IU. *After-School Programs and Activities: 2005.* Washington, DC: National Center for Education Statistics; 2006. Available at: http://nces.ed.gov/pubs2006/2006076.pdf. Accessed March 15, 2012
47. Beets MW, Beighle A, Erwin HE, Huberty JL. After-school program impact on physical activity and fitness. *Am J Prev Med.* 2009;36(6):527-537
48. Pate RR, O'Neill JR. After-school interventions to increase physical activity among youth. *Br J Sports Med.* 2009;43(1):14-18
49. Barbeau P, Johnson MH, Howe CA, Allison J, Davis CL, Gutin B, Lemmon CR. Ten months of exercise improves general and visceral adiposity, bone, and fitness in black girls. *Obesity.* 2007;15(8):2077-2085
50. Herman JR, Parker SP, Brown BJ, Sieve YJ, Denney BA, Walker SJ. After-school gardening improves children's reported vegetable intake and physical activity. *J Nutr Educ Behav.* 2006;38(3):201-202
51. Lubans D, Morgan P. Evaluation of an extra-curricular school sport programme promoting lifestyle and lifetime activity for adolescents. *J Sports Sci.* 2008;26(5):519-529
52. Robinson TN, Killen JD, Kraemer HC, Wilson DM, Matheson DM, Haskell WL, Pruitt LA, Powell TM, Owens AS, Thompson NS, Flint-Moore NM, Davis GJ, Emig KA, Brown RT, Rachon J, Green S, Varady A. Dance and reducing television viewing to prevent weight gain in African-American girls: the Stanford GEMS pilot study. *Ethn Dis.* 2003;13(1S1):S65-77
53. Story M, Sherwood NE, Himes JH, Davis M, Jacobs DR Jr, Cartwright Y, Smyth M, Rochon J. An after-school obesity prevention program for African-American girls: the Minnesota GEMS pilot study. *Ethn Dis.* 2003;13(1S1):S54-64
54. Weintraub DL, Tirumalai EC, Haydel KF, Fujimoto M, Fulton JE, Robinson TN. Team sports for overweight children: the Stanford Sports to Prevent Obesity Randomized Trial (SPORT). *Arch Pediatr Adolesc Med.* 2008;162(3):232-237
55. Gortmaker SL, Lee RM, Mozaffarian RS, Sobol AM, Nelson TF, Roth BA, Weicha JL. Effect of an after-school intervention on increases in children's physical activity. *Med Sci Sports Exerc.* 2012;44(3):450-457
56. Trost SG, Rosenkranz RR, Dzewaltowski D. Physical activity levels among attending after-school programs. *Med Sci Sports Exerc.* 2008;40(4):622-629
57. Beets MW, Huberty J, Beighle A. Physical activity of children attending afterschool programs: research- and practiced-based implications. *Am J Prev Med.* 2012;42(2):180-184
58. Nigg C, Geller K, Adams P, Hamada M, Hwang P, Chung R. Successful dissemination of fun 5-a physical activity and nutrition program for children. *Transl Behav Med.* 2012;2(3):1-10
59. National Council on Youth Sports. Report on trends and participation in organized youth sports, 2008. Available at: http://www.ncys.org/pdfs/2008/2008-ncys-market-research-report.pdf. Accessed March 13, 2012
60. Sabo D, Veliz P. *Go Out and Play: Youth Sports in America.* East Meadow, NY: Women's Sports Foundation; 2008. Available at: http://www.ncys.org/publications/2008-go-out-and-play.php. Accessed April 8, 2012

61. Katzmarzyk PT, Malina RM. Contribution of organized sports participation to estimated daily energy expenditure in youth. *Pediatr Exerc Sci.* 1998;10(4):378-386
62. Leek D, Carlson JA, Cain KL, Henrichon S, Rosenberg D, Patrick K, Sallis JF. Physical activity during youth sports practices. *Arch Pediatr Adolesc Med.* 2011;165(4):294-299
63. Bocarro JN, Kanters MA, Cerin E, Floyd MF, Casper JM, Suau LJ, McKenzie TL. School sport policy and school-based physical activity environments and their association with observed physical activity in middle school children. *Health Place.* 2012;18(1):31-38
64. Kanters M, Bocarro J, Edwards M. School sport policy analysis: Examining policy changes to increase the impact of after-school sports and facilities on physical activity. Raleigh, NC: Parks, Recreation & Tourism Management; 2011.
65. Davison KK, Werder JL, Lawson CT. Children' s active commuting to school: current knowledge and future directions. *Prev Chronic Dis.* 2008;5(3):1-11
66. Faulkner GEJ, Buliung RN, Flora PK, Fusco C. Active school transport, physical activity levels and body weight of children and youth: a systematic review. *Prev Med.* 2009; 48(1):3-8
67. Martin SL, Lee SM, Lowry R. National prevalence and correlates of walking and bicycling to school. *Am J Prev Med.* 2007;33:98-105
68. McDonald NC. Active transportation to school. *Am J Prev Med.* 2007;32(6):509-516
69. McDonald NC. Critical factors for active transportation to school among low-income and minority students: evidence from the 2001 National Household Travel Survey. *Am J Prev Med.* 2008;34:341-344
70. Safe Routes to School National Partnership. School siting: location affects the potential to walk or bike. Available at: http://www.saferoutespartnership.org/state/bestpractices/schoolsiting. Accessed March 7, 2012
71. Kerr J, Rosenberg D, Sallis JF, Saelens BE, Frank LD, Conway TL. Active commuting to school: associations with environment and parental concerns. *Med Sci Sports Exer.* 2006;38(4):787-794
72. Boarnet MG, Anderson CL, Day K, McMillan T, Alfonzo M. Evaluation of the California safe routes to school legislation. *Am J Prev Med.* 2005;28(2S2):134-140
73. Vernez Moudon A, Stewart O. Moving forward: Safe Routes to School Progress in five states. Washington State Department of Transportation, 2012. http://www.wsdot.wa.gov/research/reports/fullreports/743.3.pdf. Accessed August 24, 2012
74. Lovasi GS, Hutson MA, Guerra M, Neckerman KM. Built environments and obesity in disadvantaged populations. *Epidemiol Rev.* 2009;31:7-20
75. Spengler JO, Ko YJ, Connaughton DP. Scale development: Perceived barriers to public use of school recreational facilities. *Am J Health Behav.* 2012;36(3):311-318
76. Spengler JO, Carroll MS, Connaughton DP. Policies to promote the community use of schools: a review of state recreational user statuses. *Am J Prev Med.* 2010;39(1):81-88
77. Brink LA, Nigg CR, Lampe SMR, Kingston BA, Mootz AL, van Vliet W. Influence of schoolyard renovations on children' s physical activity: the learning landscapes program. *Am J Public Health.* 2010;100(9):1672-1678
78. National Initiative for Children' s Healthcare Quality. Childhood Obesity Action Network. Available at: http://www.nichq.org/register_coan.html. Accessed April 10, 2012

Adolesc Med 023 (2012) 511–528

Media Use and Sedentary Behavior in Adolescents: What Do We Know, What Has Been Done, and Where Do We Go?

Daheia J. Barr-Anderson, PhD, MSPH[a*],
Susan B. Sisson, PhD, CHES[b]

[a]*Department of Epidemiology and Biostatistics, Norman J. Arnold School of Public Health, University of South Carolina, 921 Assembly Street, Room 135, Columbia, SC 29208, USA*
[b]*Department of Nutritional Sciences, University of Oklahoma Health Sciences Center, P.O. Box 26901, Oklahoma City, OK 73126, USA*

INTRODUCTION

In 1950, at the dawn of the television (TV) age, an advertisement publicizing the benefits of TV was published (Table 1). With the end of World War II came the mass production of TVs, additional disposable income, and increased leisure time. Motorola was the first company to sell an affordable TV for American households,[1] making what would soon become one of America's favorite pastimes available in the comfort of the home.

Since its beginning, TV was marketed in terms of potential benefits for youth and families—leading to academic success, increased quality time as a family, and improved management of youth behavior. However, as the years progressed, TV (and other media outlets) may not have lived up to those original lofty claims. Although there are actual and perceived benefits of TV and media, there are also less desirable consequences, which will be explored in this article. Researchers, parents, and physicians need to be abreast of the current evidence to support the pros and cons of time spent viewing TV and other screen media.

In this article, we present the evidence available for the use of media (including TV and other sources) on promoting sedentary behavior in youth ages 10 to 18

*Corresponding author.
E-mail address: dbarrand@mailbox.sc.edu (D. J. Barr-Anderson).

 ISSN 1934-4287

Table 1
Adapted from a newspaper print advertisement.

Source: *New York Daily News.* September 5, 1950.

How Television Benefits Your Children

An advertisement for television from the 1950s emphatically proclaims how TV can improve behavior at home and grades at school!

Gets homework done promptly!

"Homework first – television second" is the simple rule that solved the problem in thousands of homes AND has made children more interested in school work. "Television," says the *New York Times,* "can be enjoyed in healthy moderation in the same way as sports or movie-going, but only the mother and father can make certain this will be the case."

Home, sweet TV home!

One of TV's many blessings – keeping a small fry out of mischief…and out of mother's hair! "Taking away television from children who 'act up' is a punishment that really works," writes an authority on child psychology. "The very thought of missing some pet program turns little lions into lambs. And, incidentally, those favorite programs in the late afternoon are the world's finest magnet for getting tardy youngsters home on time."

Will television strengthen family ties?

Many authorities on family and children agree that TV brings families together for good, clean entertainment right in the home. With a wide variety of wholesome programs, parents can select the TV shows that are best for their families.

TV provides family entertainment in the home and many benefits both in and outside of the home.

years. These years of development are particularly important to consider as a period during which physical activity levels have been shown to decline drastically and sedentary behaviors become more common. The term *media* is not consistently defined in the literature; however, for the purpose of this chapter, *media* includes live or recorded TV/movies, computer use, and video game use, because these are the types of media most commonly studied in adolescents and the ones most likely to contribute to sedentary behavior. We have also chosen to use the term *sedentary* in reference to all waking behaviors characterized by an energy expenditure of less than or equal to 1.5 METs while in a sitting or reclining posture.[2]

We begin with an overview of media use and then examine its association with obesogenic risk factors, such as poor diet and physical inactivity. Factors that contribute to increased media use are also explored, followed by a review of evidence-based interventions designed to reduce screen time. The article concludes with a discussion on what is not yet known about this topic and future directions for research. Although it is the most common and the primary focus here, we illustrate that TV viewing is not the only media-related sedentary behavior in which adolescents spend time. Therefore, assessing only TV viewing as a measure of overall sedentary behavior may not paint an accurate picture of overall lifestyle patterns.[3]

MEDIA USE RATES

Recommendations for media use among youth were initially established in 2001[4] and updated 10 years later[5] after an extensive review of research addressing the potential impact of media on various health and behavioral outcomes. Although the new guidelines also focus on the promotion of increased caloric intake through food marketing and advertising toward youth, the recommendation that parents limit their adolescent children's daily total screen media time to less than 2 hours of noneducational programming remained the same. Despite these long-standing recommendations for limiting screen time exposure, adolescents are using more media (eg, TV/DVD, video games, music, Internet) today than ever before. Data from the 2003 and 2007 National Survey of Children's Health (NSCH) show the number of children and adolescents meeting the American Academy of Pediatrics TV viewing recommendations of not more than 2 hours/day decreased from 84% to 78%.[6]

Time Spent Watching TV, Videos, and DVDs

Among the various types of media consumption, TV use is the highest. Rates of TV viewing among youth are available back to the year 1949.[7] More than 60 years ago, children ages 6 to 12 years reported watching an average of a little more than 3 hours of TV per day and adolescents ages 13 to 19 years reported 2.5 hours. A review of more than 90 studies and 500 samples from 1949 to 2004 showed that TV viewing remained fairly stable over the decades with the average young person watching approximately 1.8 to 2.8 hours per day, depending on age and sex.[8] The Kaiser Family Foundation 2005 report on youth media use presented slightly higher estimates of time spent watching TV: 3.25 hours for youth ages 8 to 14 years, and slightly more than 2.5 hours for youth ages 15 to 18 years.[9] However, over a 5-year period, the amount of time spent watching TV skyrocketed by 50%. In 2010, the Kaiser Family Foundation surveyed a nationally representative sample of 2002 youth and estimated that the average young person spends 4.5 hours per day viewing TV, with adolescents ages 11 to 18 years spending more time watching TV than children ages 8 to 10 years.[10] As time spent watching TV continues to increase in adolescents, some observations about context and excess have been made. Studies have found that adolescents spend more time in screen-related behaviors on weekends versus weekdays[11-14] and more than 30% of US high school students report daily TV use of 3 or more hours.[15,16]

Time Spent Using Other Media and Simultaneous Use of Different Types of Media

Multitasking (ie, using more than 1 type of media at the same time) is common among youth and contributes to almost 11 hours of media exposure (ie, total amount of media content a young person consumes each day). The highest exposures result from watching live or recorded TV, listening to music, using the computer, and playing video games.[10] Focus groups of children aged 10 to 11 years have reported on their behavior related to using multiple screen devices simultaneously. Multiscreen viewing is common among this age group and usually involves TV as a background diversion while focusing on a laptop, smartphone, or another handheld device. These children found multiscreen viewing to be enjoyable, a way to avoid having to watch advertisements, and a way to occupy time while waiting for a program to load on another device.[17]

Increasing use of time with various media outlets is not completely surprising, as the number, variety, and types of household media devices have increased in recent decades. Almost all American households own at least 1 TV, and more than 70% of adolescents have a TV in their bedrooms.[10] Three-fourths of American adolescents own a cell phone, and with their expanded functionality, most adolescents also listen to music, play games, text friends, surf the Internet, and access social networks on their phones.[18]

According to the 2010 Kaiser Family Foundation study on media use, on average, 8- to 18-year-olds are exposed to 2.5, 1.5, and 1.25 hours per day of music, computer, and video games, respectively. This represents more than an hour increase in overall media use between 2005 and 2010.[9] There are significant differences for total media exposure by age, race, and sex; youth age 8 to 10 years are exposed to less than 8 hours of media, whereas 11- to 14- and 15- to 18-year-olds reported almost 12 and 11.5 hours, respectively, of daily media exposure. White youth reported 4.5 fewer hours of daily media exposure than black or Hispanic youth (8.5, 13, and 13 hours, respectively), and boys were exposed to approximately 1 additional hour of media than girls (11.25 hours compared to 10.25 hours).

MEDIA USE AND ASSOCIATED HEALTH AND PSYCHOSOCIAL RISKS

Media Use, Obesity, and Metabolic Syndrome

It is well established that overweight and obesity have drastically increased over the past couple of decades in children and adolescents with media-related sedentary activities, such as TV viewing, computer use, and video games, cited as possible contributors. One such example is data from the National Longitudinal Study of Adolescent Health (Add Health), a prospective cohort study of more than 20,000 US students in grades 7 to 12 followed into adulthood. Add Health data show that reduced screen time (TV and video viewing) is cross-sectionally associated with lower obesity in females and longitudinally associated with lower obesity for both males and females, with a stronger influence for females.[19]

Moderate-to-vigorous physical activity (MVPA) has been established as a protective determinant of cardiometabolic risk factors (ie, obesity, hypertension, dyslipidemia, and glucose intolerance) in children and adolescents, but little work has examined the effect of sedentary behavior, and specifically media use, on these risk factors. Youth ages 6 to 19 years from NHANES 2003 to 2004 and

2005 to 2006 datasets were assigned a cardiometabolic risk score based on their composite risk factors. High TV use, defined as 4 or more hours a day, was associated with high cardiometabolic risk factors, but a similar association was not observed for high computer use. Children who watched TV for more than 4 hours per day were 2.5 times more likely to have a high cardiometabolic risk factor score than those who watched for less than 1 hour per day.[20]

Media Use and Energy Balance

There is a discrepancy in studies reporting physical activity and sports participation as a correlate (or not) with excessive TV viewing. Some studies report that youth, generally boys, are very physically active, but also engage in a large amount of screen time.[21-23] It is possible that physical activity does not "displace" time spent viewing TV. Although, it is logical that youth engaged in multiple activities outside the home, including, but not limited to sports, would have fewer available hours to watch TV at home than those youths not involved in extracurricular activities. Additionally, this may or may not have an impact on overall sedentary behaviors and energy expenditure, as TV viewing may not be an accurate surrogate for overall sedentary time,[3] and adolescents have been reported to spend large amounts of time in nonmedia-related sedentary behaviors such as social activities.[24,25]

During the time spent engaging in sedentary media use, not only do adolescents expend little energy,[26] but they are exposed to numerous advertisements for products high in calories, including fast food, high-fat and high-sugar foods, and sugar-sweetened beverages[27] that can influence the type and amount of food desired, requested, and consumed.[28] These factors may result in fostering unhealthy perceptions about food and nutrition[29] and promote weight gain. A recent review on sedentary behavior and dietary intake examined 26 studies with 72 independent samples.[30] Both longitudinal and cross-sectional studies found that sedentary behavior, which was commonly defined in these studies as screen time, was associated with poor dietary intake, including low fruit and vegetable consumption and high consumption of energy-dense, nutrient-poor snack foods and drinks, fast food, fried foods, and fat.

Media Use and Other Behaviors

Because present day media is more sophisticated than it was just 10 years ago, it can serve as a powerful educational tool or have potentially harmful effects on youth. Exposure to varied types of media can encourage language and reading skills in young children,[31] make health information accessible, enhance social connectedness, and promote modeling of positive behaviors.[32,33] However, recent reviews have documented the ill effects of media-based sedentary behavior among youth: Sedentary behavior has a negative effect on sleep, attention, and interpersonal relationships,[34] as well as body composition, fitness, self-esteem, social behavior, and academic achievement.[35]

The negative effect of media on youth may be exacerbated because instead of studying or sleeping, youth are spending more time using media, which can have an effect on their behaviors and beliefs.[33] A recent hip hop song entitled "Is Anybody Out There" by K'Naan (featuring Nelly Furtado) speaks of the ills associated with youth staying inside, playing video games, and being in isolation:

Grew up mad and antisocial

Hated outdoors, always in playing Madden™

Adam was lonely

SOCIAL-ECOLOGICAL FACTORS INFLUENCING TV/MEDIA USE

The number of published studies examining the social-ecological correlates of media and sedentary behaviors has grown in recent years. Health behaviors are complex; to have the greatest effect on behavior, interventions should address multiple spheres of influence, including home, community, school, and municipal policies.[36] Since 2004 there have been 5 published reviews[11-14,37] on the correlates of sedentary behavior in adolescents with one focusing solely on TV viewing.[11]

Understanding the correlates of sedentary behavior in adolescents, which has predominantly focused on TV viewing time, is important, particularly for the development of interventions. Correlates of time spent engaged in sedentary behaviors are not necessarily the same as those related to time spent in physical activity,[38] and adolescents can engage in high volumes of sedentary behavior as well as high volumes of MVPA.[22] As noted in the Phases of Research by Sallis et al[39] that has been adapted to sedentary behavior by Salmon et al[12] (Table 2), Phase III of research in behavioral epidemiology includes the identification of factors associated cross-sectionally and longitudinally with sedentary behavior. Identification of these factors leads scientists, health promotion researchers, physicians and nonphysician clinicians into Phase IV, which includes the evaluation of interventions to change sedentary behavior. As has been identified by Salmon et al,[12] opportunities for much future research lies in the development of interventions targeting sedentary behaviors. However, before those interventions can be developed, more research addressing known and modifiable social-ecological correlates of media use in adolescents is warranted. Summary and discussion of these varied correlates is presented in this section, based on the concentric spheres of influence in the social-ecological model: individual (which includes demographic characteristics), family and home environment, and community and school environments.[40] Since no studies have examined policy influences on media behaviors, this sphere of the social-ecological model has been omitted.

Table 2
Phases of Sedentary Behavior Research

	Focus of Phase	Current gaps in evidence
Phase I	Establish links between sedentary behavior and health	Dose–response issues (informing public health recommendations) Overall sedentary time and health Sedentary behaviors (other than screen time) and health Relative contributions of sedentary behaviors, MVPA, nonexercise activity thermogenesis, and sleep (full 24-hour movement exposure) to health indicators Tracking of sedentary behaviors Longer-term health consequences
Phase II	Establish valid and reliable measures for assessing sedentary behavior	Proxy- and self-reported survey measures Validity of accelerometer cut-points for sedentary behaviors (eg, <100 counts per minute) Validity of new technology to assess sitting time (eg, inclinometers, activPALs) Measures of mediators of change in sedentary behavior
Phase III	Identify factors associated cross-sectionally and longitudinally with sedentary behavior	Application and development of behavioral theories for sedentary behavior Longitudinal associations Correlates of sedentary behaviors other than screen time
Phase IV	Evaluate interventions to change sedentary behavior	Targeted interventions in various settings (eg, more community-based, primary care, family, transport, after-school care) Effectiveness of strategies to reduce young people's overall sedentary (sitting) time Different population groups (eg, ethnic groups, age groups, boys and girls) Identify mediators and moderators of change in sedentary behavior Examination of post-intervention behavior change maintenance
Phase V	Translate research into practice	Translational research studies Process evaluation (ie, identify determinants of program adoption) Identify methods for dissemination, adoption, implementation, maintenance, and reach

Source: Salmon J. Health risks, correlates, and interventions to reduce sedentary behavior in young people. *Am J Prev Med*. 2011;41(2):197-206. Reprinted with permission.

Individual-Level Correlates

The most consistent individual-level correlates of higher volumes of TV viewing and sedentary behavior include older age, nonwhite ethnicity, and lower socioeconomic status.[11-14] However, age and sex seem to be more important for non-Hispanic white adolescents because they were not significant correlates in nationally representative samples of non-Hispanic black and Hispanic American youth.[16] Other correlates that have been associated with higher volumes of TV viewing and screen-related sedentary behaviors include between-meal snacking;[41] watching TV during meals;[41,42] depression;[2] higher levels of child autonomy or decision-making;[43,44] less negative attitude toward excessive screen time;[3, 45,46] more negative attitude towards physical activity;[46] and liking TV.[44] Having spiritual and religious beliefs on health behaviors showed an association with lower volumes of TV viewing.[38]

Psychological factors including cognitive function, self-perception, and emotional support showed no association with TV viewing habits as summarized by Gorely et al[11] although most of these studies were conducted before 2000 and a recent study has provided evidence to the contrary.[47] Lower self-efficacy for decreasing TV time was associated with higher odds of exceeding 2 hours/day of screen time in adolescent girls, but not boys.[47] The number of studies addressing individual-level correlates of excessive screen time and TV viewing is rapidly growing. While a strong understanding of how age, race, sex, and socioeconomic status are related to screen time is beneficial, scientific literature examining modifiable, individual-level characteristics of adolescents is particularly needed. Some of these modifiable individual characteristics may include behaviors such as participation in extracurricular activities as well as attitudes and psychosocial parameters (eg, believing that TV is unhealthy, self-efficacy to decrease TV time).

Family and Home-Level Correlates

The most consistent family and home-level correlates of higher volumes of TV viewing and sedentary behavior include more hours of TV viewing by parents, lower education level of parents, single-parent status, number of small-screens in the home (ie, TV, computers, etc.), and the placement of a TV in the child's bedroom.[11-14] Not only are parental viewing habits associated with child viewing habits, but co-viewing (ie, time spent watching TV together) is also related to excessive adolescent screen time.[41,47,48] Having a TV in the bedroom has been further associated with higher risk of overweight status,[49,50] problematic social behaviors, and a number of other undesirable behavioral risk factors such as disengagement in school[50] and poor dietary habits.[51]

Other family and home-level correlates that have been associated with lower TV viewing volumes include family TV viewing rules;[45,48,52-54] parental support and encouragement of physical activity;[55-56] parents knowing their child's friends;[52] having more regular family meals;[52] eating fewer family meals in front of the TV;[42] higher family income;[46] not owning a video gaming device;[46] and having higher access to physical activity equipment.[44] Parental concern for excessive TV viewing was directly associated with TV viewing volume in adolescents (ie, greater concern was associated with higher TV time),[57] but parental self-efficacy for increasing physical activity was inversely associated with screen time in Australian adolescents.[58] An analysis exploring mediators between the home environment and TV viewing in adolescents reported that intention to watch TV, and TV viewing habits and attitudes explained approximately 55% of this relationship.[53] As has been demonstrated, there are a variety of family and home correlates that are associated with TV viewing in adolescents. These can be used to identify families at risk as well as incorporated into interventions designed to decrease sedentary lifestyle behaviors. Future research is needed to develop understanding of precisely how consistent correlates such as family habit and parental TV viewing can be modified and the most effective approaches to do so.

Neighborhood and Community-Level Correlates

The most consistent neighborhood and community-level correlate of higher volumes of adolescent TV viewing is residence in an urban versus suburban location.[11,12,14] The presence of hills in the neighborhood,[59] lower neighborhood income,[60,61] and lower connectedness/higher nuisance[61] have also been associated with higher volumes of TV viewing in adolescents. Sisson et al[52] hierarchically examined social-ecological correlates of excessive TV viewing in American children and adolescents and reported that, when considered independently, rural residence, no neighborhood support, and lower perceived neighborhood safety were associated with more TV time. However, when individual and family variables were included, only rural residence was associated with higher TV viewing time.[52] This finding could potentially explain why many studies do not show strong relationships between screen time and neighborhood and community correlates; the more distal environment is important, but to a lesser degree than individual characteristics and the home environment.

It is also worth noting that in a recent study comparing environmental correlates of obesogenic behaviors across ethnic groups, neighborhood-level factors (i.e. parental perception of neighborhood safety, number of neighborhood amenities and detractions) were associated with excessive TV viewing only among non-Hispanic white children and adolescents (6-18 years).[16] Understanding not only that there are differences in correlates of obesogenic behaviors as they relate to a specific target population, but specifically what they are and how best they can be integrated into tailored behavioral interventions is an area of much needed future research.

Summary of Social-Ecological Correlates of TV Use

As reported earlier in this article, a variety of correlates were examined in relation to TV viewing behaviors in adolescents. Some of the more consistent correlates include age, sex, race, presence of a TV in the bedroom, and parental TV viewing behaviors;[11-14] but this may in part be because of the regularity with which these variables are included in analyses. It is also worth highlighting that many of these correlates cannot be modified in interventions (ie, age, sex, race, socioeconomic status). The understanding of these nonmodifiable correlates can be used to develop and tailor specifically targeted interventions to at-risk populations. However, the inclusion of parameters that could foreseeably be modified, such as self-efficacy, placement of TVs in the home, family patterns, and perceived neighborhood safety in these tailored interventions may be a productive area for future research and exploration.

INTERVENTIONS ADDRESSING TV/MEDIA USE IN ADOLESCENTS

Following the publication of the first widely publicized randomized controlled trial to reduce TV viewing in approximately 200 children (3rd-4th grades) in California schools,[62] there have been many intervention studies targeting reduced screen time and overall sedentary behavior in children and adolescents. These studies have targeted populations of different ages; utilized various intervention delivery methods, delivery locations, and theoretical foundations; and were designed to specifically address various health behaviors such as TV viewing only or TV viewing along with physical activity and healthy eating. Since 2008, there have been 3 reviews[12,63,64] and 2 meta-analyses[65,66] summarizing the findings of these varied interventions. Four of the 5 summary papers[12,63,64,66] have examined overall sedentary behavior, not specifically TV viewing or media use. However, it is noteworthy that most of the reported interventions focused on TV viewing rather than overall sedentary time or sitting.[12,63,64,66]

In sum, these reviews and meta-analyses report that evaluated interventions targeting reduced screen time have mostly reported small, albeit statistically significant effects.[12,63-66] However, as noted in Biddle et al,[66] small individual effects may have a large population health effect if implemented on a broad scale.

Intervention Settings

Interventions aimed at reducing TV viewing have been conducted in a variety of environments.[12,63-66] Most interventions have been conducted in a school setting or partnered with schools to reach children and parents (eg, sending newsletters home) rather than modifying characteristics of the school environment.[12,64] However, other environments such as community centers, clinics, and homes have also been utilized.[12,63-66] There has been some evidence for the emphasis on including families rather than simply adolescents;[12,64] this may be particularly effective because the physical and social environment of the home and family can heavily influence the TV viewing habits of youth.[16,52]

Use of Behavioral Theory and Strategies

In addition to the range of environments in which TV viewing interventions have occurred, there is a wide variety of behavioral theories and strategies that have been utilized (Fig 1). The Guide to Community Preventive Services, Task Force on Community Preventive Services[67] identifies 4 levels of intervention (information only, behavioral strategies, environmental, and policy) that align with the concentric levels of influence addressed in the Social-Ecological Model (see Fig 1).[36] None of the identified interventions have addressed the policy level.[65] Although information and behavior change strategies were regularly used, only a few studies reported changes to the physical environment via the use of electronic TV time monitors.[65] Furthermore, the use of behavior change theory is inconsistent between studies; the most regularly reported theories include: social cognitive theory, theory of reasoned action/theory of planned behavior, transtheoretical model, and behavioral choice theory.[65] It is worth noting that there is no clear evidence to support the preferential use of one theory or model and they are often used in conjunction with one another.

Selected behavioral strategies and interventions utilized in adolescent populations are discussed next, and include examples from Switch-Play,[68] Take Action!,[69] Health in Adolescents (HEIA),[70] Switch-2-Activity,[71] and Get Moving![72] Active video games have been used to increase physical activity[73] and may potentially be used to substitute for traditional seated video games. Active video games have been shown to be effective at increasing energy expenditure,[74,75] although not necessarily to the same level of intensity as playing the actual sport.[75] TV time monitors have been used in a few studies; each reported a decrease in total TV viewing time.[69,76,77]

Most of the studies were classroom-based[68,70-72] and included lessons on health and benefits of activity and reducing sedentary and TV time,[70,72] self-monitoring,[68,71] behavioral contracting,[68,71] reinforcement,[68] discussions on intelligent TV viewing,[68] advocacy to reduce TV viewing,[68] and parental fact sheets and newsletters.[70] Only Switch-2-Activity[68] included data regarding intervention fidelity such that most teachers did modify the intervention in some way and that 71% of teachers delivered only 4 out of 6 lessons. Two studies[69,77] were home-based and both included the electronic TV time monitors (which turned off after a predetermined amount of time), although the Take Action! study[69] was much longer in duration than Epstein et al[77] (1 year vs. 9 weeks). Take Action![69] also included monthly group sessions; newsletters; a variety of behavioral strategies, including goal setting, self-monitoring, and reinforcement; in addition to regular support telephone calls from intervention staff.

Outcomes of these studies are fairly similar—the interventions were effective at decreasing TV viewing;[72,77] however, there are some nuances that deserve highlighting. Take Action![69] did not report a decrease in adolescent screen time over the 12-month intervention and children in Switch-Play[68] actually increased their viewing time. However, physical activity also increased in the Switch-Play participants,[68] unlike other interventions (Get Moving![72] and unnamed intervention by Epstein[77]), which report that physical activity does not increase concomitantly with reductions in sedentary behaviors.[72,77] It is also noteworthy, that Take Action![69] did report a decrease in TV viewing in households and in adults.

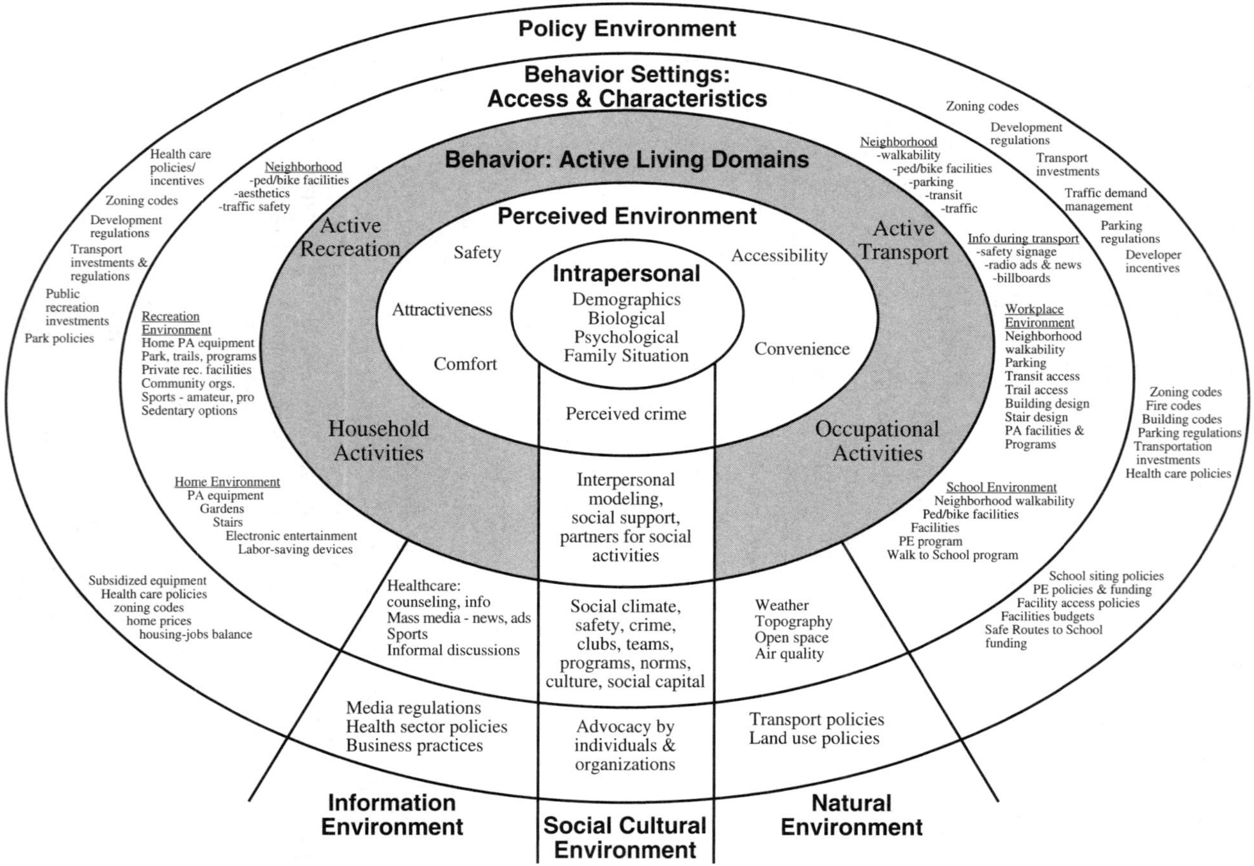

Fig 1. Ecological model of 4 domains of active living
Source: Sallis JF, Cervero RB, Ascher W, et al. An ecological approach to creating active living communities. *Annu Rev Pub Health*. 2006;27:297-322. Reprinted with permission.

It is likely the lack of significant intervention effect was the result of a decrease in TV viewing in both intervention and control adolescents.[69] HEIA[70] reported a decrease of approximately 20 minutes/day of TV/DVD use in girls but not boys, whereas Switch-2-Activity[71] reported a favorable decrease in TV viewing (of about 20 minutes) in boys, but not in girls. Get Moving[72] was the only intervention to specifically target a minority population, Latina girls. Similar to HEIA[70] and Switch-2-Activity,[71] there was an approximate 20 to 30 minute per day decrease in sedentary behaviors, although the specific instrument used to measure sedentary behavior differed slightly. Overall, the findings from these behavioral interventions targeting adolescents are encouraging, with an average reduction of approximately 20 minutes/day in screen-related behaviors.

CONCLUSION

Years of research have been conducted to better understand the relationship of media use to other behaviors and ultimately to health outcomes. The evidence is convincing that media use may have an impact on the eating and sedentary behaviors of adolescents, resulting in excessive weight gain. Throughout this article, we have portrayed what is known about media use, associated undesirable behaviors, environmental correlates and actions that have been taken (ie, interventions) to address its use. We now would like to speculate on a few areas in which future research is needed to further understand and conceptualize the effects of media use on the health of adolescents. First, although media has some adverse effects on youth, it can also be a powerful educational tool and a source for increasing knowledge and access to the wider world than would be available without its use. More research and education is needed to determine the appropriate use of media by adolescents. Secondly, as is evident in this article, the media types most studied are TV, video games, and computers. More research is needed regarding the effects of other media, such as cell phone use, and multiuse of screen devices, involving use of a single device for different purposes (eg, a smartphone being used to make/receive phone calls, watch TV/movies, and read a book, but not simultaneously). Lastly, because adolescents regularly multitask and use 2 or more forms of screen media at a time, we need to develop methods to better measure and understand multitasking. An improved understanding of multitasking is needed to inform interventions to reduce this behavior and subsequently decrease overall screen time. Because there is some evidence that interventions can effectively decrease undesirable media use in adolescents, we speculate further on necessary next steps for designing and evaluating interventions.

Future Directions for Intervention Research

Despite the number of interventions published that aim to reduce media use, there are some areas in need of future research that warrant discussion. As noted throughout the article, most studies have focused on younger children, so more work is needed to specifically address media use by adolescents. This could be particularly beneficial for public health because adolescents are amongst the most sedentary of Americans.[79] Adolescent populations are more likely to exceed the American Academy of Pediatrics recommendation for TV viewing (2 hours/day) compared to younger age groups[79] and spend 8 to 8.5 hours per day using media.[10] Within adolescent populations, more research is needed to clarify the most effective strategies needed to reach various groups such as boys versus girls; different socioeconomic strata; and various ethnic, cultural, and racial groups. One specific focus of intervention strategies that particularly warrants investigation is the family/home environment; a qualitative study noted that parents would like to decrease children's TV time but are unsure about how to address this issue or tackle the associated barriers.[80]

Future evaluations of interventions should use increased rigor (eg, use of sound theoretical frameworks), report on the fidelity of administration, and enhance methods for behavioral assessment. Methodological publications as well as process evaluations and long-term follow-ups are needed to increase the rigor of interventions as well as to identify screen time behavior moderators and mediators and determine the critical ingredients and settings for interventions that effectively reduce time spent watching TV. In addition to methodological considerations for intervention design and fidelity, measurement of specific behaviors of interest is an area where more research energy can be focused. Bryant et al[81] reported that most studies on children and adolescents that assess TV viewing have used a self-report or proxy-report system and that few of these instruments have been tested for validity and reliability. A combination of objective monitoring and time-use diaries or self-report, to specify precise behaviors, would likely be most sensitive to behavioral changes and the most accurate means for determining time spent in TV viewing and other sedentary pursuits. Furthermore, cost analyses are needed to determine the cost-benefit of specific intervention strategies.

ACKNOWLEDGMENTS

We would like to thank Ashley E. Anderson who helped with the collection and assimilation of these articles.

References

1. Black MM, Siegel EH, Abel Y, Bentley ME. Home and videotape intervention delays early complementary feeding among adolescent mothers. *Pediatrics.* 2001;107(5):E67
2. Sedentary Behaviour Research Network. Letter to the editor: standardized use of the terms "sedentary" and "sedentary behaviours." *Appl Physiol Nutr Metab.* 2012;37(3):540-542
3. Biddle SJ, Gorely T, Marshall SJ. Is television viewing a suitable marker of sedentary behavior in young people? *Ann Behav Med.* 2009;38(2):147-153
4. American Academy of Pediatrics: Children, adolescents, and television. *Pediatrics.* 2001;107(2):423-426
5. Strasburger VC. Children, adolescents, obesity, and the media. *Pediatrics.* 2011;128(1):201-208
6. Sisson SB, Broyles ST, Brittain D, Short K. Variations in obesogenic behaviors in U.S. children across geographic regions from 2003-2007. *Open J Prev Med.* 2011;1(2):25-33

7. Riley JW, Cantwell FV, Ruttiger KF. Some observations on the social effects of television. *Public Opin Q.* 1949;13(2):223-234
8. Marshall SJ, Gorely T, Biddle SJ. A descriptive epidemiology of screen-based media use in youth: a review and critique. *J Adolesc.* 2006;29(3):333-349
9. Rideout VJ, Roberts DF, Foehr UG. *Generation M: Media in the Lives of 8-18 Year-Olds.* Menlo Park, CA: Henry J. Kaiser Family Foundation; 2005
10. Rideout VJ, Foehr UG, Roberts DF. *Generation M2: Media in the Lives of 8- to 18-Year Olds.* Menlo Park, CA: Kenry J. Kaiser Family Foundation; 2010
11. Gorely T, Marshall SJ, Biddle SJ. Couch kids: correlates of television viewing among youth. *Int J Behav Med.* 2004;11(3):152-163
12. Salmon J. Health Risks, correlates, and interventions to reduce sedentary behavior in young people. *Am J Prev Med.* 2011;41(2):197-206
13. Van Der Horst K, Paw MJ, Twisk JW, Van Mechelen W. A brief review on correlates of physical activity and sedentariness in youth. *Med Sci Sports Exerc.* 2007;39(8):1241-1250
14. Pate RR, Mitchell JA, Byun W, Dowda M. Sedentary behaviour in youth. *Br J Sports Med.* 2011;45(11):906-913
15. Youth Risk Behavior Surveillance Summaries - United States. Atlanta, GA: Centers for Disease Control and Prevention; 2010
16. Sisson SB, Broyles ST. Social-ecological correlates of excessive TV viewing: difference by race and sex. *J Phys Act Health.* 2012 Mar;9(3):449-55; article first published online 2011 May 11
17. Jago R, Sebire SJ, Gorely T, Cillero IH, Biddle SJ. "I'm on it 24/7 at the moment": a qualitative examination of multi-screen viewing behaviours among UK 10-11 year olds. *Int J Behav Nutr Phys Act.* 2011;8:85
18. Lenhart A, Ling R, Campbell S, Purcell K. *Teens and Mobile Phones.* Pew Research Center: University of Michigan; 2010
19. Boone JE, Gordon-Larsen P, Adair LS, Popkin BM. Screen time and physical activity during adolescence: longitudinal effects on obesity in young adulthood. *Int J Behav Nutr Phys Act.* 2007;4:26
20. Carson V, Janssen I. Volume, patterns, and types of sedentary behavior and cardio-metabolic health in children and adolescents: a cross-sectional study. *BMC Public Health.* 2011;11:274
21. Fairclough SJ, Boddy LM, Hackett AF, Stratton G. Associations between children's socioeconomic status, weight status, and sex, with screen-based sedentary behaviours and sport participation. *Int J Pediatr Obes.* 2009;4(4):299-305
22. Jago R, Anderson CB, Baranowski T, Watson K. Adolescent patterns of physical activity differences by gender, day, and time of day. *Am J Prev Med.* 2005;28(5):447-452
23. Olds T, Wake M, Patton G, Ridley K, Waters E, Williams J, et al. How do school-day activity patterns differ with age and gender across adolescence? *J Adolesc Health.* 2009;44(1):64-72
24. Gorely T, Marshall SJ, Biddle SJ, Cameron N. The prevalence of leisure time sedentary behaviour and physical activity in adolescent girls: An ecological momentary assessment approach. *Int J Pediatr Obes.* 2007;2(4):227-234
25. Gorely T, Biddle SJ, Marshall SJ, Cameron N. The prevalence of leisure time sedentary behaviour and physical activity in adolescent boys: an ecological momentary assessment approach. *Int J Pediatr Obes.* 2009;4(4):289-298
26. Klesges RC, Shelton ML, Klesges LM. Effects of television on metabolic rate: potential implications for childhood obesity. *Pediatrics.* 1993;91(2):281-286
27. Institute of Medicine. *Preventing Childhood Obesity: Health in the Balance.* Washington, DC: The National Academies Press; 2005
28. Institute of Medicine. *Food Marketing to Children and Youth: Threat or Opportunity?* Washington, DC: The National Academies Press; 2006
29. Byrd-Bredbenner C, Grasso D. Health, medicine, and food messages in television commercials during 1992 and 1998. *J Sch Health.* 2000;70(2):61
30. Pearson N, Biddle SJ. Sedentary behavior and dietary intake in children, adolescents, and adults: a systematic review. *Am J Prev Med.* 2011;41(2):178-188
31. Linebarger DH, Walker D. Infants' and toddlers' television viewing and language outcomes. *Am Behav Sci.* 2005;48(5):624-645

32. Hogan MJ, Strasburger VC, eds. *Media and Prosocial Behavior in Children and Adolescents.* Mahwah, NJ: Lawrence Erlbaum; 2008
33. Strasburger VC, Jordan AB, Donnerstein E. Health effects of media on children and adolescents. *Pediatrics.* 2010;125(4):756-767
34. Jolin EM, Weller RA. Television viewing and its impact on childhood behaviors. *Curr Psychiatry Rep.* 2011;13(2):122-128
35. Tremblay MS, Leblanc AG, Kho ME, Saunders TJ, Larouche R, Colley RC, et al. Systematic review of sedentary behaviour and health indicators in school-aged children and youth. *Int J Behav Nutr Phys Act.* 2011;8:98
36. Sallis JF, Cervero RB, Ascher W, Henderson KA, Kraft MK, Kerr J. An ecological approach to creating active living communities. *Annu Rev Public Health.* 2006;27:297-322
37. Lawman HG, Wilson DK. A review of family and environmental correlates of health behaviors in high-risk youth. *Obesity (Silver Spring).* 2012;20(6):1142-1571; article first published online 26 Jan, 2012
38. Schmitz KH, Lytle LA, Phillips GA, Murray DM, Birnbaum AS, Kubik MY. Psychosocial correlates of physical activity and sedentary leisure habits in young adolescents: the Teens Eating for Energy and Nutrition at School study. *Prev Med.* 2002;34(2):266-278
39. Sallis JF, Owen N, Fotheringham MJ. Behavioral epidemiology: a systematic framework to classify phases of research on health promotion and disease prevention. *Ann Behav Med.* 2000;22(4):294-298
40. Fisher EB, Walker EA, Bostrom A, Fischhoff B, Haire-Joshu D, Johnson SB. Behavioral science research in the prevention of diabetes: status and opportunities. *Diabetes Care.* 2002;25(3):599-606
41. Granich J, Rosenberg M, Knuiman MW, Timperio A. Individual, social, and physical environment factors associated with electronic media use among children: sedentary behavior at home. *J Phys Act Health.* 2011;8(5):613-625
42. Saelens BE, Sallis JF, Nader PR, Broyles SL, Berry CC, Taras HL. Home environmental influences on children's television watching from early to middle childhood. *J Dev Behav Pediatr.* 2002;23(3): 127-132
43. Jago R, Page A, Froberg K, Sardinha LB, Klasson-Heggebo L, Andersen LB. Screen-viewing and the home TV environment: the European Youth Heart Study. *Prev Med.* 2008;47(5):525-529
44. Hume C, van der Horst K, Brug J, Salmon J, Oenema A. Understanding the correlates of adolescents' TV viewing: a social ecological approach. *Int J Pediatr Obes.* 2010;5(2):161-168
45. He M, Piche L, Beynon C, Harris S. Screen-related sedentary behaviors: children's and parents' attitudes, motivations, and practices. *J Nutr Educ Behav.* 2010;42(1):17-25
46. He M, Harris S, Piche L, Beynon C. Understanding screen-related sedentary behavior and its contributing factors among school-aged children: a social-ecologic exploration. *Am J Health Promot.* 2009;23(5):299-308
47. Hoyos Cillero I, Jago R, Sebire S. Individual and social predictors of screen-viewing among Spanish school children. *Eur J Pediatr.* 2011;170(1):93-102
48. Granich J, Rosenberg M, Knuiman M, Timperio A. Understanding children's sedentary behaviour: a qualitative study of the family home environment. *Health Educ Res.* 2010;25(2):199-210; article first published online 2008 May 22
49. Adachi-Mejia AM, Longacre MR, Gibson JJ, Beach ML, Titus-Ernstoff LT, Dalton MA. Children with a TV in their bedroom at higher risk for being overweight. *Int J Obes (Lond).* 2007;31(4):644-651
50. Sisson SB, Broyles ST, Newton RL Jr, Baker BL, Chernausek SD. TVs in the bedrooms of children: does it impact health and behavior? *Prev Med.* 2011;52(2):104-108
51. Barr-Anderson DJ, van den Berg P, Neumark-Sztainer D, Story M. Characteristics associated with older adolescents who have a television in their bedrooms. *Pediatrics.* 2008;121(4):718-724
52. Sisson SB, Broyles ST, Baker BL, Katzmarzyk PT. Television, reading, and computer time: correlates of school-day leisure-time sedentary behavior and relationship with overweight in children in the U.S. *J Phys Act Health.* 2011;8(Suppl 2):S188-197
53. Te Velde SJ, van der Horst K, Oenema A, Timperio A, Crawford D, Brug J. Parental and home influences on adolescents' TV viewing: a mediation analysis. *Int J Pediatr Obes.* 2011;6(2-2):e364-372
54. Barradas DT, Fulton JE, Blanck HM, Huhman M. Parental influences on youth television viewing. *J Pediatr.* 2007;151(4):369-373, 373.e1-4

55. Leatherdale ST, Wong SL. Modifiable characteristics associated with sedentary behaviours among youth. *Int J Pediatr Obes.* 2008;3(2):93-101
56. Bauer KW, Nelson MC, Boutelle KN, Neumark-Sztainer D. Parental influences on adolescents' physical activity and sedentary behavior: longitudinal findings from Project EAT-II. *Int J Behav Nutr Phys Act.* 2008;5:12
57. Pearson N, Salmon J, Crawford D, Campbell K, Timperio A. Are parental concerns for child TV viewing associated with child TV viewing and the home sedentary environment? *Int J Behav Nutr Phys Act.* 2011;8(1):102
58. Smith BJ, Grunseit A, Hardy LL, King L, Wolfenden L, Milat A. Parental influences on child physical activity and screen viewing time: a population based study. *BMC Public Health.* 2010;10:593
59. Norman G, Schmid B, Sallis J, Calfas K, Patrick K. Psychosocial and environmental correlates of adolescnt sedentary behaviors. *Pediatrics.* 2005;116:908-916
60. MacLeod KE, Gee GC, Crawford P, Wang MC. Neighbourhood environment as a predictor of television watching among girls. *J Epidemiol Community Health.* 2008;62(4):288-292
61. Kim J, Liu J, Colabianchi N, Pate RR. The effect of perceived and structural neighborhood conditions on adolescents' physical activity and sedentary behaviors. *Arch Pediatr Adolesc Med.* 2010; 164(10):935-942
62. Robinson TN. Reducing children's television viewing to prevent obesity: a randomized controlled trial. *JAMA.* 1999;282(16):1561-1567
63. Kamath CC, Vickers KS, Ehrlich A, McGovern L, Johnson J, Singhal V, et al. Clinical review: behavioral interventions to prevent childhood obesity: a systematic review and metaanalyses of randomized trials. *J Clin Endocrinol Metab.* 2008;93(12):4606-4615
64. Leung MM, Agaronov A, Grytsenko K, Yeh MC. Intervening to reduce sedentary behaviors and childhood obesity among school-age youth: a systematic review of randomized trials. *J Obes.* 2011;2012:685430
65. Maniccia DM, Davison KK, Marshall SJ, Manganello JA, Dennison BA. A meta-analysis of interventions that target children's screen time for reduction. *Pediatrics.* 2011;128(1):e193-210
66. Biddle SJ, O'Connell S, Braithwaite RE. Sedentary behaviour interventions in young people: a meta-analysis. *Br J Sports Med.* 2011;45(11):937-942
67. Zaza S, Wright-De Agüero LK, Briss PA, Truman BI, Hopkins DP, Hennessy MH, et al. Data collection instrument and procedure for systematic reviews in the Guide to Community Preventive Services. Task Force on Community Preventive Services. *Am J Prev Med.* 2000;18(1 Suppl):44-74
68. Salmon J, Ball K, Hume C, Booth M, Crawford D. Outcomes of a group-randomized trial to prevent excess weight gain, reduce screen behaviours and promote physical activity in 10-year-old children: switch-play. *Int J Obes (Lond).* 2008;32(4):601-612
69. French SA, Gerlach AF, Mitchell NR, Hannan PJ, Welsh EM. Household obesity prevention: Take Action—a group randomized trial. *Obesity (Silver Spring).* 2011;19(10):2082-2088
70. Bjelland M. Changes in adolescents' intake of sugar-sweetened beverages and sedentary behaviour: results at 8 month mid-way assessment of the HEIA study - a comprehensive, multi-component school-based randomized trial. *Int J Behav Nutr Phys Act.* 2011;8:63
71. Salmon J, Jorna M, Hume C, Arundell L, Chahine N, Tienstra M, et al. A translational research intervention to reduce screen behaviours and promote physical activity among children: Switch-2-Activity. *Health Promot Int.* 2011;26(3):311-321
72. Spruijt-Metz D, Nguyen-Michel ST, Goran MI, Chou CP, Huang TT. Reducing sedentary behavior in minority girls via a theory-based, tailored classroom media intervention. *Int J Pediatr Obes.* 2008;3(4):240-248
73. Ni Mhurchu C, Maddison R, Jiang Y, Jull A, Prapavessis H, Rodgers A. Couch potatoes to jumping beans: a pilot study of the effect of active video games on physical activity in children. *Int J Behav Nutr Phys Act.* 2008;5:8
74. Maddison R, Mhurchu CN, Jull A, Jiang Y, Prapavessis H, Rodgers A. Energy expended playing video console games: an opportunity to increase children's physical activity? *Pediatr Exerc Sci.* 2007;19(3):334-343
75. Graf DL, Pratt LV, Hester CN, Short KR. Playing active video games increases energy expenditure in children. *Pediatrics.* 2009;124(2):534-540

76. Mhurchu CN, Roberts V, Maddison R, Dorey E, Jiang Y, Jull A, et al. Effect of electronic time monitors on children's television watching: pilot trial of a home-based intervention. *Prev Med.* 2009;49(5):413-417; article first published online Sep 8, 2009
77. Epstein LH, Roemmich JN, Cavanaugh MD, Paluch RA. The motivation to be sedentary predicts weight change when sedentary behaviors are reduced. *Int J Behav Nutr Phys Act.* 2011;8:13
78. Matthews CE, Chen KY, Freedson PS, Buchowski MS, Beech BM, Pate RR, et al. Amount of time spent in sedentary behaviors in the United States, 2003-2004. *Am J Epidemiol.* 2008;167(7):875-881
79. Sisson SB, Church TS, Martin CK, Tudor-Locke C, Smith SR, Bouchard C, et al. Profiles of sedentary behavior in children and adolescents: the US National Health and Nutrition Examination Survey, 2001-2006. *Int J Pediatr Obes.* 2009;4(4):353-359
80. Jordan AB, Hersey JC, McDivitt JA, Heitzler CD. Reducing children's television-viewing time: a qualitative study of parents and their children. *Pediatrics.* 2006;118(5):e1303-1310
81. Bryant MJ, Lucove JC, Evenson KR, Marshall S. Measurement of television viewing in children and adolescents: a systematic review. *Obes Rev.* 2007;8(3):197-209

Adolesc Med 023 (2012) 529–543

Integrating Messages from the Eating Disorders Field into Obesity Prevention

Dianne Neumark-Sztainer, PhD, MPH, RD*

Professor, Division of Epidemiology and Community Health, School of Public Health, University of Minnesota, 1300 South Second Street, Suite 300, Minneapolis, MN 55454

Weight-related problems, including unhealthy weight control behaviors, binge eating, overweight and obesity, and eating disorders, are prevalent in youth. Furthermore, many young people exhibit more than one of these problems. Therefore, it is essential to consider how to simultaneously work toward the prevention of a broad range of weight-related problems in youth. Dieting, body dissatisfaction, weight talk, and weight-related teasing are commonly addressed risk factors within eating disorder prevention interventions, whereas low levels of physical activity and high intakes of foods high in fat and sugar are commonly addressed within interventions aimed at obesity prevention. Empirical data to be presented in this article demonstrate why risk factors such as dieting and body dissatisfaction, which are typically addressed within the eating disorder field, need to also be addressed within the obesity field. Although dieting and body dissatisfaction strongly predict weight gain over time, these findings are not always taken into account in the design of obesity interventions for youth. Possible reasons as to why risk factors such as dieting, body dissatisfaction, and weight stigmatization may be not adequately addressed within interventions addressing obesity are discussed. Suggestions for how physicians and other nonphysician clinicians might link messages from the fields of both eating disorders and obesity into their work with youth are provided. Finally, the potential for work on mindfulness and yoga to decrease risk factors for both eating disorders and obesity are explored.

WHERE DO THE DATA COME FROM? AN OVERVIEW OF PROJECT EAT

Most of the data discussed in this paper are drawn from the Project EAT (Eating and Activity in Teens and Young Adults) studies. Therefore, Project EAT is briefly described here. Project EAT was implemented to explore a broad spec-

*Corresponding author.
E-mail address: neumark@epi.umn.edu (D. Neumark-Sztainer).

 ISSN 1934-4287

trum of eating and weight-related problems in adolescents and to identify risk and protective factors for these outcomes. In contrast to many other studies, it included a comprehensive assessment of factors of possible relevance for both obesity and eating disorders. Given the population-based nature of the study, the focus was not on the assessment of clinical eating disorders such as anorexia nervosa and bulimia nervosa, but rather on the more prevalent disordered eating behaviors such as unhealthy weight control practices and binge eating. Additionally, height and weight were measured and both dietary intake and physical activity were assessed. Factors hypothesized to be relevant to both disordered eating and obesity, such as body satisfaction, weight talk (eg, encouragement to diet), weight teasing, family meals, dietary intake, and physical activity were selected for inclusion in the study. The study population included a high percentage of adolescents from low socioeconomic and ethnically/racially diverse backgrounds. Thus, findings from the study have relevance to youth who are at greatest risk for obesity, for whom interventions and public policies are needed.

The study includes a longitudinal component (Projects EAT-I, II, and III) in which approximately 2300 adolescents were followed for a 10-year period as they entered young adulthood. Middle school and high school adolescents were originally drawn from 31 public schools in the Minneapolis/St. Paul, Minnesota, metropolitan area. A second component of the study (EAT 2010) involved the recruitment of a new cohort of approximately 2800 adolescents from 20 schools in the same geographic area in 2010. EAT 2010 included an exploration of the family, peer, school, and neighborhood influences on weight-related problems in youth. Social cognitive theory[1,2] and an ecological framework[3,4] informed the selection of variables assessed in Project EAT; the theoretical framework guiding the study, specifically EAT 2010, is shown in Figure 1. Further details on the Project EAT studies can be found in previous publications.[5-8] Additionally, the Project EAT Web site includes information on study procedures, details on study variables, a list of all publications, and copies of surveys included in the different study arms (http://www.sph.umn.edu/eat).

WHY ADDRESS WEIGHT-RELATED PROBLEMS?

Weight-related problems are highly prevalent among adolescents. Table 1 shows the prevalence of a spectrum of weight-related problems, including unhealthy weight control behaviors, binge eating, overweight and obesity, and eating disorders. Data for weight control behaviors, binge eating, and overweight/obesity are from EAT 2010, while the data on eating disorders are from a compilation of studies. As seen in Table 1, most youth have some type of weight-related problem. Furthermore, although some adolescents may only have 1 problem (eg, only overweight without engaging in unhealthy weight control practices or binge eating), many adolescents exhibit more than 1 weight-related problem. For example, findings from Project EAT have shown that overweight youth are at high risk for engaging in unhealthy weight control practices.[5,9] In Project

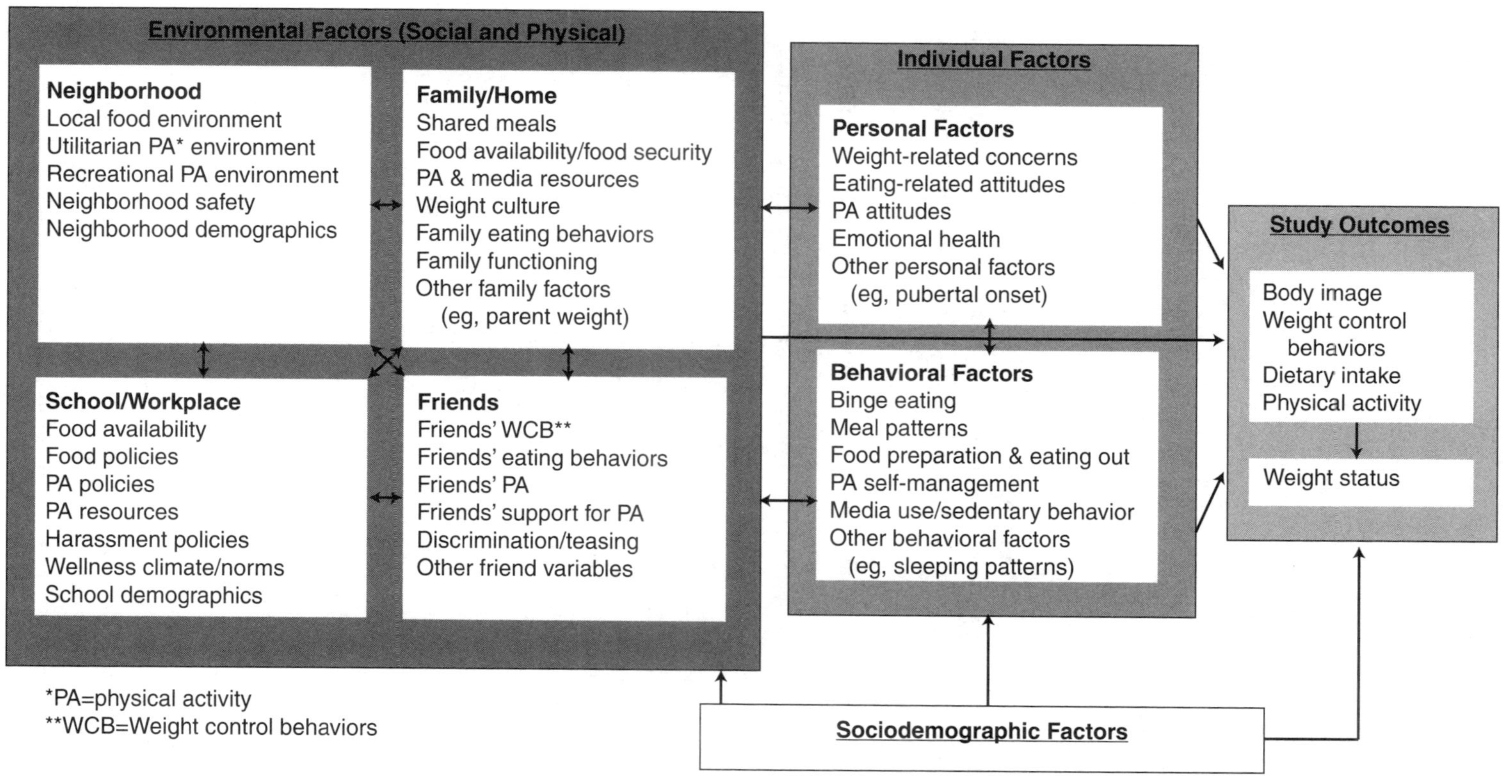

Fig 1 Theoretical Framework Guiding the Project EAT studies (specifically EAT 2010)

Table 1
Prevalence of weight-related problems in adolescents

	Girls	Boys
Unhealthy weight control behaviors	50%	38%
Dieting behaviors	46%	31%
Extreme weight control behaviors	7%	4%
Binge eating behaviors	10%	6%
Obesity	19%	26%
Overweight	20%	16%
Binge eating disorder	3-5%	1-3%
Bulimia nervosa	1-3%	<1%
Anorexia nervosa	0.5%	<0.2%

EAT-I, unhealthy weight control behaviors (ie, fasting, eating little food, using a food substitute, skipping meals, and smoking cigarettes for weight control purposes) were used by 50% of average weight girls, 69% of overweight girls, and 76% of obese girls.[5]

Much has been written about the importance of obesity prevention, given its high prevalence and associations with detrimental health consequences. However the numbers shown in Table 1 illustrate that our prevention efforts need to be broader in scope. The high prevalence and serious behavioral, psychosocial, and physical consequences associated with disordered eating and eating disorders indicate the importance of working toward the prevention of a broad spectrum of weight-related problems.[10-13] Austin has noted that eating disorders must be addressed within public health approaches targeting childhood obesity.[14] In Canada, a national meeting of researchers, practitioners, and policy makers met and wrote up a comprehensive report addressing the need for finding common ground between the fields of eating disorders and obesity to promote health.[15] Ideally, we can identify and implement strategies that have the potential to prevent a broad spectrum of weight-related problems by targeting risk factors of relevance to obesity, eating disorders, and disordered eating behaviors such as unhealthy weight control practices and binge eating.[10,11,16]

DIETING: GOOD OR BAD FOR WEIGHT MANAGEMENT?

Given the high percentage of youth who are overweight, and the high prevalences of dieting and the use of unhealthy weight control behaviors by adolescents, it is important to understand whether these behaviors are helpful or harmful with regard to weight management. Although dieting has long been a target of eating disorder prevention efforts, it has received less attention within the obesity field. Indeed, dieting or "going on a diet" is often touted as the solution to obesity and a common behavior adopted by individuals interested in losing weight. The dieting business is a huge enterprise that offers a variety of different diet plans with promises of weight loss ranging from moderate to extreme.

Findings from a recent analysis of 10-year longitudinal data from Project EAT clearly indicated that dieting is anything but the solution to excessive weight gain over time.[7] Participants were asked if they had gone on a diet in the past year to lose weight. Dieting was found to predict large weight gains during the transition from adolescence to young adulthood and the magnitude of the associations are clearly cause for public health concern. Study participants who engaged in dieting at both baseline and 5-year follow-up (ie, persistent dieters) had gained significantly more weight at 10-year follow-up compared to those who did not diet in analyses adjusted for sociodemographic characteristics and baseline body mass index (BMI).

Specifically, females who were persistent dieters increased their BMI by 4.3 units over the 10-year study period as compared to an increase of only 2.4 BMI units among the nondieters. Among males, persistent dieters increased their BMI by 7.0 units as compared to an increase of 3.4 units in nondieters. Of concern, similar patterns were found among youth who were overweight at baseline. For example, females who were overweight at baseline increased their BMI by 4.5 units as compared to an increase of only 1.6 BMI units among girls who were overweight at baseline but did not diet throughout the study period. Similar trends were found for the use of unhealthy weight control behaviors, such as skipping meals, trying to eat very little, using food substitutes, and taking diet pills. These findings represent huge differences given that they were found within a population-based sample. Furthermore, given the diverse nature of the population, findings suggest the relevance of dieting and the use of unhealthy weight control behaviors as important risk factors for obesity in ethnically/racially diverse young people.

These findings are in agreement with findings from other longitudinal studies, which have also found that dieting predicts weight gain, rather than weight loss over time.[17-22] This body of literature strongly points to a need to steer young people away from dieting. Although the avoidance of dieting behaviors has always been a key message within the eating disorder field, these data indicate the importance of adopting a similar message within the obesity field. Rather than thinking in terms of "dieting" or "going on a diet," children and adolescents should be encouraged to engage in healthful eating and physical activity patterns that can be sustained over time and may vary in accordance with one's social situation (eg, out with friends) or emotional frame of mind (eg, when feeling down). Additionally, youth should be taught to listen to internal signs of hunger and satiety; exposed to reasonable portion sizes; and provided with home, school, and neighborhood environments that make engaging in healthful behaviors the default pattern.

Given the current environment that often provides ready access to large amounts of foods that are high in calories, it can be a struggle to totally grasp how one can avoid dieting behaviors to avoid excessive weight gain. Herman et al have suggested a shift toward decreasing overeating tendencies as an alternative to dietary restraint,[23] whether these tendencies include binge eating in response to emotional stresses or overeating in the presence of large portion sizes. This suggestion is based on research showing that dietary restraint may lead to increased disinhibition and overeating in the presence of large portion sizes.[24,25] In this type of approach, a physician or nonphysician clinician (eg, dietitian, nurse, psychologist) could help children and adolescents identify situations in which overeating tends to occur and work with them to find strategies to prevent excess calorie intake such as relaxation techniques, physical activity, reaching out for social support, or the consumption of more nutrient-dense foods. As discussed later in this article, a yoga practice provides one strategy for helping individuals to be more in touch with their bodies and thus recognize signs of hunger and satiety. Additionally, a regular yoga practice can help in reducing overall stress, which can be a trigger for overeating. Although strong evaluations are needed to test the effectiveness and acceptability of these strategies as alternatives to dieting, the empirical data, showing that dieting is prevalent in youth and predicts large weight gains over time, clearly demonstrate that efforts must be made to help youth avoid dieting for weight management.

WHAT ABOUT BODY DISSATISFACTION?

Similar to dieting, body dissatisfaction is one of the key risk factors for eating disorders and a prime target addressed within eating disorder prevention efforts.[26] Less clear is how to address body image within the obesity field. One could argue that it is important for overweight youth to be dissatisfied with their bodies as a first step to change. Alternatively, it could be argued that adolescents who feel badly about their bodies find it difficult to engage in self-nurturing behaviors. Two studies that utilized the Project EAT longitudinal data provide support for the latter argument and suggest that body dissatisfaction does not motivate young people to engage in healthier behaviors and increases risk for weight gain over time.[27,28]

The first study examined 5-year longitudinal associations between body satisfaction and the use of both health-promoting (eg, physical activity, fruit and vegetable intake) and health-compromising behaviors (eg, unhealthy weight control practices and binge eating).[28] The aim was to gather information to assess whether low body satisfaction motivates youth to engage in healthier behaviors or, alternatively, serves as an impediment to a healthier behavioral repertoire. Lower levels of body satisfaction at baseline predicted more health-compromising behaviors, such as unhealthy weight control behavior and binge eating, and fewer health promoting behaviors, such as physical activity, at 5-year follow-up. For example, in analyses adjusting for sociodemographic characteristics, BMI, and physical activity at baseline, girls with low levels of baseline body satisfaction reported 3.9 hours of physical activity a week at 5-year follow-up, whereas girls with high levels of body satisfaction reported 4.5 hours of activity. In response to the question, “Does body satisfaction matter?” results suggested that body satisfaction does matter and interventions are needed to help youth feel better about their bodies.

The second study addressed the question, "How is body satisfaction related to changes in BMI in overweight adolescent girls?"[27] The focus was on overweight youth, given that it could be argued that overweight youth should feel dissatisfied with their bodies to motivate change. BMI changes as a function of baseline body satisfaction were examined in analyses that adjusted for sociodemographic characteristics and baseline BMI. The findings, which are quite striking, are shown in Figure 2. Whereas girls with high levels of body satisfaction at baseline increased their BMI by 1 unit over a 5-year period, girls with low levels of body satisfaction increased their BMI by 3 units on average.

Findings from these studies strongly suggest the importance of addressing body satisfaction within interventions aimed at obesity prevention. Balance needs to be achieved between helping youth feel better about their bodies and also helping them realize the importance of developing healthful eating and physical activity behaviors to achieve a weight that is most healthful for them. This is not an easy message to deliver. In New Moves, a school-based intervention with high school adolescent girls at risk for obesity and other weight problems, girls decreased their use of unhealthy weight control behaviors and increased their level of body satisfaction.[29-32] Intervention strategies included a supportive physical education classroom for the girls, sessions that emphasized a non-dieting approach to healthful eating, group work on countering media and peer influences likely to have a negative effect on body image, and individual motivational interviewing sessions. In addition to the positive

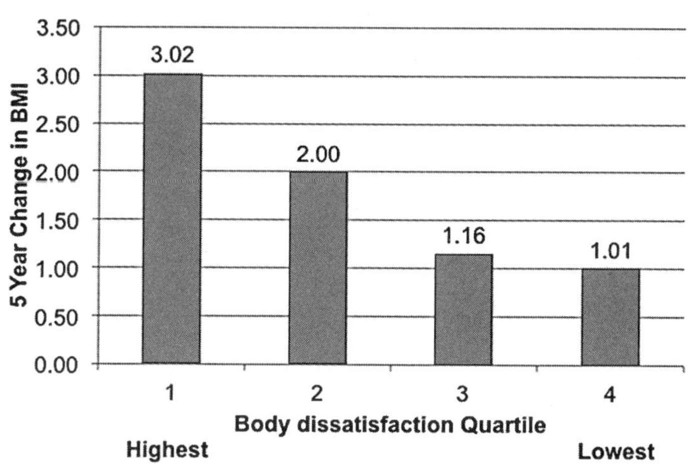

Fig 2. Adjusted mean BMI change between Time 1 and Time 2, by Time 1 body satisfaction quartile, in overweight adolescent girls. Source: van den Berg P, Neumark-Sztainer D. Fat 'n happy 5 years later: is it bad for overweight girls to like their bodies? *J Adolesc Health.* 2007;41: 415-417. Reprinted with permission.

changes seen with regard to body image and the use of unhealthy weight control practices, the girls showed some increases in their overall physical activity. However, the girls did not show a significant decrease in their BMI or percent body fat as compared to girls in the control condition. Further work is needed to develop interventions that are effective in preventing a broad array of weight-related problems in youth.

DOES IT HELP FOR PARENTS TO DISCUSS WEIGHT WITH THEIR ADOLESCENT CHILDREN?

Within the eating disorders field, there is a lot of emphasis on avoiding weight talk at home, whether this involves talking about one's weight, encouraging one's child to diet as a weight management strategy, or more overt weight-related teasing in which comments perceived by adolescents as derogatory are made by family members. An important question regards the relevance of weight talk at home for obesity risk. Are parents of overweight children talking with their children about healthful eating, physical activity, and weight? Does weight teasing occur in the homes of youth? And do any of these types of conversations infer benefits for youth in terms of weight management?

Within the obesity field, concern has been expressed that some parents may not recognize that their overweight children are actually overweight. In response, actions such as weighing children in schools and sending report cards home,[33-37] or developing campaigns that alert parents to the health consequences of childhood obesity and the need to act, are being implemented.[38] However, there are little data to support that actual knowledge about one's child's weight status leads to healthier parent actions. In Project EAT, we examined whether parents of overweight adolescents, who accurately perceived that their children were overweight, provided a more supportive environment for their children in terms of the types of foods available at home; opportunities for physical activity; and encouragement to engage in healthier eating behaviors, more physical activity, and dieting for weight control purposes.[39] This analysis was conducted in a random subset of adolescents whose parents also participated in the study. Results indicated few differences between the groups. In fact, the only difference between the families was that parents who accurately reported that their children were overweight were more likely to encourage their children to diet, as compared to parents of overweight children who did not report that their children were overweight. Of concern, encouragement to diet predicted larger weight gains in these children 5 years later. This study was not an intervention study; thus implications for interventions that involve informing parents about their children's weight status need to be made cautiously. Nevertheless, these results suggest that it is not enough to inform parents about their children's overweight status; in fact, this information on its own could be harmful. Furthermore, parents need to hear that weight talk at home that is meant to be helpful (ie, encouragement to diet) may be counterproductive to weight management in youth.

Another type of weight talk worthy of consideration here is weight-related teasing. Within the obesity field, weight teasing is certainly not promoted as a strategy for obesity prevention or treatment, but those working with overweight youth may not realize that being teased about one's weight actually is a strong predictor of weight gain over time. In Project EAT, longitudinal analyses found that adolescents who were teased by family members about their weight were at significantly greater risk for being overweight 5 years later, even after adjusting for baseline weight status and sociodemographics.[13] Similarly, in another large study of adolescents, the Growing Up Today Study, Haines and colleagues found that hurtful weight-related comments made by parents longitudinally predicted overweight status in adolescent girls.[20] Thus, there is great concern that campaigns in which overweight children are negatively portrayed could increase the risk for weight mistreatment by others, which is likely to be counterproductive to obesity prevention and to increase risk for other psychosocial outcomes.

WHY ARE DIETING, BODY DISSATISFACTION, AND WEIGHT TALK OFTEN NOT ADDRESSED IN OBESITY INTERVENTIONS?

Following a recent presentation on the topic of integrating eating disorder and obesity prevention, one of the physicians in the audience asked why factors such as dieting, body dissatisfaction, and weight talk are not routinely addressed within obesity interventions. Given the strong associations described in the previous sections, it would seem as though primary aims within both obesity prevention and treatment programs should be to (1) ensure that youth avoid dieting behaviors; (2) engage youth in activities to help them feel better about their bodies; and (3) surround youth with supportive environments in which harmful weight talk does not happen. Indeed, Austin has appropriately labeled this inattention to risk factors for eating disorders as "the blind spot in the drive for childhood obesity prevention."[14]

One reason that dieting, body dissatisfaction, and weight talk are not adequately addressed within obesity prevention and treatment interventions may be that we do not totally understand the relationships between these factors and weight gain over time, and we may not believe that these associations are of a causal nature. It is easier to grasp that children are becoming overweight because they are drinking more sweetened beverages, eating fewer vegetables, and being less physically active and address these behaviors directly. It is likely that youth engage in dieting behaviors as a substitute to healthier behaviors that can be maintained over a long period. Although further research is needed to understand why dieting, body dissatisfaction, and weight talk predict weight gain over time, the strong associations previously described cannot be ignored. Furthermore, the strong empirical associations found between dieting and weight gain are in accordance with testimonials of overweight adults who describe a history of failed diets that contributed to ongoing weight gain over time. Existing data strongly suggest that it is worthwhile to help youth avoid dieting behaviors, feel better about their bodies, and be exposed to environments in which weight talk is minimal and does not include weight-related teasing. Interventions with such aims are not only likely to prevent excessive weight gain, but also to decrease risk for eating disorders and improve overall feelings of well-being in young people.

The development of integrated approaches is essential in our work with youth. More challenging is finding effective approaches that integrate principles from the eating disorders field into the obesity field. The next section includes a description of some ideas for physicians and nonphysician clinicians working within health care settings. Additionally, through my personal practice and an intensive study of yoga, I have begun to think about the potential that a yoga practice has in addressing risk factors of relevance to a broad spectrum of weight-related problems. These ideas are presented in the final section of this chapter.

INTEGRATED APPROACHES TO PREVENTION: WHAT CAN PHYSICIAN AND NONPHYSICIAN CLINICIANS DO?

Research suggests that the type of language used to discuss weight-related topics is important to youth and their families.[40] Physician and nonphysician clinicians are increasingly concerned about the high prevalence of obesity in youth, with many also expressing questions about how to address obesity without increasing an adolescent's risk for eating disorders or an unhealthy preoccupation with weight. The data described in this article suggest that by discouraging the use of dieting behaviors, helping youth feel better about themselves and their bodies, and working with families to avoid harmful weight talk at home, youth may actually decrease their risk for both obesity and eating disorders. What might this look like within a short health care visit? Some suggestions are included in Table 2. For a more thorough description, the reader is referred to a previous publication.[41]

A next step may be to develop a framework whereby the points raised in Table 2 could be implemented on a regular basis into clinic visits or addressed via a physician-led health team approach. For example, it may be appropriate for the physician to assess weight status, engagement in unhealthy weight control behaviors, body image concerns, and exposure to weight-related teasing and other forms of weight mistreatment. Although mild problems can be addressed within the health care visit (eg, a discussion about the ineffectiveness of dieting), more severe problems might best be addressed within a group program run by an interdisciplinary team. Evaluations of different types of approaches are needed to ensure their effectiveness, sustainability, and acceptability to youth and their families.

YOGA: AN ANCIENT PRACTICE WITH POTENTIAL RELEVANCE FOR ADDRESSING MORE MODERN WEIGHT-RELATED PROBLEMS

The practice of yoga offers potential for the integration of messages from the fields of eating disorders and obesity via the reduction of risk factors and the enhancement of protective factors for the broad spectrum of weight-related

Table 2
Recommendations for physicians and nonphysician clinicians

Recommendation:	Some suggested actions:
Discourage dieting and unhealthy weight control behaviors	Talk about how dieting is often a short-term behavior and how research shows that dieting predicts large weight gains over time. Discuss alternative behaviors that youth can engage in over a sustained period of time. Ask about foods that youth enjoy and physical activities that they find to be fun and are easily accessible to them.
Promote a positive body image	Recognize that adolescents are sensitive about their bodies, particularly overweight youth. Ask adolescents they feel about their bodies. What do they like? How are they good to themselves? Use appropriate language; research suggests that terms such as *weight* (eg, I'm concerned about the health implications of your weight) are preferred over *overweight* and certainly *obese*.[40]
Provide a place for teens to discuss weight mistreatment	Ask teens if they have been teased about their weight/body or experienced weight-related mistreatment. For overweight youth, assume that some type of weight mistreatment has occurred. Let youth know that any type of weight mistreatment is not acceptable, nor funny, and explore strategies for responding and reducing exposure. If level of weight mistreatment is high, refer to appropriate caretaker (eg, social worker, psychologist) who may have more time and skills to address.
Work with adolescent and family to decrease weight talk at home	Discuss the negative implications of weight talk—even when comments are well intentioned. Practice alternatives to weight talk at home. Discuss alternative ideas to help adolescent engage in healthy behaviors (eg, family meals, involvement in physical activity). Stress that it is much more effective to change the home environment to make healthier eating and physical activity behaviors easier than to discuss these behaviors and engage in weight talk. Make it absolutely clear that weight-related teasing is never funny and can have serious implications for physical and psychological health. Provide appropriate resources for parents (eg, books, Web sites, or support groups).

problems. Yoga may be able to help young people feel better about their bodies, be more in touch with their feelings of hunger and satiety, and find healthy strategies for dealing with stress. Three principles from the practice of yoga are presented here as starting points for the discussion on how yoga may be incorporated within interventions utilizing an integrated approach to preventing a broad spectrum of weight-related problems.

The first principle is *asana*, which is the physical practice and postures of yoga, and the component with which individuals tend to be most familiar. An *asana* practice may range from being very still to very active. For example, a physical practice might involve seated and resting poses that are held for periods of time and allow for stretching, relaxation, and internal reflection. In contrast, a more active physical practice might involve a mixture of sun salutations in which the individual is engaging in moderate to vigorous activities and strenuous holding poses that build strength in different parts of the body. Often an *asana* practice involves a mixture of both restful and vigorous movements, but may be greatly altered in accordance with the needs and physical abilities of different people, and with an individual's needs on any given day. If taught within an environment that is comfortable for people of different shapes, sizes, and skill levels, and if adapted to meet the varying physical needs and abilities of participants, a physical yoga practice can offer a strategy for people to move in a manner that works for them. This physical practice has the potential to help individuals feel good about their bodies and lead to a desire for self-care via appropriate movement and more healthful eating patterns. On a practical level, the physical practice of yoga can be done in a small space, provided that a suitable space that offers some privacy can be found within one's home or within a clinical setting.

The second principle of yoga with potential relevance to both eating disorders and obesity prevention is *pranyama*, which is the breath work of yoga. Paying attention to one's breath, and engaging in different breathing techniques can help in monitoring one's emotional state, decreasing stress, and remaining present. Thus, an individual can learn to monitor feelings of stress or anxiety throughout the day by noticing if one's breath is quicker than normal. And one can engage in a *pranyama* practice to deal with these feelings of stress or anxiety. Given that excessive eating (eg, binge eating) or excessive restrictive behaviors may both be triggered by feelings related to stress or anxiety, it is important to monitor these feelings and to have tools to deal with them. Ideally, one would engage in a *pranyama* practice on a regular basis to prevent extreme changes in one's emotions and unhealthy reactions to these emotions throughout the day. Alternatively (or additionally) one could potentially learn to use these strategies when a stressful situation arises to deal with this situation in a manner that is not harmful to one's self. For example, perhaps instead of immediately binge eating as a result of stress, or overeating when coming home from school, one might train oneself to first take 5 minutes to engage in mindful slow breathing, which might decrease the need to binge, reduce the amount of food consumed, or lead to the selection of healthier foods.

The third principle to be discussed here is that of *ahimsa*, or nonviolence toward oneself and others. This principle extends well beyond physical violence to include more subtle thoughts (eg, negative thoughts about one's body) and actions (eg, engaging in unhealthy weight control practices or teasing others about their weight) and offers a potential framework for getting youth to modify both thought and actions related to various weight-related problems. Adolescents who engage in negative thoughts about themselves, use unhealthy weight control practices, and consume large amounts of foods high in calories and low in nutrients may benefit from learning about the practice of *ahimsa* and modifying their thoughts and actions to avoid self-harm. Similarly youth and family members engaging in harmful weight talk and weight teasing are not practicing *ahimsa* in that they may be hurting others. It is important to develop new strategies to address topics related to obesity and eating disorders because new and different approaches may gather the interest of youth.

Many questions arise in thinking about if and how to incorporate yoga, and the previously discussed 3 principles, into interventions that utilize an integrated approach to the prevention of weight-related problems in youth. Clearly further work is needed to explore questions such as: Are these practices suitable for all youth, and if not, for whom? How can these principles be incorporated into youth interventions to make them attractive to youth and enhance their effectiveness in reducing weight-related problems? How might we utilize the principles and practice of yoga with families, within school-based programs, at community settings, or within clinical settings? How and where can physician and nonphysician clinicians be trained to utilize these principles or find those who are trained and work together as a team? And how effective are such approaches in addressing different weight-related problems? These are questions that I am currently beginning to explore. This exploration is leading me to believe that the practice of yoga, or the incorporation of some of its principles into our work with youth, has the potential to offer another toolbox that is suitable for some youth and some physicians as we work to prevent and reduce the prevalence of eating and weight-related problems in youth.

CONCLUSIONS

In summary, it is essential to consider the broad spectrum of weight-related problems in working with youth, given their high prevalence, health consequences, and overlap within persons. The existence of shared risk factors allows for the development of interventions of relevance to obesity, eating disorders, and disordered eating behaviors. Empirical data from longitudinal studies clearly demonstrate that risk factors for eating disorders such as dieting, body dissatisfaction, and exposure to weight-related teasing are also strong risk factors for excessive weight gain over time. These findings indicate that obesity prevention interventions and policies should aim to reduce these risk factors. Clearly new strategies are needed for addressing obesity in youth that are effective, engaging, and free of unintended harmful consequences. Additional research is needed to evaluate the feasibility and effectiveness of proposed strategies for integrated interventions.

References

1. Bandura A. *Social Foundations of Thought and Action: A Social Cognitive Theory*. Englewood Cliffs, NJ: Prentice-Hall, Inc.; 1986
2. McAlister AL, Perry CL, Parcel GS. How individuals, environments, and health behaviors interact: Social Cognitive Theory. In: Glanz K, Rimer BK, Viswanath K, eds. *Health Behavior and Health Education: Theory, Research, and Practice*. 4th ed. San Francisco, CA: Jossey-Bass; 2008:169-188

3. Sallis JF, Owen N, Fisher EB. Ecological models of health behavior. In: Glanz K, Rimer BK, Viswanath K, eds. *Health Behavior and Health Education: Theory, Research, and Practice*. 4th ed. San Francisco, CA: Jossey-Bass; 2008:465-485
4. Story M, Kaphingst KM, Robinson-O'Brien R, Glanz K. Creating healthy food and eating environments: Policy and environmental approaches. *Annu Rev Public Health*. 2008;29:253-272
5. Neumark-Sztainer D, Story M, Hannan PJ, Perry CL, Irving LM. Weight-related concerns and behaviors among overweight and non-overweight adolescents: implications for preventing weight-related disorders. *Arch Pediatr Adolesc Med*. 2002;156(2):171-178
6. Larson NI, Neumark-Sztainer D, Story M, van den Berg P, Hannan PJ. Identifying correlates of young adults' weight behavior: survey development. *Am J Health Behav*. 2011;35:712-725
7. Neumark-Sztainer D, Wall M, Story M, Standish AR. Dieting and unhealthy weight control behaviors during adolescence: associations with 10-year changes in body mass index. *J Adolesc Health*. 2012;50(1):80-86
8. Neumark-Sztainer D, Wall MM, Larson N, et al. Secular trends in weight status and weight-related attitudes and behaviors in adolescents from 1999 to 2010. *Prev Med*. 2012;54(1):77-81
9. Neumark-Sztainer D, Wall M, Story M, Sherwood NE. Five-year longitudinal predictive factors for disordered eating in a population-based sample of overweight adolescents: implications for prevention and treatment. *Int J Eat Disord*. 2009;42(7):664-672
10. Neumark-Sztainer D. Obesity and eating disorder prevention: an integrated approach? *Adolesc Med*. 2003;14:159-173
11. Neumark-Sztainer D. Can we simultaneously work toward the prevention of obesity and eating disorders in children and adolescents. *Int J Eat Disord*. 2005;38:220-227
12. Haines J, Neumark-Sztainer D. Prevention of obesity and eating disorders: a consideration of shared risk factors. *Health Educ Res*. 2006;21:770-782
13. Neumark-Sztainer D, Wall M, Haines J, Story M, Sherwood NE, van den Berg P. Shared risk and protective factors for overweight and disordered eating in adolescents. *Am J Prev Med*. 2007;33:359-369
14. Austin SB. The blind spot in the drive for childhood obesity prevention: bringing eating disorders prevention into focus as a public health priority. *Am J Public Health*. 2011;101(101):e1-4
15. Obesity and Eating Disorders: Seeking common ground to promote health: A national meeting of researchers, practitioners, and policy makers. Paper presented at: Obesity and Eating Disorders Symposium; November, 2007; Calgary, Alberta, Canada. http://www.ocoped.ca/DNN/PDF/Obesity_eating_disorders_2007.pdf. Accessed November 2, 2012
16. Neumark-Sztainer D. The interface between the eating disorders and obesity fields: moving toward a model of shared knowledge and collaboration. *Eat Weight Disord*. 2009;14(1):51-58
17. Viner RM, Cole TJ. Who changes body mass between adolescence and adulthood? Factors predicting change in BMI between 16 year and 30 years in the 1970 British Birth Cohort. *Int J Obes*. 2006;30(9):1368-1374
18. Chaput JP, Leblanc C, Perusse L, Despres JP, Bouchard C, Tremblay A. Risk factors for adult overweight and obesity in the Quebec Family Study: have we been barking up the wrong tree? *Obesity (Silver Spring)*. 2009;17(10):1964-1970
19. Field AE, Austin SB, Taylor CB, et al. Relation between dieting and weight change among preadolescents and adolescents. *Pediatrics*. 2003;112(4):900-906
20. Haines J, Kleinman KP, Rifas-Shiman SL, Field AE, Austin SB. Examination of shared risk and protective factors for overweight and disordered eating among adolescents. *Arch Pediatr Adolesc Med*. 2010;164(4):336-343
21. Tanofsky-Kraff M, Cohen ML, Yanovski SZ, et al. A prospective study of psychological predictors of body fat gain among children at high risk for adult obesity. *Pediatrics*. 2006;117:1203-1209
22. Stice E, Presnell K, Shaw H, Rohde P. Psychological and behavioral risk factors for obesity onset in adolescent girls: a prospective study. *J Consult Clin Psychol*. 2005;73(2):195-202
23. Herman CP, van Strien T, Polivy J. Undereating or eliminating overeating? *Am Psychol*. 2008;63(3):202-203
24. Polivy J, Herman CP, Deo R. Getting a bigger slice of the pie. Effects on eating and emotion in restrained and unrestrained eaters. *Appetite*. 2010;55(3):426-430

25. Bryant EJ, King NA, Blundell JE. Disinhibition: its effects on appetite and weight regulation. *Obesity Rev.* 2008;9(5):409-419
26. Levine MP, Smolak L. *The Prevention of Eating Problems and Eating Disorders: Theory, Research, and Practice.* Mahwah, NJ: Lawrence Erlbaum Associates; 2006
27. van den Berg P, Neumark-Sztainer D. Fat 'n happy 5 years later: is it bad for overweight girls to like their bodies? *J Adolesc Health.* 2007;41:415-417
28. Neumark-Sztainer D, Paxton SJ, Hannan PJ, Haines J, Story M. Does body satisfaction matter? Five-year longitudinal associations between body satisfaction and health behaviors in adolescent females and males. *J Adolesc Health.* 2006;39:244-251
29. Neumark-Sztainer D. New Moves Online. 2009. Available at: http://www.newmovesonline.com. Accessed November 2, 2012
30. Neumark-Sztainer D, Flattum C, Feldman S, Petrich C. Striving to prevent obesity and other weight-related problems in adolescent girls: The New Moves approach. In: O'Dea JA, Eriksen M, eds. *Childhood Obesity Prevention - International Research, Controversies, and Interventions.* New York: Oxford University Press; 2010
31. Neumark-Sztainer D, Flattum CF, Story M, Feldman S, Petrich CA. Dietary approaches to healthy weight management for adolescents: The New Moves model. *Adolesc Med.* 2008;19(3):421-430
32. Neumark-Sztainer D, Friend SE, Flattum CF, et al. New Moves-Preventing weight-related problems in adolescent girls: a group-randomized study. *Am J Prev Med.* 2010;39(5):421-432
33. Should schools issue a "health report card," reporting a child's body mass index, as Arkansas plans to do? *Journal of Physical Education, Recreation & Dance.* 2004;75(3):10-12
34. Chomitz VR, Collins J, Kim J, Kramer E, McGowan R. Promoting healthy weight among elementary school children via a health report card approach. *Arch Pediatr Adolesc Med.* 2003;157(8):765-772
35. Evans EW, Sonneville KR. BMI report cards: will they pass or fail in the fight against pediatric obesity? *Curr Opin Pediatr.* 2009;21(4):431-436
36. Forman SF, Woods ER. BMI report cards: do they make the grade? *Curr Opin Pediatr.* 2009;21(4):429-430
37. Ikeda JP, Crawford PB, Woodward-Lopez G. BMI screening in schools: helpful or harmful? *Health Educ Res.* 2006;21(6):761-769
38. Children's Healthcare of Atlanta Inc. Strong4Life Campaign. 2012. Available at: strong4life.com. Accessed November 2, 2012.
39. Neumark-Sztainer D, Wall M, Story M, van den Berg P. Accurate parental classification of their overweight adolescents' weight status: does it matter? *Pediatrics.* 2008;121:e1495-1502
40. Puhl RM, Peterson JL, Luedicke J. Parental perceptions of weight terminology that providers use with youth. *Pediatrics.* 2011;128(4):e786-793
41. Neumark-Sztainer D. Preventing obesity and eating disorders in adolescents: what can health care providers do? *J Adolesc Health.* 2009;44(3):206-213

Adolesc Med 023 (2012) 544–570

Interventions for Treating Overweight and Obesity in Adolescents

Alberta S. Kong, MD, MPH*[a], Jeanne Dalen, PhD[b], Sylvia Negrete, MD[a], Sarah G. Sanders, MS, RN[a], Patricia C. Keane, MS, RD[a], Sally M. Davis, PhD[a]

[a]*Department of Pediatrics, University of New Mexico School of Medicine, MSC 10 5590, 1 University of New Mexico, Albuquerque, NM*
[b]*Oregon Research Institute, 1715 Franklin Blvd., Eugene, OR 97403*

INTRODUCTION

The prevalence of overweight and obesity has increased dramatically in adolescents over the past 30 years with current estimates at 34%.[1] Overweight is defined as at or greater than a body mass index (BMI) of 85th percentile, and obesity is defined as at or greater than a BMI of 95th percentile according to the 2000 sex-specific BMI-for-age growth charts from the Centers for Disease Control and Prevention (CDC).[2] Within the past few decades, the percentage of American adolescents 12 to 19 years of age who are obese has increased more than 3-fold from 6% to 18%.[3] Obesity during adolescence is the single best predictor of adult obesity and ensuing health complications, including type 2 diabetes, heart disease, and premature death.[4, 5] Furthermore, conditions that were historically adult entities are now highly prevalent in obese adolescents, with up to 44% having metabolic syndrome[6] and 30% having pre-diabetes.[7] To prevent obesity-related health consequences, treatment of adolescent overweight and obesity is critical. The American Academy of Pediatrics (AAP) recommends a 4-stage approach for treatment of adolescents (Tables 1 and 2).[8] Components within the stages range from general recommendations of lifestyle modification to medication and surgery. This article provides a review of the current literature on interventions that have demonstrated efficacy in the treatment of adolescent overweight and obesity. Intervention categories covered in this review include dietary, physical activity, behavioral multicomponent, pharmacological, and surgical approaches that can be used to meet the AAP 4-stage approach.

*Corresponding author.
E-mail address: akong@salud.unm.edu (A. S. Kong).

 ISSN 1934-4287

Table 1
American Academy of Pediatrics 4-stage approach to weight management for adolescents

Stages	Components	Suggested Professional
1. Prevention Plus	Recommend ≥5 servings of fruits and vegetables/day. ≤2 hours of screen time/day; no television where child sleeps. Minimize or eliminate sugar-sweetened beverages. Address eating behaviors (eg, eating away from home, daily breakfast, family dinners, and skipping meals). Recommend ≥1 hour of physical activity/day. Amount of physical activity may need to be graded for children who are sedentary; they may not achieve 1 hour/day initially. Involve entire family. Acknowledge cultural differences.	Primary care provider or trained professional staff member (eg, registered nurse)
2. Structured weight management	Develop plan with family for balanced-macronutrient diet emphasizing small amounts of energy-dense foods. Because this diet provides less energy, ensure that protein is high quality and sufficient to prevent loss of muscle mass. Increase structure of daily meals and snacks. Reduce screen time to ≤1 hour/day. Increase time spent in physical activity (≥60 minutes of supervised active play/day). Instruct patient and/or parent in monitoring (eg, screen time, physical activity, dietary intake, and restaurant logs) to improve adherence. Perform medical screening (eg, vital signs, assessment tools, and laboratory tests).	Registered dietician or physician/nurse practitioner
3. Comprehensive multidisciplinary intervention	Distinguished from stage 2 by more frequent patient/provider contact, more active use of behavioral strategies, more formal monitoring, and feedback regarding progress to improve adherence. Multidisciplinary approach is essential. Components of multidisciplinary behavioral weight control programs include: Moderate/strong parental involvement for children < 12 years of age; parental involvement should decrease gradually as adolescents increase in age; Assessments of diet, physical activity, and weight (body fat) before treatment and at specified intervals thereafter to evaluate progress; Structured behavioral program that includes at least food monitoring, short-term diet and activity goal setting, and contingency management; Parent/caregiver training to improve home food and activity environments; and Structured dietary and physical activity interventions that improve dietary quality and result in negative energy balance.	Multidisciplinary team with expertise in childhood obesity, including behavioral counselor (eg, social worker, psychologist, trained nurse practitioner, or other mental health care provider), registered dietician, and exercise specialist. Alternative could be dietician and behavioral counselor based in primary care office, along with outside, structured, physical activity program (eg, team sports, YMCA, or Boys and Girls Club program). For areas without services, consider innovative program (eg, telemedicine).
4. Tertiary care intervention	Continued diet and physical activity counseling plus consideration of meal replacements, very-low-energy diet, medication, and surgery	Same as above

Table 2
American Academy of Pediatrics staged treatment of adolescent overweight and obesity

BMI percentile	Starting Stage	Weight Goal	Duration in Stage
85th-94th (overweight)	Prevention Plus	Weight maintenance until BMI <85th percentile or slowing of weight gain, as indicated by downward trend in BMI curve.	Advance to more intensive level of intervention depending on responses to treatment, age, health risks, and motivation. Advance to stage 2, structured weight management, after 3-6 months if increasing BMI percentile or persistent medical condition. A child in Prevention Plus stage with BMI that has tracked in the same percentile over time with no medical risks may have a low risk for excess body fat; therefore, may continue obesity prevention strategies and not advance treatment stages.
95th-98th	Prevention Plus or structured weight loss (depending on age, degree of obesity, health risks, and motivation)	Weight loss until BMI <85th percentile, with no more than average of 2 lbs/week. If greater loss is noted, monitor patient for causes of excessive weight loss.	Advance to more intensive level of intervention depending on responses to treatment, age, health risks, and motivation. Advance to stage 2, structured weight management, after 3-6 months if increasing BMI percentile or persistent medical condition.
≥99th	Stage 1, 2, or 3 (depending on age, degree of obesity, health risks, and motivation)	Weight loss not to exceed average of 2 lbs/week. If greater loss is noted, monitor patient for causes of excessive weight loss.	Advance to more intensive levels of intervention depending on responses to treatment, age, health risks, and motivation of patient and family. Advance from stage 3 (comprehensive multidisciplinary intervention) to stage 4 (tertiary care) after 3-6 months if comorbidity present and patient not showing improvement; patients may warrant tertiary care evaluation to determine next level of treatment.

DIET

Dietary Recommendations for Adolescents

The United States Department of Agriculture (USDA) 2010 Dietary Guidelines for Americans offers general recommendations for a healthy diet based on age, gender, and activity level.[9] Calorie ranges for sedentary adolescents aged 13 to 18 years are 1600 to 1800/day for females and 2000 to 2400/day for males, with acceptable macronutrient distribution ranges (AMDR) expressed as a percentage of total calories: 10% to 30% from protein, 45% to 65% from carbohydrates, 25% to 30% from fat with less than 10% from saturated fat, and 25 to 31 grams of fiber per day. Suggested food patterns that meet recommended calorie ranges are provided in Table 3.

The USDA has released MyPlate and related materials, which translate the Dietary Guidelines into more understandable messages and practical applications for consumers. Primary care physicians and consumers alike may access specific calorie and meal patterns, as well as tracking and goal-setting tools, at http://www.choosemyplate.gov/.

The Academy of Nutrition and Dietetics (AND), formerly the American Dietetic Association, Pediatric Weight Management Guidelines recommend a multi-component weight management program that includes an individualized nutrition prescription, based on individual energy needs and macronutrient (fat, protein, carbohydrate) distribution.[10] A prescribed or structured diet plan has been shown to be more desirable among adolescents than an unstructured dietary plan.[11] AND further recommends no less than a 1200 calorie/day diet with medical monitoring and coordination with a registered dietitian (RD). This approach has been associated with short and longer-term (more than 1 year) improvements in BMI and body composition in adolescents.[10]

Recent Randomized Controlled Trials with a Primarily Dietary Component

Recent randomized controlled trials (RCTs) of dietary interventions with BMI as the primary outcome include calorie-restricted diets with varying distribution of macronutrients. Diet prescriptions for weight loss in adolescents are typically 1200 to 1500 calories or reduced calorie based on individually calcu-

Table 3
Suggested food patterns for sedentary adolescents

	1600-1800 calorie diet	2000-2400 calorie diet
Fruits	1.5 cups	1.5-2 cups
Vegetables	2-2.5 cups	2.5-3 cups
Grains	5-6 ounces	6-8 ounces
Whole grains[a]	2.5-3 ounces	3-4 ounces
Protein foods	5 ounces	5-6.5 ounces
Dairy[b]	3 cups	3 cups
Oils	22-24 grams	24-31 grams
SoFAS	8-9% of calories	9-14% of calories

[a]Half of all grains should be whole grains
[b]After age 2 years, nonfat (skim) or low-fat milk are recommended
Abbreviations: SoFAS = Solid fats and added sugars

lated energy needs. Many follow a variety of macronutrient distribution patterns (eg, low carbohydrate/low fat, high carbohydrate/low fat) (Table 4).

The protein-sparing modified fast is a high protein/low carbohydrate (HPLC) diet and is considered to be useful for preserving lean body mass during weight loss, which would be of particular importance with still-developing obese adolescents, where loss of lean body mass would be detrimental for development. It is only to be used for short-term weight management (no longer than 10 weeks) and under the supervision of a medical team specializing in pediatric obesity. A RCT with severely obese (BMI ≥99th percentile) adolescents was conducted to evaluate the effects of a HPLC diet without caloric restriction compared with a caloric-controlled, low fat (LF) diet.[12] Both groups were directed to participate in at least 30 minutes a day of vigorous physical activity. A decrease in BMI z-score was found in both groups at the end of the 13-week intervention with a greater reduction in the HPLC group. At 36-week follow-up, although weight was lower than baseline in both groups, group differences were no longer significant. It is worth noting that both groups had high attrition rate. Of the 46 subjects who initiated the diets, 18 HPLC and 15 LF subjects completed the 13-week intervention with 50% attrition in both groups by the 36-week follow-up.

Another study evaluating diets with various macronutrient content found that all tested diet regimens were associated with a significant reduction in BMI.[13] The 12-week intervention included 55 obese Israeli adolescents aged 12 to 18 years randomized to 1 of 3 diets of 1200 to 1500 calories: (1) low carbohydrate/low fat, (2) low carbohydrate/high fat, or (3) high carbohydrate/low fat. At the end of the 12-week intervention period, all participants were placed on a HCLF maintenance diet with follow-up every 3 months for the remaining 9 months. At 52 weeks, the overall decrease from baseline was still significant. There was no difference between diet groups. Dropout rate was 21.8%, and after 1 year, the compliance rate to the maintenance diet was 52.7% with no differences seen across diet groups.

Table 4
Common macronutrient distribution of diets

	Carbohydrate	Protein	Fat
AMDR	45-60%	10-30%	25-30%
LCLF	20%	50%	30%
LCHF	20%	20%	60%
HCLF	50-60%	20%	30%

Abbreviations: AMDR =Acceptable Macronutrient Distribution Ranges; LCLF = Low Carbohydrate, Low Fat; LCHF = Low Carbohydrate, High Fat; HCLF = High Carbohydrate, Low Fat

Reduced glycemic load diets have also been suggested as an effective dietary approach for treatment of adolescent obesity, although the evidence is stronger for overall energy restriction, particularly in the long term.[10] A RCT in Argentina with 86 obese hyperinsulinemic adolescents assigned to a 16-week, 1400 calorie diet (60% carbohydrate, 20% protein, and 20% fat distribution) with either a low-glycemic index/low-insulin response (LIR) diet or a conventional diet (CD)[14] documented a mean decrease in BMI of 3.9 kg/m^2. The LIR diet consisted of low-glycemic index carbohydrates (which have been shown to delay digestion and improve satiety) with separation of carbohydrate and protein foods across different meals, as combinations of these foods have been shown to increase the postprandial insulin response. No significant difference was found in BMI between groups; however, mean reduction of waist circumference and insulin resistance was greater in the LIR group than in the CD group. Attrition rate was only 12.7%, and adherence to both diets was good.

In general, adhering to a calorie-restricted diet, regardless of macronutrient distribution, reduces BMI among adolescents in clinical trials. However, adolescents choose foods within the social context of family and peer groups, and within their school and neighborhood environments. Understanding these influences on dietary adherence is important and may help anticipate and address challenges to individualized dietary prescriptions. It is important to note that none of the previously discussed studies had follow-up beyond 1 year.

PHYSICAL ACTIVITY

There is a general consensus that physical activity (PA) alone is not sufficient for effective weight loss.[15] Nevertheless, PA is an essential component of treatment programs,[16] as both short- and long-term PA programs provide positive effects.[17-19] Recent research provides insights for exercise prescription, including the type, intensity, frequency, and duration that are most beneficial for change in BMI and body composition. Guidelines of PA required for health maintenance in adolescents are listed in Table 5.

Type

Type of exercise can be divided into 2 major categories: aerobic and resistance training. Aerobic activities are those in which the large muscles of the body are moved in a rhythmic fashion, such that cardiorespiratory fitness is improved (eg, running, swimming, aerobic dance). Resistance exercises require muscular force over and above that required for usual daily activities. Resistance exercise and muscle-strengthening activities are synonymous. Examples include lifting weights and using resistance bands. Bone-strengthening activities are those that bear weight through the long bones and can fall under either aerobic or resistance types of training. Table 6 lists examples of aerobic and resistance training activities suitable for adolescents. Both aerobic training [20-23] and resistance train-

Table 5
Physical activity guidelines for adolescents

Recommendations	Organizations
60 minutes daily moderate or vigorous physical activity	AAP[a], CDC[b], President's Council[c], USDA[d], DHHS[e], Surgeon General[f]
Include vigorous intensity at least 3 days/week	AAP[g], CDC[b], President's Council[c], USDA[d], DHHS[e], Surgeon General[f]
Include bone-strengthening at least 3 days/week	CDC[b], President's Council[c], USDA[d], DHHS[e], Surgeon General[f]
Include muscle-strengthening at least 3 days/week	CDC[b], President's Council[c], USDA[d], DHHS[e]
Total media time ≤1-2 hours/day of quality programming	AAP[g]
Total noneducational screen time ≤2 hours/day	AAP[h]

[a]American Academy of Pediatrics Policy Statement 2006 Active Healthy Living: Prevention of childhood obesity through increased physical activity. Available at: http://pediatrics.aappublications.org/content/117/5/1834.ful.html
[b]Centers for Disease Control and Prevention Youth Physical Activity Guidelines. Available at: http://www.cdc.gov/healthyyouth/physicalactivity/guidelines.htm
[c]President's Council on Fitness, Sports and Nutrition. Available at: http://fitness.gov/
[d]United States Department of Agriculture. Available at: http://www.choosemyplate.gov/physical-activity/amount.html
[e]United States Department of Health and Human Services Physical Activity Guidelines for Americans. Available at: http://www.health.gov/PAguidelines/
[f]United States Surgeon General. Available at: http://www.surgeongeneral.gov/library/obesityvision/obesityvision2010.pdf
[g]American Academy of Pediatrics - Expert Panel on Integrated Guidelines for Cardiovascular Health and Risk Reduction in Children and Adolescents: Summary Report. Available at: http://pediatrics.aappublications.org/content/128/Supplement_5/S213.full.html
[h]American Academy of Pediatrics Policy Statement 2011 Children, Adolescents, Obesity, and the Media. Available at: http://pediatrics.aappublications.org/content/128/1/201.full.html

ing[24,25] show positive results in decreasing weight and/or body fat measures in recent studies as well as improvements in other indices (such as insulin sensitivity and plasma lipid level) with and without change in body composition.[17,23,26] Three recent studies have found that combined aerobic training and resistance training are more effective than either alone.[18,27,28]

Active video games (AVG) for increasing PA are being examined since they can pique interest, provide challenge, and can be done in relative privacy. A recent study showed a small positive impact on BMI,[29] while another study found that adolescents lost interest in the AVG and discontinued optional use by the end of the 4-week program.[30] In a 12-week naturalistic intervention study, children (BMI 50th to 99th percentile) who received active video games did not increase their overall physical activity as compared to children receiving inactive video games.[31] A study that compared a virtual cycling game to cycling to music demonstrated that music was just as effective as the game in producing results.[32] Finally, 3 studies have shown that energy expenditure with AVG varies from

Table 6
Sample exercises for adolescents

Type	Aerobic	Resistance or Muscle Strengthening	Bone Strengthening
Brisk walking (3 miles per hour)	√		√
Running	√		√
Jumping rope	√		√
Swimming	√		
Dancing	√		√
Bicycling	√		
Skating (including skate board, long board, ice skates, roller blades, etc.)	√		
Skiing and snow boarding	√		
Sports (including basketball, football, soccer, tennis)	√		√
Group aerobic exercise (including kick boxing, LA Boxing, aerobic dance, etc.)	√		√
Active video games such as Wii Fit and Kinect	√		
Lifting weights (including free weights, weight machines, and body weight exercises)		√	√
Resistance band exercises		√	√
Climbing (eg, at a climbing gym with proper safety equipment)		√	
Pilates		√	
Yoga		√	√
Martial arts classes		√	√

light to moderate and up to vigorous intensity.[33-35] Although AVG show promise, it may be best to use them as an introduction to exercise, and not as the main component of an extended activity program.

Studies of other specific types of exercise such as martial arts[36] are limited, and body composition results have not been conclusive. One study found that energy cost of exercise was similar between all activities (swimming, games, sports, strength/stability circuit) except for walking which was significantly lower.[37] School-based interventions are effective at increasing PA in adolescents;[38,39] however they have not shown consistent positive effects on BMI.[40] In a meta-analysis of school-based intervention studies in children ages 5 to 18 years, the 12 RCTs that were included showed a nonsignificant difference in the change in BMI (weighted mean difference 0.01 kg/m^2, 95% CI −0.14 to 0.14).[40]

In summary, aerobic training combined with resistance training may be the most effective in terms of weight and fat loss, and active video games show potential as an adjunct method. The specific type of activity is not as important as the time spent being active.

Intensity

Moderate to vigorous physical activity (MVPA) is the range of intensity most frequently recommended by professional organizations. Moderate intensity equates to PA that raises the heart rate and breaks a sweat, whereas vigorous intensity PA causes a higher heart rate and breathing that is hard and fast.[41] Another method recommended by the CDC to determine intensity is a "talk test." If one can talk but not sing during the activity, the exercise is moderate; if one cannot say more than a few words without pausing for breath, the intensity level is vigorous.[41] In the scientific community, intensity is often defined by metabolic equivalents (METs). METs express oxygen uptake relative to resting oxygen uptake.[42] One MET is the amount of energy expended by a person sitting quietly. Commonly, the adjectives light, moderate, and vigorous are equated with the following METs for PA intensity: Light is less than 3 METs, moderate is 3.0 to 6.0 METs, and vigorous is greater than 6 METs.[42]

Of special interest for obesity treatment, exercise at low intensity favors fat oxidation (ie, the use of fat stores rather than glucose for creation of energy).[43] Also, low-intensity exercise allows for longer duration, and therefore increased energy expenditure.[43] Current studies in exercise for adolescent obesity treatment are divided between low-intensity (maximum fat oxidation level, or 40% VO_{2max}), and high-intensity (70% VO_{2max}) exercise. Similar to Gutin's findings in 2002,[44] that no differences in body composition were found between moderate- and high-intensity training, effective weight loss and change in body composition occur with both types of programs: those designed for low-intensity exercise[45-48] and those focused on high-intensity.[22,24]

Frequency and Duration

Current guidelines for treatment programs recommend that obese adolescents engage in PA for at least 1 hour each day.[8,49] Although body composition was not evaluated, Saavedra found in a meta-analysis that aerobic exercise programs for obese children that were 3 sessions per week for more than 60 minutes each, for more than 12 weeks, were most effective at improving aerobic fitness.[20] Studies cited in the current article that were successful at changing body composition through physical activity utilized programs that ranged from 2 to 4 times per week, 45 to 60 minutes per session, and varied in duration from 8 weeks to 1 year.

Decreasing Sedentary Time

In recent years, sedentary time has become a topic of interest separate from PA time. Accruing large amounts of sedentary time causes health risks regardless of amount of PA. Tremblay and colleagues completed a meta-analysis of studies that aimed to decrease sedentary behavior in youth ages 5 to 17 years.[50] Across 8 RCTs there was an effect of $-0.89 kg/m^2$ (95% CI of -1.67 to -0.11, $p = 0.03$)

in mean BMI in the intervention group. Most studies focused on time spent watching TV as the indicator for sedentary behavior. Analyses of 170 studies (including the 8 RCTs, as well as intervention, longitudinal, and cross-sectional studies) showed that sedentary time is associated with overweight and obesity in a dose-response manner; greater than 2 hours per day of TV time was found to be associated with increased risk, and additional time increases the risk. Other health factors addressed in the meta-analyses included fitness, metabolic syndrome, and cardiovascular disease risk factors; self-esteem; social behavior; and academic achievement. Each of these factors was improved with decreased sedentary time; however, only 1 of the 93 studies analyzed was a RCT.

Factors Influencing Participation in Physical Activity

Perhaps one of the most important and challenging factors in prescribing exercise for obese adolescents is ensuring regular and sustained participation. Self-confidence and self-efficacy are 2 key factors that can affect participation.[51,52] Parents can also play a major role in participation. Sola and colleagues found that continued participation in a 12-month PA program was related to the parent physically participating.[19] In addition, PA level of the parent may influence adolescent participation.[53,54]

Future Directions

PA for the attainment of positive body composition outcomes tends to be the focus of obesity treatment programs. However, other health outcomes may be just as or more important than body composition for adolescents. Two recent reviews have emphasized this notion. In a meta-analysis by Ekelund and colleagues, higher MVPA time was associated with better cardiovascular risk factors in children and adolescents, aged 4 to 18 years.[55] PA can also have a positive effect on insulin resistance[56] and on satiety factors in obese adolescents.[55] In light of the effect that PA has on multiple health indicators, increasing the amount of PA time for the obese adolescent results in improved health regardless of whether it contributes to weight loss.

BEHAVIORAL MULTICOMPONENT LIFESTYLE PROGRAMS

Though dietary and PA approaches may improve weight outcomes in the short term, interventions for adolescent obesity seem more effective when strategies are combined, rather than when used in isolation.[58-61] Interventions that combine diet, exercise, and other weight-related behavior change have been documented in numerous randomized controlled trials and meta-analyses to be superior to minimal or no-treatment control groups.[59,62,63] Consequently, lifestyle interventions currently represent the most successful treatment for adolescent obesity[49,62,64] and are the recommended mode of treatment by the US Preventive Services Task Force.[63] Lifestyle interventions utilize a multicomponent approach and typically include the use of behavioral components and cognitive skill building to foster sustained behavioral change.[49,65]

Behavioral Therapy

Behaviorally based therapies (BT) stress the development of new eating and exercise habits and provide specific strategies for changing the adolescent's environment.[64] Among treatment programs and RCTs, several behavioral change components have been shown to support healthy weight control and generally include stimulus control strategies, self-monitoring, and reinforcement.[49,65-69] Stimulus control techniques involve limiting exposure to triggers for the unhealthy behavior and typically include strategies for restructuring the home to encourage healthy behaviors and limiting unhealthy behaviors associated with eating and activity[64] (eg, eating more slowly, eating in one designated area, limiting "junk food" available in the house).[70] Additionally, self-monitoring by means of maintaining records of behaviors that support or impede weight loss efforts[70] and generating contracts that consist of self-selected goals assist with recognizing and reinforcing desirable behaviors.[62]

Cognitive Behavioral Therapy

Though the behavioral components in weight-loss interventions are central, research suggests that the inclusion of cognitive treatment components may result in increased treatment effectiveness.[62,66] Cognitive behavioral therapy (CBT) strategies attempt to address cognitive distortions regarding body image and eating, instruction in self-monitoring, problem-solving techniques, motivational issues, and focus on specific weight-loss goals and barriers to healthy behavior.[70] CBT aims to assist individuals to identify negative, self-defeating thoughts and to replace them with more accurate, positive statements.[71,72] This is considered essential as the widespread prevalence of psychological distress in obese populations is thought to be a key factor in the inability to maintain dietary changes and subsequent weight loss. For example, overweight adolescents report engaging in significantly more emotional binge-eating behaviors and experiencing lower self-esteem, lower self-concept, and higher rates of psychosocial difficulties than their non-overweight peers.[73,74] Furthermore, higher levels of depressive and anxiety symptoms and lower self-esteem in overweight adolescents have been associated with less healthy beliefs about their ability to engage in a healthy lifestyle.[75]

A number of RCTs examining the efficacy of CBT have reported significant improvements in weight status,[51,76,77] with 2 including follow-up beyond 12 months.[76,77] Jelalian and colleagues reported similar improvements in weight when comparing CBT and adventure therapy with CBT and aerobic exercise, but it was not possible to determine whether the practical exercise components had more of an effect than the CBT program itself.[51] Mellin and colleagues found that adolescents treated with CBT had significant improvements in their relative weight and related behaviors compared with a no treatment control group.[77] Braet and associates compared 3 delivery methods of CBT to a placebo and reported a significantly greater weight reduction with CBT that did not differ between delivery modes. However, their findings were limited by the fact that the subjects in the placebo group were not randomly allocated but, rather, consisted of people who were unable to attend the other treatment sessions.[76] Another RCT used a slightly different approach in that it compared cognitive therapy (CT), as opposed to CBT, with BT and a control treatment.[66] Although improved BMIs were shown over the 10-week treatment period, BT was superior to CT and the control treatment. However, these results were not followed up to assess whether the weight loss was maintained.

Overall, though the use of multicomponent interventions for the treatment of obesity is well supported in the literature, there remains a lack of consistency among studies that impedes comparisons across various treatment programs.[78] Thus, currently the evidence is not entirely clear on the best multicomponent program for addressing overweight and obesity in adolescents. Specific components and best delivery methods of interventions that are the most efficacious have not yet been identified.

Setting and Intensity of Programs

The amount of weight change associated with lifestyle interventions in adolescents varies by intervention intensity and setting.[79] The greatest level of weight loss found in a systematic review conducted by Whitlock and coworkers was seen in a 10-month residential program (3250 hours) with 76 youth aged 10 to 17 years. Average weight of participants in the intervention group decreased from 75% obese to 24%, whereas those on a waiting list increased 6%.[80]

Lifestyle interventions in the school setting can produce short-term improvements in weight. However, there is limited evidence supporting that these improvements can be maintained over the 12 months following the end of treatment. In the meta-analysis conducted by Whitlock and colleagues,[79] a pooled estimate of BMI from school obesity intervention trials with students ages 6 to 14 years was -0.82 kg/m^2 (CI $= -1.18, -0.46$) lower in those treated compared with those in the control group. These trials conducted in the school setting reported 0.4 to 2.07 kg/m^2 difference in the mean BMI change between intervention and control groups at 6 to 12 months. The pooled estimate translates to about a 4 pound difference for a 12-year-old boy or girl (assuming growth of 2 inches or less). For a 16-year-old girl, this BMI difference equals about 4.5 to 5 pounds and for a 16-year-old boy, this would be about 5 to 6 pounds. School obesity interventions included were of moderate intensity, defined as 26 to 75 hours of contact.

Comprehensive behavioral interventions of medium- to high-intensity (defined as $>$ 25 hours of contact) were identified as the most effective.[63] High intensity interventions in specialty health care settings (eg, pediatric obesity referral clinics) resulted in a 1.9 to 3.3 kg/m^2 difference in mean BMI change 6 to 12 months following treatment when compared with controls. For a 12-year-old boy or girl this would translate to 16.6 to 17.75 pounds difference under the same growth assumptions. For girls aged 16 years, this BMI difference would be about 20 pounds and 22 to 23 pounds for boys aged 16 years with 2 inches of growth or less.

Family Involvement

Most treatment programs for adolescents focus on individual-level interventions with varying degrees of parental participation. However, adolescent eating behaviors are not developed in a vacuum but are vastly influenced by family and culture. Thus, incorporating the family system into obesity interventions has been identified as an important strategy for sustained behavioral change and creating programs to improve parenting behaviors relevant to obesity is considered to be a highly promising strategy.[81,82] Though there is a consistent body of literature indicating that high levels of parental involvement lead to greater weight loss with overweight children,[82,83] the optimal approach of parental involvement in adolescent treatment programs has not been well elucidated because of a small body of research that reflects conflicting results.[84-87] However, most recent meta-analyses indicate that parents should be viewed as key players and central agents of change in the treatment of weight-related problems.[16,88]

Motivational Interviewing

Over the past 10 years, there has been considerable interest by physicians and nonphysician clinicians in the use of motivational interviewing (MI) to promote behavior change within multicomponent weight loss programs.[89-91] MI has been defined as a directive, client-centered counseling style for eliciting behavior change by helping clients explore and resolve ambivalence.[92-94] The underlying tenets of MI assume that change is more likely to be affected by internal motivation, rather than external information.[92] The key goal of the intervention is to increase the importance of change from the clients' perspective, along with their confidence in successfully changing, without the therapist advocating change. As such, this model is seen as a direct contrast to the traditional patient education models that rely heavily on direct questioning and providing information and advice given in the hope of changing behavior.[95]

Experts assert that MI should be conceived as a platform for treatment delivery rather than the primary treatment modality,[96] and thus, research has tried to determine how best to integrate MI within standard cognitive and behavioral weight-loss strategies. Although MI has shown promise in the adult obesity literature as effecting positive lifestyle change, little is known about the effectiveness of MI with adolescents, and research studies have reflected mixed results.[89,92,97]

In the Dietary Intervention Study in Children, adolescents who received 1 in-person MI session and 1 follow-up session showed a significant reduction in the proportion of calories from fat and dietary cholesterol, and overall dietary adherence scores improved at 3-month follow-up.[98] However, recent studies examining the additive benefits of MI have failed to replicate significant findings. For example, Flattum and colleagues conducted a preliminary study with 20 overweight 16- to 18-year-old females.[99] The 18-week pilot study looked at the efficacy of 7 individual MI sessions to develop weight management goal setting. Although attendance was high and 90% of adolescents set at least 2 weight management goals, results did not clearly identify any effects on overweight or obesity. These same results were reflected in a 2011 follow-up study conducted by the same authors evaluating the feasibility and effectiveness of the MI-based individual counseling component of New Moves, a school-based program designed to prevent weight-related problems in adolescent girls.[100] This is in accordance with other recent studies showing no additive effects on health outcomes by adding an MI component to the intervention.[101-103]

In summary, the studies reviewed here indicate that MI might be feasible with overweight adolescents. However, currently there is insufficient data to determine the efficacy of MI for the prevention or treatment of adolescent obesity. More research is needed to ultimately understand whether MI is effective for adolescent obesity outcomes in studies that include larger sample sizes and standardization regarding MI implementation and training practices.[92]

PHARMACOLOGIC THERAPY FOR OBESE ADOLESCENTS

The Expert Committee on the Prevention, Assessment, and Treatment of Child and Adolescent Overweight and Obesity panel recommends pharmacologic intervention in the fourth stage of weight management, when lifestyle interventions have been unsuccessful.[49] Pharmacologic treatment has not been extensively studied in children and adolescents; however, 3 medications may be useful in combination with diet, PA, and behavioral modification. These are orlistat, metformin, and sibutramine.[104] Results of clinical trials are outlined in Tables 7 and 8. Sibutramine, a central serotonin and norepinephrine reuptake inhibitor that is associated with increased satiety, showed promising results in adolescents.[105,107] However, in October 2010 the manufacturer recalled sibutramine after researchers found an increase in myocardial infarction and stroke risk in the Sibutramine Cardiovascular Outcomes Trial (SCOUT Trial).[108,109]

Orlistat

Orlistat is the only medication currently approved by the US Food and Drug Administration (FDA) for the treatment of obesity in adolescents (12-16 years).[110] Orlistat is a fat absorbing inhibitor that blocks the absorption of about 30% of the fat contained in a meal by inhibiting gastric and pancreatic lipase,

Table 7
Clinical trials of orlistat in children and adolescents

Author/Country	N	Duration (months)	Age (years)	Dosage	Type of trial	BMI change	+Lifestyle
Ozkan et al, 2004, Turkey[111]	42	5-15	10-16	120 mg tid	Randomized, open-label, controlled	-4.2 kg/m^2 (vs. control)	Yes
Chanoine et al, 2005, US/Canada[112]	539	12	12-16	120 mg tid	Randomized, double-blind, placebo-controlled	-0.9 kg/m^2 (vs. placebo)	Yes
Maahs et al, 2006, US[113]	40	6	14-18	120 mg tid	Randomized, double-blind, placebo-controlled	-0.5 kg/m^2 (vs. placebo, nonsignificant)	Yes

Abbreviations: BMI = body mass index; tid = three times daily

Table 8
Clinical trials of metformin in children and adolescents

Author/Country	N	Duration (months)	Age (years)	Dosage	Type of trial	BMI change	+Lifestyle
Freemark et al, 2001, US[115]	29	6	12-19	500 mg bid	Nonrandomized, double-blind, placebo-controlled	−1.3% (vs. baseline)	No
Kay et al, 2001[116]	24	2	Mean age 15.65 years	850 mg bid	Randomized, double-blind, placebo-controlled	Weight change −2.7 kg (vs. placebo)	Yes
Srinivasan et al, 2006, Australia[117]	28	6	9-18	1 g bid	Randomized, double-blind, placebo-controlled	−1.26 kg/m^2 (vs. placebo)	No
Atabek et al, 2008, Turkey[118]	120	6	9-17	500 mg bid	Randomized, double-blind, placebo-controlled	−1.8 kg/m^2 (vs. placebo)	Yes
Love-Osborne et al, 2008, US[119]	85	6	12-19	500 mg qid-850 mg bid	Randomized, double-blind, placebo-controlled	−0.8 kg/m^2 (vs. placebo)	Yes
Wilson et al, 2010, US[120]	77	12	13-18	2 g qd	Randomized, double-blind, placebo-controlled	−0.9 kg/m^2 (vs. placebo)	Yes
Yanovski et al, 2011, US[121]	6	6	6-12	1 g bid	Randomized, double-blind, placebo-controlled	−1.09 kg/m^2 (vs. placebo)	Yes

Abbreviations: bid = twice daily; BMI = body mass index; qd = daily; qid = four times daily

thereby inducing weight loss. The undigested fat is excreted in the stool and may be associated with some gastrointestinal side effects such as flatulence with leakage, oily stools, and decrease in plasma fat-soluble vitamin levels. Adhering to a reduced-fat diet can reduce these adverse side effects.[104]

Orlistat decreases BMI by 0.5 to 4.2 kg/m^2 in adolescents when compared to placebo or control in RCTs (see Table 7).[111-113] The largest RCT of orlistat to date was done by Chanoine and colleagues.[112] In this multicenter trial, 539 obese adolescents (aged 12-16 years), at 32 centers in the US and Canada, received orlistat (n = 357) or placebo (n = 182) for 1 year. In addition, all subjects received exercise counseling, behavioral therapy, and a hypocaloric diet that was intended to provide 30% of calories from fat, 50% from carbohydrate, and 20% from protein, (assigned caloric intake ranged from 1400-1800 kcal/d for boys and 1200-1600 kcal/d for girls). Both treatment groups had a decrease in BMI up to 12 weeks during the intervention. Thereafter, BMI stabilized with orlistat but increased beyond baseline with placebo. Specifically, of the 349 subjects that completed the study, BMI decreased from baseline by 0.55 kg/m^2 with orlistat but increased by 0.31 kg/m^2 with placebo at 1 year. Furthermore, researchers found that early weight loss up to 12 weeks predicted a favorable outcome in both treatment groups but was more than twice as likely to occur in the orlistat group. Therefore, the addition of orlistat may be an effective adjunct to lifestyle modification for weight loss, but should be re-evaluated at 3 months of treatment to identify subjects who do not respond favorably and discontinue treatment.[114]

It is important to note that in another double-blind RCT, 40 obese adolescents (aged 14-18 years) received orlistat or placebo for 6 months in addition to a hypocaloric diet and behavioral modification. Statistical difference in BMI was not noted between groups.[113]

An updated systematic review for the US Preventive Services Task Force noted that long-term follow-up of weight loss after active treatment with orlistat has never been conducted in adolescents. However, they concluded that a combined behavioral-pharmacological intervention may be useful for obese adolescents, especially if future research confirms that weight loss is maintained after pharmacologic treatment ends.[63]

Metformin

Metformin is a biguanide that has been approved by the FDA for the treatment of type 2 diabetes mellitus and has been evaluated in small clinical trials for weight loss in obese children and adolescents (see Table 8).[115-121] Metformin reduces hepatic glucose production, decreases plasma insulin, enhances insulin sensitivity (in muscle, liver, and fat), inhibits fat cell lipogenesis, and may reduce food intake by increasing glucagon-like peptide, which is an appetite suppressing substance found in the brain and intestine. Most adolescents tolerate this drug, and side effects are usually dose-related and include gastrointestinal side effects such as abdominal discomfort, diarrhea, nausea, and flatulence.[104,110,122]

Studies have documented the beneficial effects of metformin on BMI, fasting serum glucose, insulin, and improved lipid profiles in hyperinsulinimic[115] and normoglycemic[116] obese adolescents. Furthermore, Srinivasan and colleagues,[117] in a randomized, double-blind, crossover trial of 28 obese children (aged 9-18 years) with clinical suspicion of insulin resistance, found that metformin had a greater treatment effect over placebo for weight (-4.35 kg, $p = 0.02$), BMI (-1.26 kg/m^2, $p = 0.002$), and waist circumference (-2.8cm, $p = 0.003$). Other RCTs have demonstrated similar BMI reduction ranging from -0.8 to -1.8 kg/m^2 when 6 months[118,119,121] and 12 months[120] of metformin therapy was added to a lifestyle intervention.

In summary, clinical trials support that metformin is safe and well tolerated with minimal gastrointestinal side effect, and that it results in a modest decrease in BMI (-0.8 to -1.8 kg/m^2) in obese children and adolescents, when combined with lifestyle modification. However, larger, longer-term studies are needed to establish its role in the treatment of obese adolescents.[123] Currently, metformin has not been approved by the FDA for the treatment of obese adolescents.

BARIATRIC SURGICAL INTERVENTIONS FOR SEVERE OBESITY

It is estimated that about 4% of children and adolescents in the US have a BMI *greater than or equal to* the 99th percentile, defined as severe obesity. Furthermore, 88% of these children remain severely obese as adults with a BMI of greater than 35 kg/m^2.[4] Because of the increasing number of adolescents with severe obesity who are not responsive to behavioral or pharmacologic interventions, expert panels have made recommendations regarding when to consider bariatric surgery.[49,124] Updated bariatric surgery selection criteria for adolescents have been proposed by Pratt and coworkers (Table 9).[125] Current AAP expert panel recommendations on when to consider bariatric surgery in adolescents are based on the 2004 Inge and colleagues selection criteria.[49,124]

Bariatric surgical procedures have been described by Xanthakos and collaborators.[126] Early evidence has been documented for 2 bariatric surgical procedures for weight loss in adolescents. First is the Roux-en-Y Gastric Bypass (RYGB), which dates back to the 1960s for adults and 1980s for adolescents in the United States. RYGB restricts food intake by creating a small gastric pouch and also reduces food absorption via bypass of the proximal small intestine. The second most commonly performed bariatric surgical procedure is laparoscopic adjustable gastric banding (LAGB), which since 1998 is a new investigational procedure. Preliminary, short-term data suggests that LAGB may be a safe alternative, with fewer nutritional risks than RYGB. The LAGB is a restrictive procedure in which a silicone band is placed around the entire upper portion of the stomach,

Table 9
Criteria for bariatric surgery in adolescents

	2004 Criteria[124]	2009 Updated Criteria[125]
Body Mass Index (BMI)	BMI ≥40 kg/m^2 with a serious comorbidity such as: • Type 2 diabetes mellitus • Obstructive sleep apnea • Pseudotumor cerebri	BMI ≥35 kg/m^2 with a major comorbidity such as: • Type 2 diabetes mellitus • Moderate or severe obstructive sleep apnea • Pseudotumor cerebri • Severe or progressive steatohepatitis
	BMI ≥50 kg/m^2 with other comorbidities such as: • Hypertension • Dyslipidemia • Nonalcoholic steatohepatitis • Significantly impaired activities of daily living • Other less serious comorbidities	BMI ≥40 kg/m^2 with a mild comorbidity such as: • Hypertension • Dyslipidemia • Mild obstructive sleep apnea • Insulin resistance • Glucose intolerance • Impaired quality of life or impaired activities of daily living • Other mild comorbidities
Eligibility Criteria	Skeletal maturity: generally ≥13 years of age for girls and ≥15 years of age for boys	Skeletal maturity: must have completed at least 95% of skeletal maturity based on radiographic evidence Tanner stage: IV or V (unless bariatric surgery is indicated earlier because of severe comorbidities)
	Lifestyle changes: • Failed weight loss efforts for ≥6 months in a behavior-based treatment program • Must be capable and willing to adhere to nutritional guidelines postoperatively	Lifestyle changes: • Demonstrate ability to understand what dietary and physical activity changes will be required postoperatively
	Psychosocial: • Must have emotional and cognitive maturity to demonstrate decisional capacity and provide informed assent to surgical treatment • Have a supportive family environment • Demonstrate commitment to comprehensive medical and psychologic evaluations both before and after surgery	Psychosocial: • Must have evidence for mature decision making, with understanding of benefits and potential risks of surgery • Must have evidence for appropriate social support without evidence of neglect or abuse • If a psychiatric condition is present (eg, depression, anxiety, binge eating disorder), it is under treatment • Evidence that the patient and family have the ability and motivation to comply with recommended treatments pre- and post-operatively

Contraindications for Bariatric Surgery	• Medically correctable cause of obesity • Ongoing substance abuse problem (within the preceding year) • A medical, psychiatric, or cognitive condition that impairs decision-making capacity or prevents adherence to postoperative dietary and medication regimens • Current lactation, pregnancy, or planned pregnancy within 18 months of procedure • Inability of the patient or family to comprehend the surgical risks and need for lifelong postoperative medical and nutritional monitoring

creating a tiny pouch where food empties from the esophagus to the upper stomach. This procedure has not been FDA approved for patients younger than 18 years.[125,127] Although RYGB is still considered the standard of care for weight loss surgery in adolescents with severe obesity, a California retrospective population cohort analysis between 2005 and 2007 found a 7-fold rate increase in LAGB and a corresponding decrease in RYGB surgeries performed in adolescents.[128]

A recent meta-analysis[127] concluded that bariatric surgery in adolescents may induce weight loss and improve or cure medical comorbidities such as diabetes, hypertension, dyslipidemia, sleep apnea, musculoskeletal conditions, and asthma. However, limited evidence was found supporting enhanced quality of life, and no evidence was found to determine whether bariatric surgery extends life in adolescents. Furthermore, bariatric surgery such as the RYGB has the potential for life-threatening conditions, including death, shock, pulmonary embolism, severe malnutrition, immediate postoperative bleeding, and gastrointestinal obstruction, with the most reported complication being protein-calorie malnutrition and micronutrient deficiency. With LAGB, reoperations were performed for band slippage, gastric dilation, hiatal hernia, intragastric band migration, tubing crack, psychological intolerance of the band, and cholecystitis, with the most reported complication being band slippage. For optimal effectiveness, adolescents who undergo bariatric surgery require careful evaluation before surgery and must adhere to lifelong nutritional, multivitamin and mineral supplementation guidelines to prevent severe complications.[49,124,125,127] Compared with adults, adolescent patients may have less adherence to postsurgical dietary regimens, nutritional supplements, and physical activity recommendations.[129]

Bariatric surgery recommendations for adolescents are largely based on cohort studies, nonrandomized clinical trials, case reports, expert opinion, and clinical observations. One prospective randomized controlled trial exists in the current literature. In this study, 50 adolescents (aged 14-18 years) with BMI greater than 35 were recruited from a community in Melbourne, Australia, and randomized to either a supervised lifestyle intervention or LAGB. Patients were followed for 2 years and LAGB participants lost a mean of 34.6 kg (95% CI, 30.2-39.0) compared to a mean loss of 3 kg (95% CI, 2.1-8.1) in the lifestyle group. Twenty-one

(84%) in the LAGB compared to 3 (12%) in the lifestyle group lost more than 50% of excess weight, corrected for age. Associated benefits included risk reduction of diabetes, cardiovascular disease, and improvement in quality of life.[130]

In summary, bariatric surgical interventions for weight loss are not a quick fix. Short-term data has shown some benefits in severely obese adolescents, but there is a paucity of long-term data. To address this, a NIH-funded, multicenter prospective Teen-Longitudinal Assessment of Bariatric Surgery (Teen-LABS) and associated ancillary studies are underway.[131]

CONCLUSION

In this report, we reviewed recently published interventions for treating overweight and obesity in adolescents. On close examination of current studies, it becomes clear that treatment of overweight and obese adolescents is extremely complex and challenging. Recent studies related to the consequences of obesity, such as in an article reporting on the TODAY study to treat type 2 diabetes in adolescents,[132] point out just how complex treatment is once a teen develops diabetes. The finding of high treatment failure rates in adolescents with type 2 diabetes illustrates the critical need to treat overweight and obese teens to prevent them from developing the disorder. An editorial commenting on the TODAY study[133] describes this treatment complexity and recommends public-policy approaches and broader environmental changes to support healthier lifestyles. Although we reviewed various efficacious treatment approaches for treating overweight and obesity on an individual level, we should be reminded that prevention and treatment requires a coordinated and integrated effort that should include not only individual changes but also intrapersonal, community, social, policy, and major changes in the environment to effectively address childhood and adolescent obesity.

References

1. Ogden CL, Carroll MD, Kit BK, Flegal KM. Prevalence of obesity and trends in body mass index among US children and adolescents, 1999-2010. *JAMA.* 2012;307(5):483-490
2. Kuczmarski RJ, Ogden CL, Guo SS, et al. 2000 CDC growth charts for the United States: Methods and development. *Vital Health Stat 11.* 2002(246):1-190
3. Ogden CL, Carroll MD, Curtin LR, Lamb MM, Flegal KM. Prevalence of high body mass index in US children and adolescents, 2007-2008. *JAMA.* 2010;303(3):242-249
4. Freedman DS, Mei Z, Srinivasan SR, Berenson GS, Dietz WH. Cardiovascular risk factors and excess adiposity among overweight children and adolescents: the Bogalusa Heart Study. *J Pediatr.* 2007;150(1):12-17 e12
5. Institute of Medicine. *Accelerating Progress in Obesity Prevention: Solving the Weight of the Nation.* Washington, DC: National Academies Press; 2012
6. Cook S, Auinger P, Li C, Ford ES. Metabolic syndrome rates in United States adolescents, from the National Health and Nutrition Examination Survey, 1999-2002. *J Pediatr.* 2008;152(2):165-170
7. Li C, Ford ES, Zhao G, Mokdad AH. Prevalence of pre-diabetes and its association with clustering of cardiometabolic risk factors and hyperinsulinemia among U.S. adolescents: National Health and Nutrition Examination Survey 2005-2006. *Diabetes Care.* 2009;32(2):342-347

8. Spear BA, Barlow SE, Ervin C, et al. Recommendations for treatment of child and adolescent overweight and obesity. *Pediatrics.* 2007;120 (Suppl 4):S254-288
9. U.S. Department of Agriculture. Dietary Guidelines for Americans. 2010. Available at: http://www.cnpp.usda.gov/dgas2010_policydocument.htm. Accessed November 5, 2012
10. American Dietetic Association. Pediatric Weight Management Evidence-Based Nutrition Practice Guideline. 2007. Available at: www.adaevidencelibrary.com. Accessed November 5, 2012
11. Truby H, Baxter KA, Barrett P, et al. The Eat Smart Study: a randomised controlled trial of a reduced carbohydrate versus a low fat diet for weight loss in obese adolescents. *BMC Public Health.* 2010;10:464
12. Krebs NF, Gao D, Gralla J, Collins JS, Johnson SL. Efficacy and safety of a high protein, low carbohydrate diet for weight loss in severely obese adolescents. *J Pediatr.* 2010;157(2):252-258
13. Demol S, Yackobovitch-Gavan M, Shalitin S, Nagelberg N, Gillon-Keren M, Phillip M. Low-carbohydrate (low & high-fat) versus high-carbohydrate low-fat diets in the treatment of obesity in adolescents. *Acta Paediatr.* 2009;98(2):346-351
14. Armeno ML, Krochik AG, Mazza CS. Evaluation of two dietary treatments in obese hyperinsulinemic adolescents. *J Pediatr Endocrinol Metab.* 2011;24(9-10):715-722
15. Khan UI, Collier M. Medical interventions in adolescent obesity. *Adolesc Med.* 2008;19(3):406-420, viii
16. McGovern L, Johnson JN, Paulo R, et al. Clinical review: treatment of pediatric obesity: a systematic review and meta-analysis of randomized trials. *J Clin Endocrinol Metab.* 2008;93(12):4600-4605
17. Maggio AB, Aggoun Y, Martin XE, Marchand LM, Beghetti M, Farpour-Lambert NJ. Long-term follow-up of cardiovascular risk factors after exercise training in obese children. *Int J Pediatr Obes.* 2011;6(2-2):e603-610
18. de Mello MT, de Piano A, Carnier J, et al. Long-term effects of aerobic plus resistance training on the metabolic syndrome and adiponectinemia in obese adolescents. *J Clin Hypertens (Greenwich).* 2011;13(5):343-350
19. Sola K, Brekke N, Brekke M. An activity-based intervention for obese and physically inactive children organized in primary care: feasibility and impact on fitness and BMI A one-year follow-up study. *Scand J Prim Health Care.* 2010;28(4):199-204
20. Saavedra JM, Escalante Y, Garcia-Hermoso A. Improvement of aerobic fitness in obese children: a meta-analysis. *Int J Pediatr Obes.* 2011;6(3-4):169-177
21. Ingul CB, Tjonna AE, Stolen TO, Stoylen A, Wisloff U. Impaired cardiac function among obese adolescents: effect of aerobic interval training. *Arch Pediatr Adolesc Med.* 2010;164(9):852-859
22. Tjonna AE, Stolen TO, Bye A, et al. Aerobic interval training reduces cardiovascular risk factors more than a multitreatment approach in overweight adolescents. *Clin Sci (Lond).* 2009;116(4):317-326
23. Kim ES, Im JA, Kim KC, et al. Improved insulin sensitivity and adiponectin level after exercise training in obese Korean youth. *Obesity (Silver Spring).* 2007;15(12):3023-3030
24. Benson AC, Torode ME, Fiatarone Singh MA. The effect of high-intensity progressive resistance training on adiposity in children: a randomized controlled trial. *Int J Obes (Lond).* 2008;32(6):1016-1027
25. Naylor LH, Watts K, Sharpe JA, et al. Resistance training and diastolic myocardial tissue velocities in obese children. *Med Sci Sports Exerc.* 2008;40(12):2027-2032
26. Hernan Jimenez O, Ramirez-Velez R. [Strength training improves insulin sensitivity and plasma lipid levels without altering body composition in overweight and obese subjects]. *Endocrinol Nutr.* 2011;58(4):169-174
27. Davis JN, Tung A, Chak SS, et al. Aerobic and strength training reduces adiposity in overweight Latina adolescents. *Med Sci Sports Exerc.* 2009;41(7):1494-1503
28. Heyman E, Toutain C, Delamarche P, et al. Exercise training and cardiovascular risk factors in type 1 diabetic adolescent girls. *Pediatr Exerc Sci.* 2007;19(4):408-419
29. Maddison R, Foley L, Ni Mhurchu C, et al. Effects of active video games on body composition: a randomized controlled trial. *Am J Clin Nutr.* 2011;94(1):156-163
30. Radon K, Fürbeck B, Thomas S, et al. Feasibility of activity-promoting video games among obese adolescents and young adults in a clinical setting. *J Sci Med Sport.* 2011;14(1):42-5.

31. Baranowski T, Abdelsamad D, Baranowski J, et al. Impact of an active video game on healthy children's physical activity. *Pediatrics.* 2012;129(3):e636-642
32. Adamo KB, Rutherford JA, Goldfield GS. Effects of interactive video game cycling on overweight and obese adolescent health. *Appl Physiol Nutr Metab.* 2010;35(6):805-15
33. Graves LE, Ridgers ND, Williams K, Stratton G, Atkinson G, Cable NT. The physiological cost and enjoyment of Wii Fit in adolescents, young adults, and older adults. *J Phys Act Health.* 2010;7(3):393-401
34. Bailey BW, McInnis K. Energy cost of exergaming: a comparison of the energy cost of 6 forms of exergaming. *Arch Pediatr Adolesc Med.* 2011;165(7):597-602
35. White K, Schofield G, Kilding AE. Energy expended by boys playing active video games. *J Sci Med Sport.* 2011;14(2):130-134
36. Tsang TW, Kohn MR, Chow CM, Fiatarone Singh MA. Kung fu training improves physical fitness measures in overweight/obese adolescents: the "martial fitness" study. *J Obes.* 2010;pii:672751; article first published online Jun 7
37. Thiel C, Vogt L, Claussnitzer G, Banzer W. Energy cost of youth obesity exercise modes. *Int J Sports Med.* 2011;32(2):142-146
38. van Sluijs EM, McMinn AM, Griffin SJ. Effectiveness of interventions to promote physical activity in children and adolescents: systematic review of controlled trials. *BMJ.* 2007;335(7622):703
39. Dobbins M, De Corby K, Robeson P, Husson H, Tirilis D. School-based physical activity programs for promoting physical activity and fitness in children and adolescents aged 6-18. *Cochrane Database Syst Rev.* 2009(1):CD007651
40. Harris KC, Kuramoto LK, Schulzer M, Retallack JE. Effect of school-based physical activity interventions on body mass index in children: a meta-analysis. *CMAJ.* 2009;180(7):719-726
41. Center for Disease Control and Prevention. 2008 Physical Activity Guidelines for Americans. 2008. Available at: http://www.cdc.gov/physicalactivity/everyone/guidelines/adults.html. Accessed March 6, 2012
42. American College of Sports Medicine. *ACSM's Guidelines for Exercise Testing and Prescription.* 7th ed. Philadelphia: Lippincott Williams & Wilkins; 2006
43. Heyward V. Designing Weight Management and Body Composition Programs. *Advanced Fitness Assessment and Exercise Prescription.* 5th ed. Champaign, IL: Human Kinetics; 2006
44. Gutin B, Barbeau P, Owens S, et al. Effects of exercise intensity on cardiovascular fitness, total body composition, and visceral adiposity of obese adolescents. *Am J Clin Nutr.* 2002;75(5):818-826
45. Lazzer S, Lafortuna C, Busti C, Galli R, Agosti F, Sartorio A. Effects of low- and high-intensity exercise training on body composition and substrate metabolism in obese adolescents. *J Endocrinol Invest.* 2011;34(1):45-52
46. Ben Ounis O, Elloumi M, Makni E, et al. Exercise improves the ApoB/ApoA-I ratio, a marker of the metabolic syndrome in obese children. *Acta Paediatr.* 2010;99(11):1679-1685
47. Ben Ounis O, Elloumi M, Zouhal H, et al. Effect of individualized exercise training combined with diet restriction on inflammatory markers and IGF-1/IGFBP-3 in obese children. *Ann Nutr Metab.* 2010;56(4):260-266
48. Togashi K, Masuda H, Iguchi K. Effect of diet and exercise treatment for obese Japanese children on abdominal fat distribution. *Res Sports Med.* 2010;18(1):62-70
49. Barlow SE. Expert committee recommendations regarding the prevention, assessment, and treatment of child and adolescent overweight and obesity: summary report. *Pediatrics.* 2007;120 Suppl 4:S164-192
50. Tremblay MS, LeBlanc AG, Kho ME, et al. Systematic review of sedentary behaviour and health indicators in school-aged children and youth. *Int J Behav Nutr Phys Act.* 2011;8:98
51. Jelalian E, Mehlenbeck R, Lloyd-Richardson EE, Birmaher V, Wing RR. "Adventure therapy" combined with cognitive-behavioral treatment for overweight adolescents. *Int J Obes (Lond).* 2006;30(1):31-39.
52. Daley AJ, Copeland RJ, Wright NP, Wales JK. "I can actually exercise if I want to; it isn't as hard as I thought": a qualitative study of the experiences and views of obese adolescents participating in an exercise therapy intervention. *J Health Psychol.* 2008;13(6):810-819

53. Trost SG, Kerr LM, Ward DS, Pate RR. Physical activity and determinants of physical activity in obese and non-obese children. *Int J Obes Relat Metab Disord.* 2001;25(6):822-829
54. Pescud M, Pettigrew S, McGuigan MR, Newton RU. Factors influencing overweight children's commencement of and continuation in a resistance training program. *BMC Public Health.* 2010;10:709.
55. Ekelund U, Luan J, Sherar LB, Esliger DW, Griew P, Cooper A. Moderate to vigorous physical activity and sedentary time and cardiometabolic risk factors in children and adolescents. *JAMA.* 2012;307(7):704-712
56. Tompkins CL, Moran K, Preedom S, Brock DW. Physical activity-induced improvements in markers of insulin resistance in overweight and obese children and adolescents. *Curr Diabetes Rev.* 2011;7(3):164-170
57. Balagopal PB, Gidding SS, Buckloh LM, et al. Changes in circulating satiety hormones in obese children: a randomized controlled physical activity-based intervention study. *Obesity (Silver Spring).* 2010;18(9):1747-1753
58. Lobstein T, Baur L, Uauy R. Obesity in children and young people: a crisis in public health. *Obes Rev.* 2004;5 Suppl 1:4-104
59. Oude Luttikhuis H, Baur L, Jansen H, et al. Interventions for treating obesity in children. *Cochrane Database Syst Rev.* 2009(1):CD001872
60. Butryn ML, Wadden TA, Rukstalis MR, et al. Maintenance of weight loss in adolescents: current status and future directions. *J Obes.* 2010;2010:789280
61. Epstein LH, Myers MD, Raynor HA, Saelens BE. Treatment of pediatric obesity. *Pediatrics.* 1998;101(3 Pt 2):554-570
62. Wilfley DE, Tibbs TL, Van Buren DJ, Reach KP, Walker MS, Epstein LH. Lifestyle interventions in the treatment of childhood overweight: a meta-analytic review of randomized controlled trials. *Health Psychol.* 2007;26(5):521-532
63. Whitlock EP, O'Connor EA, Williams SB, Beil TL, Lutz KW. Effectiveness of weight management interventions in children: a targeted systematic review for the USPSTF. *Pediatrics.* 2010;125(2):e396-418
64. Tsiros MD, Sinn N, Coates AM, Howe PR, Buckley JD. Treatment of adolescent overweight and obesity. *Eur J Pediatr.* 2008;167(1):9-16
65. Faith MS, Saelens BE, Wilfley DE, Allison DB. Behavioral treatment of childhood and adolescent obesity: Current status, challenges, and future directions. In: Thompson JK, Smolak L, eds. *Body Image, Eating Disorders, and Obesity in Youth: Assessment, Prevention, and Treatment.* Washington, DC: American Psychological Association; 2001
66. Herrera EA, Johnston CA, Steele RG. A comparison of cognitive and behavioral treatments for pediatric obesity. *Children's Health Care.* 2004;33(2)
67. Nemet D, Barkan S, Epstein Y, Friedland O, Kowen G, Eliakim A. Short- and long-term beneficial effects of a combined dietary-behavioral-physical activity intervention for the treatment of childhood obesity. *Pediatrics.* 2005;115(4):e443-449
68. Saelens BE, Sallis JF, Wilfley DE, Patrick K, Cella JA, Buchta R. Behavioral weight control for overweight adolescents initiated in primary care. *Obes Res.* 2002;10(1):22-32
69. Coates TJ, Jeffery RW, Slinkard LA, Killen JD, Danaher BG. Frequency of contact and monetary reward in weight loss, lipid change, and blood pressure reduction with adolescents. *Behav Ther.* 1982;13:175-185
70. Phillips JEH, Hull EE, Rofey DL. Childhood obesity: Psychological correlates and recommended therapeutic strategies. In: Bagchi D, ed. *Global Perspectives on Childhood Obesity: Current Status, Consequences and Prevention*: Waltham, MA: Academic Press; 2011
71. Butler AC, Chapman JE, Forman EM, Beck AT. The empirical status of cognitive-behavioral therapy: a review of meta-analyses. *Clin Psychol Rev.* 2006;26(1):17-31
72. Cooper Z, Fairburn CF, Hawker DM. *Cognitive-Behavioral Treatment of Obesity: A Clinician's Guide.* New York: Guilford Press; 2003
73. Neumark-Sztainer D, Story M, French SA, Hannan PJ, Resnick MD, Blum RW. Psychosocial concerns and health-compromising behaviors among overweight and nonoverweight adolescents. *Obes Res.* 1997;5(3):237-249

74. Mellin AE, Neumark-Sztainer D, Story M, Ireland M, Resnick MD. Unhealthy behaviors and psychosocial difficulties among overweight adolescents: the potential impact of familial factors. *J Adolesc Health.* 2002;31(2):145-153
75. Melnyk BM, Small L, Morrison-Beedy D, et al. Mental health correlates of healthy lifestyle attitudes, beliefs, choices, and behaviors in overweight adolescents. *J Pediatr Health Care.* 2006;20(6):401-406
76. Braet C, Winckel MV. Long-term follow-up of a cognitive behavioral treatment program for obese children. *Behav Ther.* 2000;31(1):55-74
77. Mellin LM, Slinkard LA, Irwin CE, Jr. Adolescent obesity intervention: validation of the SHAPE-DOWN program. *J Am Diet Assoc.* 1987;87(3):333-338
78. Summerbell CD, Ashton V, Campbell KJ, Edmunds L, Kelly S, Waters E. Interventions for treating obesity in children. *Cochrane Database Syst Rev.* 2003(3):CD001872
79. Whitlock EA, O'Connor EP, Williams SB, Beil TL, Lutz KW. Effectiveness of weight management programs in children and adolescents. *Evid Rep Technol Assess (Full Rep).* 2008(170):1-308
80. Braet C, Tanghe A, Bode PD, Franckx H, Winckel MV. Inpatient treatment of obese children: a multicomponent programme without stringent calorie restriction. *Eur J Pediatr.* 2003;162(6):391-396
81. Lindsay AC, Sussner KM, Kim J, Gortmaker S. The role of parents in preventing childhood obesity. *The Future of children / Center for the Future of Children, the David and Lucile Packard Foundation.* 2006;16(1):169-186
82. Golan M, Kaufman V, Shahar DR. Childhood obesity treatment: targeting parents exclusively v. parents and children. *Br J Nutr.* 2006;95(5):1008-1015
83. Kamath CC, Vickers KS, Ehrlich A, et al. Clinical review: behavioral interventions to prevent childhood obesity: a systematic review and metaanalyses of randomized trials. *J Clin Endocrinol Metab.* 2008;93(12):4606-4615
84. Brownell KD, Kelman JH, Stunkard AJ. Treatment of obese children with and without their mothers: changes in weight and blood pressure. *Pediatrics.* 1983;71(4):515-523
85. Jiang JX, Xia XL, Greiner T, Lian GL, Rosenqvist U. A two year family based behaviour treatment for obese children. *Arch Dis Child.* 2005;90(12):1235-1238
86. Nowicka P, Hoglund P, Pietrobelli A, Lissau I, Flodmark CE. Family Weight School treatment: 1-year results in obese adolescents. *Int J Pediatr Obes.* 2008;3(3):141-147
87. Wadden TA, Stunkard AJ, Rich L, Rubin CJ, Sweidel G, McKinney S. Obesity in black adolescent girls: a controlled clinical trial of treatment by diet, behavior modification, and parental support. *Pediatrics.* 1990;85(3):345-352
88. McLean N, Griffin S, Toney K, Hardeman W. Family involvement in weight control, weight maintenance and weight-loss interventions: a systematic review of randomised trials. *Int J Obes Relat Metab Disord.* 2003;27(9):987-1005
89. Burke BL, Arkowitz H, Menchola M. The efficacy of motivational interviewing: a meta-analysis of controlled clinical trials. *J Consult Clin Psychol.* 2003;71(5):843-861
90. Dunn C, Deroo L, Rivara FP. The use of brief interventions adapted from motivational interviewing across behavioral domains: a systematic review. *Addiction.* 2001;96(12):1725-1742
91. Emmons KM, Rollnick S. Motivational interviewing in health care settings. Opportunities and limitations. *Am J Prev Med.* 2001;20(1):68-74
92. Resnicow K, Davis R, Rollnick S. Motivational interviewing for pediatric obesity: Conceptual issues and evidence review. *J Am Diet Assoc.* 2006;106(12):2024-2033
93. Miller WR, Rollnick S. *Motivational Interviewing: Preparing People for Change.* 2nd ed. New York: Guilford Press; 2002
94. Prochaska JO, Butterworth S, Redding CA, et al. Initial efficacy of MI, TTM tailoring and HRI's with multiple behaviors for employee health promotion. *Prev Med.* 2008;46(3):226-231
95. Rubak S, Sandbaek A, Lauritzen T, Christensen B. Motivational interviewing: a systematic review and meta-analysis. *Br J Gen Pract.* 2005;55(513):305-312
96. Spruijt-Metz D, Barnett E, Davis J, Resnicow K. Obesity in Minorities. In: Naar-King S, Suarez M, eds. *Motivational interviewing with adolescents and young adults.* New York: The Guilford Press; 2011

97. Brennan L, Walkley J, Fraser SF, Greenway K, Wilks R. Motivational interviewing and cognitive behaviour therapy in the treatment of adolescent overweight and obesity: study design and methodology. *Contemp Clin Trials.* 2008;29(3):359-375
98. Berg-Smith SM, Stevens VJ, Brown KM, et al. A brief motivational intervention to improve dietary adherence in adolescents. The Dietary Intervention Study in Children (DISC) Research Group. *Health Educ Res.* 1999;14(3):399-410
99. Flattum C, Friend S, Neumark-Sztainer D, Story M. Motivational interviewing as a component of a school-based obesity prevention program for adolescent girls. *J Am Diet Assoc.* 2009;109(1):91-94
100. Flattum C, Friend S, Story M, Neumark-Sztainer D. Evaluation of an individualized counseling approach as part of a multicomponent school-based program to prevent weight-related problems among adolescent girls. *J Am Diet Assoc.* 2011;111(8):1218-1223
101. Davis JN, Gyllenhammer LE, Vanni AA, et al. Startup circuit training program reduces metabolic risk in Latino adolescents. *Med Sci Sports Exerc.* 2011;43(11):2195-2203
102. Davis JN, Kelly LA, Lane CJ, et al. Randomized control trial to improve adiposity and insulin resistance in overweight Latino adolescents. *Obesity (Silver Spring).* 2009;17(8):1542-1548
103. Resnicow K, Taylor R, Baskin M, McCarty F. Results of go girls: a weight control program for overweight African-American adolescent females. *Obes Res.* 2005;13(10):1739-1748
104. Rogovik AL, Chanoine JP, Goldman RD. Pharmacotherapy and weight-loss supplements for treatment of paediatric obesity. *Drugs.* 2010;70(3):335-346
105. Berkowitz RI, Wadden TA, Tershakovec AM, Cronquist JL. Behavior therapy and sibutramine for the treatment of adolescent obesity: a randomized controlled trial. *JAMA.* 2003;289(14):1805-1812
106. Berkowitz RI, Fujioka K, Daniels SR, et al. Effects of sibutramine treatment in obese adolescents: a randomized trial. *Ann Intern Med.* 2006;145(2):81-90
107. Godoy-Matos A, Carraro L, Vieira A, et al. Treatment of obese adolescents with sibutramine: a randomized, double-blind, controlled study. *J Clin Endocrinol Metab.* 2005;90(3):1460-1465
108. James WP, Caterson ID, Coutinho W, et al. Effect of sibutramine on cardiovascular outcomes in overweight and obese subjects. *N Engl J Med.* 2010;363(10):905-917
109. U.S. Food and Drug Administration (FDA). FDA drug safety communication: FDA recommends against the continued use of Meridia (sibutramine). Available at: http://www.fda.gov/Drugs/DrugSafety/ucm228746.htm. Accessed January 17, 2012
110. Greydanus DE, Bricker LA, Feucht C. Pharmacotherapy for obese adolescents. *Pediatr Clin North Am.* 2011;58(1):139-153, xi
111. Ozkan B, Bereket A, Turan S, Keskin S. Addition of orlistat to conventional treatment in adolescents with severe obesity. *Eur J Pediatr.* 2004;163(12):738-741
112. Chanoine JP, Hampl S, Jensen C, Boldrin M, Hauptman J. Effect of orlistat on weight and body composition in obese adolescents: a randomized controlled trial. *JAMA.* 2005;293(23):2873-2883.
113. Maahs D, de Serna DG, Kolotkin RL, et al. Randomized, double-blind, placebo-controlled trial of orlistat for weight loss in adolescents. *Endocr Pract.* 2006;12(1):18-28
114. Chanoine JP, Richard M. Early weight loss and outcome at one year in obese adolescents treated with orlistat or placebo. *Int J Pediatr Obes.* 2011;6(2):95-101
115. Freemark M, Bursey D. The effects of metformin on body mass index and glucose tolerance in obese adolescents with fasting hyperinsulinemia and a family history of type 2 diabetes. *Pediatrics.* 2001;107(4):E55
116. Kay JP, Alemzadeh R, Langley G, D'Angelo L, Smith P, Holshouser S. Beneficial effects of metformin in normoglycemic morbidly obese adolescents. *Metabolism.* 2001;50(12):1457-1461
117. Srinivasan S, Ambler GR, Baur LA, et al. Randomized, controlled trial of metformin for obesity and insulin resistance in children and adolescents: improvement in body composition and fasting insulin. *J Clin Endocrinol Metab.* 2006;91(6):2074-2080
118. Atabek ME, Pirgon O. Use of metformin in obese adolescents with hyperinsulinemia: a 6-month, randomized, double-blind, placebo-controlled clinical trial. *J Pediatr Endocrinol Metab.* 2008;21(4):339-348

119. Love-Osborne K, Sheeder J, Zeitler P. Addition of metformin to a lifestyle modification program in adolescents with insulin resistance. *J Pediatr.* 2008;152(6):817-822
120. Wilson DM, Abrams SH, Aye T, et al. Metformin extended release treatment of adolescent obesity: a 48-week randomized, double-blind, placebo-controlled trial with 48-week follow-up. *Arch Pediatr Adolesc Med.* 2010;164(2):116-123
121. Yanovski JA, Krakoff J, Salaita CG, et al. Effects of metformin on body weight and body composition in obese insulin-resistant children: a randomized clinical trial. *Diabetes.* 2011;60(2):477-485
122. Mosby Inc. *Mosby's Medical Dictionary,* 8th Edition. St. Louis, MO: Mosby; 2008
123. Park MH, Kinra S, Ward KJ, White B, Viner RM. Metformin for obesity in children and adolescents: a systematic review. *Diabetes Care.* 2009;32(9):1743-1745
124. Inge TH, Krebs NF, Garcia VF, et al. Bariatric surgery for severely overweight adolescents: concerns and recommendations. *Pediatrics.* 2004;114(1):217-223
125. Pratt JS, Lenders CM, Dionne EA, et al. Best practice updates for pediatric/adolescent weight loss surgery. *Obesity (Silver Spring).* 2009;17(5):901-910
126. Xanthakos SA, Daniels SR, Inge TH. Bariatric surgery in adolescents: an update. *Adolesc Med Clin.* 2006;17(3):589-612; abstract x
127. Treadwell JR, Sun F, Schoelles K. Systematic review and meta-analysis of bariatric surgery for pediatric obesity. *Ann Surg.* 2008;248(5):763-776
128. Jen HC, Rickard DG, Shew SB, et al. Trends and outcomes of adolescent bariatric surgery in California, 2005-2007. *Pediatrics.* 2010;126(4):e746-753
129. Rand CS, Macgregor AM. Adolescents having obesity surgery: a 6-year follow-up. *South Med J.* 1994;87(12):1208-1213
130. O'Brien PE, Sawyer SM, Laurie C, et al. Laparoscopic adjustable gastric banding in severely obese adolescents: a randomized trial. *JAMA.* 2010;303(6):519-526
131. Inge TH, Zeller M, Harmon C, et al. Teen-Longitudinal Assessment of Bariatric Surgery: methodological features of the first prospective multicenter study of adolescent bariatric surgery. *J Pediatr Surg.* 2007;42(11):1969-1971
132. TODAY Study Group. A clinical trial to maintain glycemic control in youth with type 2 diabetes. *N Engl J Med.* 366(24):2247-2256; article first published online Apr 29
133. Allen DB. TODAY—a stark glimpse of tomorrow. *N Engl J Med.* 2012;366(24):2315-2316

Adolesc Med 023 (2012) 571–588

Emerging Adulthood: A Critical Age for Preventing Excess Weight Gain?

Nicole A. VanKim, MPH*, Nicole Larson, PhD, MPH, RD, Melissa N. Laska, PhD, RD

Division of Epidemiology and Community Health, School of Public Health, University of Minnesota, 1300 South Second Street, Suite 300, Minneapolis, MN 55454

In recent decades, societal changes in the United States and other industrialized nations have given rise to a distinct developmental period between adolescence and adulthood.[1] This period of development during the late teens and early twenties has been termed "emerging adulthood" and is characterized by independent exploration of possible life directions without the restrictions of adolescence or the responsibilities associated with filling adult roles. Although cultural and economic factors sometimes limit the extent to which young people are able to use these years for exploration, it is common today for young people to delay entering a long-term job, marriage, or parenthood until at least their late twenties. Emerging adulthood is often marked by important transitions such as leaving home and the experience of increased autonomy with fewer household rules. At the same time, many young people this age do not have adult responsibilities such as adhering to workplace standards, maintaining a home, or caring for young children. The period of transition from adolescence to adulthood may thus be an important time for establishing health attitudes and patterns of health behavior because young people have the freedom to continue to intensify the process of identity exploration begun in their earlier teen years.

Health promotion and disease prevention efforts targeting emerging adults not only have the potential to influence the adoption of health attitudes and long-term behaviors but may also reduce immediate and future risk for adverse health outcomes. The period of emerging adulthood was once considered to be an age of optimal health and well-being; however, there is now growing recog-

*Corresponding author.
E-mail address: vank0056@umn.edu (N. A. VanKim).

 ISSN 1934-4287

nition that the transition from adolescence to adulthood is a high-risk period for the development of obesity as well as unhealthy eating and physical activity (PA) patterns. Survey data from the National Longitudinal Study of Adolescent Health (Add Health), a nationally representative cohort of young people, indicated that the prevalence of obesity doubles during the transition from adolescence to adulthood and doubles again as individuals progress from their twenties to their thirties.[2] In 2010, the US national prevalence of overweight was estimated to be 24% and the prevalence of obesity was 17% among young people ages 18 to 24 years, based on self-reported height and weight data (which has been shown to underestimate overweight and obesity prevalence).[3] Declines in overall diet quality and adverse changes in PA patterns correspondingly occur during the transition from adolescence to adulthood, and most US emerging adults fail to meet federal health guidelines.[4] Intake of fruit, vegetables, whole grains, and several vitamins and minerals are lower than recommended and nearly all individuals this age exceed the recommended maximum energy intake from solid fats, added sugars, and alcoholic beverages.[5-7] Of further concern, fewer than two-thirds of US emerging adults achieve recommended levels of moderate-to-vigorous PA (MVPA).[8] The presence of obesity and unhealthy lifestyle patterns during the emerging adult years are likely to affect reproductive outcomes[9] among those bearing children and have been associated with increased risk for chronic diseases such as diabetes and cardiovascular disease.[10,11]

Despite the importance of avoiding excess weight gain and establishing healthy eating and PA patterns in emerging adulthood, there are few guidelines for clinical care or health promotion programs in place that are specific to this distinct developmental period.[12] Emerging adults have historically had the lowest rates of health insurance coverage of any age group in the United States;[13] however, recent efforts at the state and federal levels to expand the provision of health insurance allows millions of young people to retain coverage through age 26.[12,14] To ensure that new opportunities for preventive interventions created by this large-scale policy action are not missed, evidence-based guidelines urgently need to be developed for the emerging adult years and broadly disseminated to physicians as well as community-based health professionals.

The purpose of this article is to inform such efforts by summarizing peer-reviewed studies that have examined aspects of weight-related health in emerging adulthood. More specifically, in this literature review we address (1) adverse changes in diet, eating behaviors, PA, and sedentary behavior during the transition from adolescence to adulthood; (2) disparities in weight and weight-related behaviors; (3) existing evidence from research that has evaluated obesity prevention strategies; and (4) priority areas for future research and health promotion efforts.

ADVERSE CHANGES DURING EMERGING ADULTHOOD

Dietary Intake and Eating Behaviors

Dietary quality seems to generally be poor among emerging adults in the United States, and most in this age group may not be meeting national health guidelines.[4] In addition, factors contributing to poor diet, such as unstructured meals, eating away from home, and limited meal preparation, may be challenges unique to emerging adults. Few large research initiatives have captured the emerging adult years with much specificity, though numerous studies have documented the poor dietary patterns that occur as young people age. For example, much of the work from nationally representative datasets and large surveillance systems very broadly characterize "young adulthood" as being inclusive of the second, and possibly the third, decade of life. To illustrate this point, we highlight the following series of studies.

Using data from the 2003 to 2004 National Health and Nutrition Examination Survey (NHANES), Kimmons and colleagues[15] examined young adults ages 19 to 30 years and found a median daily fruit intake of 0.3 cups and a median daily vegetable intake of 1.8 cups among this age group. This translated into 6.7% of this age group meeting national recommendations for fruit intake and 13.1% meeting recommendations for vegetable intake. Additionally, data from Project EAT (Eating and Activity in Teens and Young Adults), a 10-year longitudinal study of weight-related behaviors among adolescents transitioning into adulthood, indicated deterioration in the number of servings of fruits and vegetables consumed from middle adolescence (14-18 years old) to emerging adulthood (18-23 years old).[16]

Popkin examined 2005 to 2006 NHANES data and found that the 19- to 39-year-old age group consumed an average of 520 mL (207 kilocalories) of sugar-sweetened soft drinks or fruit drinks per day, compared with only 307 mL (122 kilocalories) among 40 to 59 year olds.[17] Thus, among this young adult age group, average consumption of these 2 types of beverages alone accounts for most recommended daily "empty calories" (ie, added sugars or solid fats) according to the US Department of Agriculture My Plate Program; these recommendations are to limit empty calories to about 300 kilocalories per day for those aged 19 to 30 years (260 calories per day for women and 330 calories per day for men).[18] Furthermore, average intake of soda or fruit juice appeared to be highest among those ages 13 to 18 and 19 to 39 years compared to other age groups.[17]

Data from wave III of the Add Health study (2001-2002) indicated that cohort participants aged 18 to 27 frequently consumed fast food, reporting an average frequency of 2.5 days per week.[19] Previous research has indicated that fast food intake as low as once per week on a regular basis may be associated with a variety of adverse health outcomes.[20-23] In addition, cohort participants reported low levels of other healthful behaviors, such as eating breakfast; mean breakfast consumption frequency was 3 times per week.[19] Findings from this study also indicated that fast food intake significantly increased and breakfast consumption significantly decreased in the cohort between wave II (ages 11-21 years) and wave III assessments.

Overall, the findings from these and other studies highlight the fact that the young adult years are characterized by poor food choices and unhealthful eating patterns. Numerous studies have noted the significant decline in dietary quality as young people age, and the emerging adult years may be a particularly critical period for these declining health behaviors.[4,16,24-26]

Emerging adulthood commonly represents a unique time of transitioning and increasing responsibility for one's day-to-day activities. Most individuals at this age are gaining extensive independence in their choices about how, what, where, and when to eat for the first time in their lives. Previous research indicates that among the emerging adult age group, away-from-home eating, infrequent home meal preparation, and unstructured eating patterns—practices that are all generally associated with unhealthy dietary outcomes—may be particular challenges contributing to poor dietary intake.[1]

In general, research has shown that meals prepared at home tend to be more healthful than commercially prepared meals.[27] Findings from Project EAT indicated that emerging adulthood is a critical age at which to establish home food preparation habits and skills. More specifically, results indicated that frequent home food preparation during emerging adulthood (19-23 years of age) was a significant predictor of better dietary quality 5 years later in the mid-to-late twenties (24-28 years), including greater intake of fruits and vegetables and less frequent intake of sugar-sweetened beverages and fast food.[28] In contrast, the frequency of home food preparation during adolescence (15-18 years) did not yield consistent associations with dietary intake at ages 24 to 28 years.[28] Of concern, given the critical nature of the emerging adult period, findings from Project EAT have also shown that most young people this age do not engage in fundamental food preparation-related behaviors on a regular basis, including buying fresh vegetables; writing a grocery list; preparing a green salad; preparing a dinner that includes chicken, fish, or vegetables; or preparing an entire dinner for 2 or more people.[29] Lack of engagement in home food preparation may represent a major obstacle to healthy eating among emerging adults.

In addition to challenges with home food preparation that need to be addressed, the emerging adult age group faces other challenges related to meal structure and routines. Existing research has highlighted the healthful attributes of structured family meals in childhood and adolescence; however, mealtime patterns likely decline in quality and structure as young people move out of their family's home and begin establishing an independent lifestyle.[30] One study of 18- to 23-year-olds found that a large proportion of meals for emerging adults were eaten alone or while engaging in activities, such as watching television, using a computer, driving, or doing other activities.[31] In this study, more than half of eating occasions also occurred with no advanced planning or prior consideration as to what would be consumed, which is consistent with other research that found a high frequency of "eating on the run" in this age group.[32] This work also indicated that many of these characteristics of less structured mealtimes are associated with unhealthful food choices and suggests that there are likely important elements of dietary habits that not only reflect the specific foods that one consumes, but also the situational characteristics of and context around the meal itself.[31] Overall, mealtime structure and routines may be critical target areas for future nutrition intervention studies among emerging adults.

Physical Activity

Limited longitudinal data from Add Health and Project EAT have shown a decrease in PA from adolescence into emerging adulthood.[33,34] Among females in the Project EAT cohort, the decrease was striking as young women reduced their MVPA from 5.1 hours per week in middle adolescence (14-18 years) to 3.5 hours per week in emerging adulthood (18-23 years).[34] It also seems that decreases in PA may begin in early adolescence (11-15 years), particularly among females;[34,35] although for males, substantial declines do not occur until the transition into emerging adulthood. More specifically, among males in Project EAT, MVPA was found to remain stable at about 6.5 hours per week throughout early and middle adolescence and then decrease to 5.1 hours per week by 18 to 23 years of age.[34] Decreases in PA continue throughout emerging adulthood before stabilizing during mid-adulthood (30-64 years).[35] It seems that changes in PA during emerging adulthood may co-occur with events such as entering committed relationships or having a child. More specifically, Caspersen and colleagues attributed the small changes in PA during mid-adulthood (30-64 years) to the stability of work and household responsibilities.[35] On the other hand, the instability of these responsibilities during young adulthood (18-29 years) may correspond with the more drastic decreases in PA during this time period.

The observed decreases in PA are notable since data from the Coronary Artery Risk Development in Young Adults Study (CARDIA), a longitudinal cohort following adults over time, have consistently documented the association between engaging in higher levels of PA during young adulthood (18-30 years) with improved health outcomes, such as less weight gain and lower blood pressure, in older ages (2, 5, 7, 10, 15, and 20 years later).[36-39] Thus, continuing to engage in PA during young adulthood may be an important behavioral component for reducing morbidity later in life.

Sedentary Behavior

Common assessments of sedentary behavior include measures of screen time, such as television viewing or computer use. Limited research has been conducted in emerging adults; however, longitudinal data from Project EAT indicated an increase in leisure-time computer use, particularly among males who reported an average of 10.4 hours/week in middle adolescence (14-18 years) and 14.2 hours/week in emerging adulthood (18-23 years).[34] Similar results were documented from Add Health data, where screen time was measured using a composite measure of television viewing, video viewing, and video or computer game use. The prevalence of meeting screen-time recommendations (ie, $<$14 hours per week for adolescents) decreased from adolescence into emerging adulthood.[33] Cross-sectional data from NHANES further indicates there might be a positive relationship between age and sedentary behavior as measured using accelerometers. That is, as adults age the amount of time spent being sedentary increases.[40]

There is a lack of studies examining the relationship between sedentary behavior and health outcomes among young adults in particular. We identified one study using CARDIA data that found that among young adults (23-35 years), those who watched television 2 to 4 hours per day had a higher prevalence of obesity compared to young adults who watched 0 to 1 hours of television per day.[41] Additional research on sedentary behavior among emerging adults is needed, especially considering the accessibility and normality of technology to this age group. Recent reports on Internet use estimated that 97% of US young adults (ages 18-29) use the Internet, which represents the highest percentage among all adult age groups (overall, 82% of adults use the Internet).[42] Related, an estimated 95% of US young adults (ages 18-34 years) own a cell phone, 57% own a desktop computer, 70% own a laptop, 74% own an iPod or mp3 player, and 63% own a game console.[42] For every device except owning a desktop computer, young adults have the highest percentage of ownership. The prevalence of technology, particularly among young adults, highlights the need to better assess and understand sedentary behaviors and their impact on health, because technology may facilitate sedentary behaviors.

DISPARITIES IN WEIGHT AND WEIGHT-RELATED BEHAVIORS

Emerging adulthood is not only a period when behavioral health declines,[4,43,44] but also when health disparities begin to accelerate.[43,45-47] Despite this, data examining emerging adult health disparities are limited. In general, weight-related disparities across race and ethnicity, socioeconomic position (SEP), and gender have been well documented in nearly all age groups.[48-50] More recently, lesbian, gay, and bisexual (LGB) populations have also been identified by the Institute of Medicine as potentially being at higher risk for obesity and weight behaviors.[51]

Race/Ethnicity

Prevalence data from NHANES has consistently documented disparities in obesity across racial and ethnic groups with non-Hispanic black females generally having the highest prevalence of overweight and obesity at almost every age.[49,50,52] Among young adults (ages 20-39 years) in 2009 to 2010, this pattern is consistent with an estimated 34.5% of non-Hispanic white males, 35.8% of non-Hispanic black males, and 30.8% of Hispanic males being obese. Among similarly aged females, 26.9% of non-Hispanic white females, 56.2% of non-Hispanic black females, and 34.4% of Hispanic females are obese.[52] Between 1999 and 2010, the prevalence of obesity significantly increased among all males and non-Hispanic black females and Mexican American females. There was no significant increase in obesity during this time frame for non-Hispanic white females.[52] Data from Add Health suggests that Asian young adults (18-26 years) may have the lowest prevalence of obesity.[43] Similar findings were also documented among a national sample of college students.[45]

Data for weight behaviors, such as PA and food consumption, are more limited when examining racial/ethnic differences. However, existing research indicates that there are differences across racial and ethnic groups among emerging adults that are important when addressing obesity and weight-related issues. In general, black females seem to have the highest risk of physical inactivity and unhealthful eating patterns.[43,44] Among other racial/ethnic groups, existing research does not demonstrate as consistent a pattern in weight behaviors.

Research documenting disparities in PA across race/ethnicity has reported mixed findings. Cross-sectional PA data on emerging adults (18-24 years) from the 2004 Behavioral Risk Factor Surveillance System (BRFSS) suggests that more non-Hispanic white males (88.3%), non-Hispanic white females (83.9%), and non-Hispanic black males (81.7%) engage in PA than Hispanic males (68.5%), Hispanic females (60.0%), and non-Hispanic black females (66.2%).[44] Similarly, data from Add Health indicated that among 18- to 26-year-old females, black females had the highest prevalence of no exercise. Furthermore, Native American females and Asian males had the lowest prevalence of no exercise.[13] In contrast to these findings, Add Health findings indicated that white males had the highest prevalence of no exercise,[43] and findings from a national sample of college students indicated that Asian females were the least likely to engage in vigorous PA and that Hispanic females were the most likely to engage in vigorous PA.[53] There were no significant differences among males by race/ethnicity as well as among black, Native American, and white females in vigorous PA.[53] Thus, it seems that black females might be less likely to engage in PA; however, for other groups findings do not demonstrate a clear and consistent disparity, although this may be in part because of differences in samples used for analysis (eg, college students only).

Research using Add Health data has also investigated racial and ethnic disparities in eating habits among young adults. Among females, black respondents ate breakfast the fewest days per week and consumed fast food the most days per week. The comparisons showed that white females ate breakfast the most days per week, and Native American females ate fast food the fewest days per week. Similarly, among males, white respondents also ate breakfast the most days per week and black respondents consumed fast food the most days per week. However, Native American males ate breakfast the fewest days per week, and Asian respondents consumed fast food the fewest days per week.[43]

Socioeconomic Position

Generally, higher SEP is associated with more favorable weight and weight behaviors;[48,54,55] yet, research on SEP and health among emerging adults is limited. For emerging adults, SEP can be a particularly difficult construct to measure, given that it is a time period of social identity development and formation.[56] For example, educational attainment is often used as a measure of SEP among emerging adults; however, given that a substantial proportion of emerging adults are enrolled in postsecondary institutions,[57] education may not yet fully or accurately capture their SEP. The inconsistency in measuring SEP among emerging adults may be one reason why findings have been mixed.[45,53,58] To demonstrate this point, a cross-sectional study of college students found that low "parental educational attainment" (specifically parents having less than a high school diploma) as a measure of SEP was associated with lower fruit and vegetable consumption, less hard and light PA, and more unhealthy weight control behaviors. Using a self-perception of "financial strain" as a measure of SEP similarly indicated that high strain was associated with less hard and light PA and more unhealthy weight control behaviors, but also a higher prevalence of binge drinking and tobacco use.[58] Furthermore, Scharoun-Lee and colleagues assessed multiple dimensions of SEP and found that 4 typologies of SEP were identified among young adults and that these typologies were most salient among females.[59] These studies provide examples of how the instability and complexities of SEP during emerging adulthood may provide added challenges to measuring SEP and also that measuring different dimensions of SEP may show divergent associations with weight-related behaviors.

Intersections of Race/Ethnicity and Socioeconomic Position

Although evidence among all adults suggests that weight and weight behaviors tend to be less favorable among black and Hispanic adults as well as those in low SEP, cross-sectional survey research has shown that the dynamics between race/ethnicity and SEP, particularly related to obesity, are intricate.[54,55] Among emerging adults in particular, longitudinal research using Add Health data has highlighted the complexities between race/ethnicity and SEP, noting that racial/ethnic disparities in obesity remain evident within each strata of SEP.[59,60] More specifically, using a life course assessment of SEP, Scharoun-Lee and colleagues found that SEP was strongly associated with the persistence of obesity from adolescence to adulthood in both males and females. Among those who experienced persistent disadvantage across the transition from adolescence to adulthood, black emerging adults experienced higher incident and persistent obesity compared to white emerging adults. Similarly, among those who experienced overall socioeconomic advantages during the transition, black emerging adults still had more incident and persistent obesity compared to white emerging adults.[60] Thus, to understand disparities in weight and weight behaviors, exploring the intersections of race/ethnicity and SEP may be a particularly important expansion to exploring disparities. In addition, studying health at the intersections of race/ethnicity and SEP may also provide a clearer context to interpret findings related to weight and behavioral disparities.

Sexual Orientation

Data specifically examining obesity or weight-related disparities according to sexual orientation among emerging adults is limited. Overall, LGB individuals may be at higher risk for unhealthy weight control behaviors and obesity, although more research in this area is needed. Longitudinal studies are particularly limited when it comes to LGB weight-related health. Only 2 longitudinal analyses were identified, both using data from the Growing Up Today Study (GUTS), a cohort study of children of the female participants in the Nurses' Health Study II. One study found that disparities in purging and binging behaviors persisted throughout adolescence into young adulthood (12-23 years) by sexual orientation for both males and females, with "mostly heterosexual" and bisexual males and females, as well as gay males, generally at greater risk of these behaviors than their heterosexual counterparts.[61] Another study using GUTS data examined longitudinal trends in weight status and found consistently higher BMI between the ages of 12 and 23, among "mostly heterosexual" and LGB females compared to heterosexual females. In contrast, among males, heterosexual males gained more weight over time compared to "mostly heterosexual" and LGB males.[62]

Although the studies using GUTS data have provided important longitudinal information on sexual orientation and weight-related health, the results may be limited to generalization because the participants are all children of nurses and thus, not representative of the overall population. In addition, the GUTS cohort has a higher proportion of white participants compared to the general population. However, research using population-based data examining prevalence of obesity and weight behaviors among emerging adults by sexual orientation is not available. More research on disparities across sexual orientation is needed, particularly among emerging adults, for whom development of sexual orientation may be a salient issue related to health.

Disparities in weight and weight behaviors are important in considering how to prevent excess weight gain among emerging adults. More specifically, emerging adulthood may be a critical period for addressing widening health disparities.

Existing research indicates that among emerging adults, disparities may exist across race/ethnicity, SEP, and sexual orientation, and that the intersections of these identities and constructs may also be pertinent in understanding and addressing disparities. Overall it appears that black, Hispanic, low SEP, and LGB emerging adults may have the highest risk of obesity and poor weight behaviors and thus, having culturally competent approaches to weight gain prevention among emerging adults is needed to prevent widening disparities and to help reduce existing disparities.

INTERVENTIONS FOR WEIGHT GAIN PREVENTION

There is a dire lack of evidence to support the development and dissemination of effective obesity prevention programs for emerging adults, particularly for young people who do not enroll at a 4-year college or university. A recent, systematic review of the scientific literature identified only 10 interventions for which the efficacy of strategies among young people in this age group have been evaluated by assessing change in weight status.[63] Although an additional 27 interventions have addressed other outcomes relevant to weight gain, including dietary intake and PA, published evaluations of the intervention strategies did not examine their effect on weight status. More than half of the interventions (n = 6 of 10) that examined change in weight, BMI, and/or body composition were in the form of university courses or seminars and nearly all tested strategies focused on individual-level delivery. Similarly, most interventions that targeted change in dietary factors or PA also took place on 4-year college or university campuses. The systematic review identified promising, individual-level strategies based on the existing evidence; however, the efficacy of these strategies in populations other than traditional postsecondary students is unknown, and there is an urgent need for the development of population-based strategies.

Of the 6 interventions that evaluated the effect of university courses or seminars on change in weight status, 5 interventions found some evidence of benefit.[63] Although effect sizes were often small and detailed descriptions of intervention components were missing from several of the published evaluation studies, the findings might be used to inform the development of strategies for future large-scale studies. Innovative aspects of the evaluated courses and seminars with positive findings included the use of academic incentives for participation, peer educators, Internet-based educational tools, and visual feedback in the form of graphs showing changes in weight. For example, one study evaluated the effect of an online course and the provision of weekly feedback on weight change in a sample of 159 healthy, first-year university students.[64] Students were randomized to 1 of 4 arms: (1) a 6-week online course; (2) weekly feedback; (3) the combination of an online course and weekly feedback; or (4) the control group. The online course used academic software to provide downloadable materials, group discussion boards, self-assessment tools, experiential activities, and homework assignments. Students in the weekly feedback and combined arms were asked to weigh themselves weekly and send the results to study staff that prepared graphs showing individualized change in weight status. The highest levels of adherence were reported for the weekly feedback only (90%) and combined (82%) arms, and those in the combined group had a lower mean BMI at postintervention compared with the control group.

The 4 other interventions for which evaluation data were collected to assess change in weight status also emphasized the potential promise of incorporating technology-driven strategies and peer support along with principles of self-regulation. Although effect sizes were also small in many cases, evidence of a beneficial effect was found for at least 1 of the arms for 3 of the 4 interventions. One illustrative study evaluated the effect of teaching young adults behavioral weight control skills (eg, self-monitoring, stimulus control, and problem solving) in a community-based sample of 65 women.[65] Participants were randomized to 1 of 3 arms: (1) 10 weekly group meetings; (2) 10 weekly mailed lessons and assignments; or (3) the control group. Control participants were given a brochure about healthy lifestyle choices but were not contacted by research staff during the intervention. All other participants regardless of assignment to the group meeting or correspondence format were given modest dietary and exercise goals and asked to set a healthy weight range determined by their baseline weight. No significant group differences were found at the 6-month follow-up; however, the average decrease in weight among participants assigned to the group meeting format was greater than the average weight change among control participants. The average decrease in weight among participants assigned to the correspondence format was similar to the average change among control participants, suggesting the likely importance of communicating with peers.

Among the additional interventions that did not assess change in weight status, 19 focused on dietary intake or diet-related factors (eg, fruit/vegetable intake, food purchasing behaviors), 7 focused on PA (eg, MVPA, muscle strengthening, and flexibility), and 1 was designed to target multiple health behaviors (eg, PA, diet, sleep, stress, substance use). The interventions incorporated a diverse range of strategies, including academic courses, telephone counseling, tailored messaging, point-of-purchase nutrition labeling in college/university cafeterias, social marketing, and cooking lessons. Although most of the studies focused on diet found some evidence of a positive effect, the PA interventions reported inconsistent results. The strategies described by these interventions need further evaluation, given the mixed findings for those designed to promote improvements in PA (3 reporting positive effects and 4 reporting mixed and/or null results) and the diversity of study designs and assessment methods used by those designed to promote better dietary intake.

In addition to the intervention research described earlier that has focused largely on individual-level strategies, there is growing evidence for the potential importance of population-based strategies. Environmental approaches that may be particularly relevant for emerging adults include those targeting away-from-home food consumption, sugar-sweetened beverage consumption, and use of preventive health care. Emerging adults have been heavily targeted by marketing campaigns from the fast food and soft drink industries over the past decade, and young people in this age group are among the highest consumers of fast-food meals and sugar-sweetened beverages.[4] Although adolescents and emerging adults use similar numbers of health care visits annually, the proportion of visits made by young adult males for preventive care is substantially lower.[66] Further, most preventive visits made by young adult females are with obstetrics and gynecology providers, with a significant proportion likely representing repeated visits for prenatal care.[66] Future research is needed to evaluate approaches among emerging adult populations such as required nutrition menu labeling in chain restaurants, proposed increases in sugar-sweetened beverage taxes, and the expansion of insurance coverage.

IMPLICATIONS FOR RESEARCH AND HEALTH PROMOTION

Based on this review of weight-related health among emerging adults, we prioritized and summarized several areas for future health research and promotion (Table 1). In the area of health research, there needs to be consistency in defining the "emerging adult" years across studies conducted in the United States and

Table 1
Research and health promotion needs related to weight-related health among emerging adults

Research Needs	Consistency in defining "emerging adulthood"
	More research among those not enrolled in traditional college and university settings, including those enrolled in 2-year community and technical colleges as well as those not attending college
	Identification of modifiable determinants of weight-related factors; specifically, mechanisms that could be targeted with intervention strategies (eg, adoption and support of food preparation skills), in addition to specific dietary and activity behaviors related to weight gain (eg, consumption of sugar-sweetened soft drinks)
	Further exploration of health disparities across a variety of identities and constructs, as well as the intersections of identities and constructs (eg, low SEP black females), to address the widening gap in health that occurs during emerging adulthood
Promotion Needs	Recognition of emerging adulthood as a unique period for health among national health objectives
	Identification of ways to enhance and evaluate institutional settings (particularly postsecondary settings) to help support healthy food choices and PA through environmental change and policy adoption, as well as national policies that facilitate health for emerging adults (eg, the Affordable Care Act, which expanded health insurance coverage to millions of young adults to age 26)
	Implementation of culturally tailored health promotion efforts that are appropriate for emerging adults, particularly for those who may be at higher risk of excessive weight gain or obesity (eg, some racial/ethnic groups, low SEP, LGB)

other industrialized nations. As highlighted throughout this article, the age ranges for emerging adulthood can vary depending on the data source or national guideline (Table 2). Uniformity in the definition of emerging adulthood would allow for greater comparability in research findings and also the ability for national guidelines to be developed for this specific age group. In addition, there is a particular need for research among emerging adults who are enrolled in 2-year community and technical colleges as well as those not attending col-

Table 2
Examples of adolescent and emerging adult age groupings used in weight-related surveillance systems, national guidelines, and professional and clinical organizations

	Age ranges (years)	
Source	Adolescence	Emerging adulthood
National Surveillance Systems		
Behavioral Risk Factor Surveillance System *(http://www.cdc.gov/brfss/)*		18-24 25-34
Youth Risk Behavior Surveillance System *(http://www.cdc.gov/yrbs/)*	9th-12th grades (approximately ages 14-18)	
National Health and Nutrition Examination Survey *(http://www.cdc.gov/nchs/nhanes.htm/)*	12-19	20+[a]
National Guidelines and Initiatives		
ChooseMyPlate *(http://www.choosemyplate.gov/)*	6-11 (children)	19-30
Dietary Guidelines for Americans 2010 *(http://health.gov/dietaryguidelines/)*	9-13 *14-18*	19-30
Dietary Reference Intakes *(http://www.nutrition.gov/smart-nutrition-101/dietary-reference-intakes-rdas)*		
Healthy People 2020 *(http://www.healthypeople.gov/)*	10-19	20-24
National Initiative to Improve Adolescent Health *(http://www.cdc.gov/healthyyouth/adolescenthealth/nationalinitiative/index.htm)*	10-24[b]	
Physical Activity Guidelines for Americans 2008 *(http://health.gov/paguidelines/)*	6-17[c]	18-64[a]
Professional and Clinical Organizations		
American Academy of Pediatrics *(http://www.healthychildren.org/)*	12-17	18-21
Society for Adolescent Health and Medicine *(http://www.adolescenthealth.org/)*	10-25[b]	

[a]Emerging adulthood is not specifically defined for these sources, rather emerging adulthood is included as part of a general adult age range
[b]Adolescence and emerging adulthood ages are grouped together
[c]Includes children in this age grouping

lege. Of the existing research, particularly related to interventions, traditional 4-year college and university representation far outweighs other settings. Related, there needs to be more rigorous evaluation of intervention strategies within various settings. The development of interventions requires the identification of modifiable weight-related factors relevant to this age group, which represents a currently understudied area. Also, health disparities research (examining across race and ethnicity, SEP, sexual orientation, and the intersections of these identities and constructs) is needed for emerging adults because evidence suggests that this may be a critical age for widening disparities. Currently, research is limited for emerging adults and further work in this area can help bolster existing knowledge on emerging adult health.

With regard to health promotion, there is currently a lack of national health objectives for emerging adults. For example, Healthy People 2020 objectives include priorities for children, adolescents, adults, and older adults, but do not yet provide objectives for emerging adults specifically. National health objectives are vital in that they provide a framework in which to focus health promotion efforts. Related to the development of health objectives, there are 2 important aspects related to emerging adulthood that should be considered. First, as described earlier, the expansion of health insurance coverage during the early twenties (i.e., the Affordable Care Act, which provides young adults up to age 26 coverage under their parents' health plan) has allowed millions of previously uninsured young adults to have continued health coverage[14] and thus, guidelines for physicians and other community-based health professionals need to be developed for this age group. This ensures that appropriate care is provided for emerging adults. Furthermore, settings such as educational institutions and the workplace may be critical environments for supporting healthy food choices and PA through population-based strategies such as environmental changes and policy adoption. Research among children and adolescents has focused on primary and secondary school environments to improve health, and postsecondary educational institutions represent a further extension of creating healthy school environments. Finally, emerging adulthood is a period for identity development and health promotion efforts should work to identify tailored strategies that address the unique needs and interests of this age group, as well as emerging adults of different races and ethnicities, SEP, sexual orientations, and any other identities.

CONCLUSION

In conclusion, emerging adulthood represents a critical age for weight gain prevention. Although existing literature focusing on this age group is limited, evidence suggests that the unique transitional nature of emerging adulthood creates opportunities for developing and maintaining healthy attitudes and behaviors as well as addressing health disparities. Despite this, little research has been conducted in this age group, particularly among those who are not attending a traditional 4-year college or university. Thus, further research and intervention development and implementation are needed specific for emerging adults to ensure health into later adulthood.

ACKNOWLEDGEMENTS

For this work, salary support for Ms. VanKim was provided by Award Number T32DK083250 from the National Institute of Diabetes and Digestive and Kidney Diseases (NIDDK). Salary support for Dr. Laska was provided by award number K07CA126837 from the National Cancer Institute (NCI). The content of this work is solely the responsibility of the authors and does not necessarily represent the official views of the NIDDK, NCI, or the National Institutes of Health. The National Institutes of Health did not play a role in designing the study, collecting the data, or analyzing/interpreting the results.

References

1. Arnett JJ. Emerging adulthood: a theory of development from the late teens through the twenties. *Am Psychol.* 2000;55(5):469-480
2. Gordon-Larsen P, The NS, Adair LS. Longitudinal trends in obesity in the United States from adolescence to the third decade of life. *Obesity.* 2010;18(9):1801-1804
3. Centers for Disease Control and Prevention. Behavioral Risk Factor Surveillance System Survey Data; 2010. Available at: www.cdc.gov/brfss. Accessed November 5, 2012
4. Nelson MC, Story M, Larson NI, Neumark-Sztainer D, Lytle LA. Emerging adulthood and college-aged youth: an overlooked age for weight-related behavior change. *Obesity.* 2008;16(10):2205-2211
5. Krebs-Smith S, Guenther P, Subar A, Kirkpatrick S, Dodd K. Americans do not meet federal dietary recommendations. *J Nutr.* 2010;140(10):1832-1838
6. Moshfegh A, Goldman J, Cleveland L. *What We Eat in America, NHANES 2001-2002: Usual Nutrient Intakes from Food Compared to Dietary Reference Intakes.* Beltsville, MD: U.S. Department of Agriculture, Agricultural Research Service; 2005
7. Moshfegh A, Goldman J, Ahuja J, Rhodes D, LaComb R. *What We Eat in America, NHANES 2005-2006: Usual Nutrient Intakes from Food and Water Compared to 1997 Dietary Reference Intakes for Vitamin D, Calcium, Phosphorus, and Magnesium.* U.S. Department of Agriculture, Agricultural Research Service; 2009
8. Centers for Disease Control and Prevention. Behavioral Risk Factor Surveillance System Survey Data. 2009. Available at: www.cdc.gov/brfss. Accessed November 5, 2012
9. Nodine P, Hastings-Tolsma M. Maternal obesity: improving pregnancy outcomes. *Am J Matern Child Nurs.* 2012;37(2):110-115
10. Lloyd-Jones DM, Liu K, Colangelo LA, et al. Consistently stable or decreased body mass index in young adulthood and longitudinal changes in metabolic syndrome components: the Coronary Artery Risk Development in Young Adults Study. *Circulation.* 2007;115(8):1004-1011
11. Truesdale K, Stevens J, Lewis C, et al. Changes in risk factors for cardiovascular disease by baseline weight status in young adults who maintain or gain weight over 15 years: the CARDIA study. *Int J Obes.* 2006;30(9):1397-1407
12. Irwin C. Young adults are worse off than adolescents. *J Adolesc Health.* 2010;46(5):405-406
13. DeNavas-Walt C, Proctor BD, Smith JC. Income, poverty, and health insurance status in the United States: 2009. U.S. Census Bureau, Current Population Reports; 2010
14. Monheit AC, Cantor JC, DeLia D, Belloff D. How have state policies to expand dependent coverage affected the health insurance status of young adults? *Health Serv Res.* 2011;46(1 Pt 2):251-267
15. Kimmons J, Gillespie C, Seymour J, Serdula M, Blanck M. Fruit and vegetable intake among adolescents and adults in the United States: percentage meeting individualized recommendations. *Medscape J Med.* 2009;11(1):26

16. Larson NI, Neumark-Sztainer D, Hannan PJ, Story M. Trends in adolescent fruit and vegetable consumption, 1999-2004 - Project EAT. *Am J Prev Med.* 2007;32(2):147-150
17. Popkin BM. Patterns of beverage use across the lifecycle. *Physiol Behav.* 2010;100(1):4-9
18. United States Department of Agriculture. http://www.ChooseMyPlate.gov
19. Niemeier HM, Raynor HA, Lloyd-Richardson EE, Rogers ML, Wing RR. Fast food consumption and breakfast skipping: predictors of weight gain from adolescence to adulthood in a nationally representative sample. *J Adolesc Health.* 2006;39(6):842-849
20. Pereira MA, Kartashov AI, Ebbeling CB, et al. Fast-food habits, weight gain, and insulin resistance (the CARDIA study): 15-year prospective analysis. *Lancet.* 2005;365(9453):36-42
21. Boutelle KN, Fulkerson JA, Neumark-Sztainer D, Story M, French SA. Fast food for family meals: relationships with parent and adolescent food intake, home food availability and weight status. *Public Health Nutr.* 2007;10(1):16-23
22. French SA, Harnack L, Jeffery RW. Fast food restaurant use among women in the Pound of Prevention study: dietary, behavioral and demographic correlates. *Int J Obes.* 2000;24(10):1353-1359
23. French SA, Story M, Neumark-Sztainer D, Fulkerson JA, Hannan P. Fast food restaurant use among adolescents. *Int J Obes Relat Metab Disord.* 2001;25(12):1823-1833
24. Lien N, Lytle LA, Klepp KI. Stability in consumption of fruit, vegetables, and sugary foods in a cohort from age 14 to age 21. *Prev Med.* 2001;33(3):217-226
25. Bauer KW, Larson NI, Nelson MC, Story M, Neumark-Sztainer D. Fast food intake among adolescents: secular and longitudinal trends from 1999 to 2004. *Prev Med.* 2009;48(3):284-287
26. Larson NI, Neumark-Sztainer D, Story M, et al. Fast food intake: longitudinal trends during the transition to young adulthood and correlates of intake. *J Adolesc Health.* 2008;43(1):79-86
27. Guthrie JF, Lin BH, Frazao E. Role of food prepared away from home in the American diet, 1977-78 versus 1994-96: changes and consequences. *J Nutr Educ Behav.* 2002;34(3):140-150
28. Laska MN, Larson NI, Neumark-Sztainer D, Story M. Does involvement in food preparation track from adolescence to young adulthood and is it associated with better dietary quality? Findings from a 10-year longitudinal study. *Public Health Nutr.* 2011:1-9
29. Larson NI, Perry CL, Story M, Neumark-Sztainer D. Food preparation by young adults is associated with better diet quality. *J Am Diet Assoc.* 2006;106(12):2001-2007
30. Neumark-Sztainer D, Larson NI, Fulkerson JA, Eisenberg ME, Story M. Family meals and adolescents: what have we learned from Project EAT (Eating Among Teens)? *Public Health Nutr.* 2010;13(7):1113-1121; article first published online Feb 10, 2010
31. Laska MN, Graham DJ, Moe SG, Lytle LA, Fulkerson JA. Situational characteristics of young adult eating occasions: a real-time data collection using Personal Digital Assistants. *Public Health Nutr.* 2010;Dec 8:1-8
32. Larson NI, Nelson MC, Neumark-Sztainer D, Story M, Hannan PJ. Making time for meals: meal structure and associations with dietary intake in young adults. *J Am Diet Assoc.* 2009;109(1):72-79
33. Gordon-Larsen P, Nelson MC, Popkin BM. Longitudinal physical activity and sedentary behavior trends: adolescence to adulthood. *Am J Prev Med.* 2004;27(4):277-283
34. Nelson MC, Neumark-Sztainer D, Hannan PJ, Sirard JR, Story M. Longitudinal and secular trends in physical activity and sedentary behavior during adolescence. *Pediatrics.* 2006;118(6):E1627-E1634
35. Caspersen CJ, Pereira MA, Curran KM. Changes in physical activity patterns in the United States, by sex and cross-sectional age. *Med Sci Sports Exerc.* 2000;32(9):1601-1609
36. Schmitz KH, Jacobs Jr. DR, Leon AS, Schreiner PJ, Sternfeld B. Physical activity and body weight: associations over ten years in the CARDIA study. *Int J Obes Relat Metab Disord.* 2000;24(11):1475-1487
37. Parker ED, Schmitz KH, Jacobs DJ, Dengel DR, Schreiner PJ. Physical activity in young adults and incident hypertension over 15 years of follow-up: the CARDIA study. *Am J Public Health.* 2007;97(4):703-709
38. Gordon-Larson P, Hou N, Sidney S, et al. Fifteen-year longitudinal trends in walking patterns and their impact on weight change. *Am J Clin Nutr.* 2009;89(1):19-26
39. Hankinson A, Daviglus M, Bouchard C, et al. Maintaining a high physical activity level over 20 years and weight gain. *JAMA.* 2010;304(23):2603-2610

40. Matthews CE, Chen KY, Freedson PS, et al. Amount of time spent in sedentary behaviors in the United States, 2003-2004. *Am J Epidemiol.* 2008;167(7):875-881
41. Sidney S, Sternfeld B, Haskell WL, et al. Television viewing and cardiovascular risk factors in young adults: the CARDIA Study. *Ann Epidemiol.* 1996;6:154-159
42. Pew Research Center's Internet & American Life Project. 2012. Available at: http://pewinternet.org/. Accessed August 9, 2012
43. Harris KM, Gordon-Larsen P, Chantala K, Udry JR. Longitudinal trends in race/ethnic disparities in leading health indicators from adolescence to young adulthood. *Arch Pediatr Adolesc Med.* 2006;160(1):74-81
44. Park MJ, Mulye TP, Adams SH, Brindis CD, Irwin Jr. CE. The health status of young adults in the United States. *J Adolesc Health.* 2006;39(3):305-317
45. Nelson TF, Gortmaker SL, Subramanian SV, Cheung L, Wechsler H. Disparities in overweight and obesity among US college students. *Am J Health Behav.* 2007;31(4):363-373
46. Nelson MC, Larson NI, Barr-Anderson DJ, Neumark-Sztainer D, Story M. Disparities in dietary intake, meal patterning, and home food environments among young adult nonstudents and 2- and 4-year college students. *Am J Public Health.* 2009;99(7):1216-1219; article first published online May 14, 2009
47. Laska MN, Pasch KE, Lust K, Story M, Ehlinger E. The differential prevalence of obesity and related behaviors in two- vs. four-year colleges. *Obesity.* 2011;19(2):453-456
48. Wang Y, Beydoun MA. The obesity epidemic in the United States—gender, age, socioeconomic, racial/ethnic, and geographic characteristics: a systematic review and meta-regression analysis. *Epidemiol Rev.* 2007;29:6-28
49. Flegal KM, Carroll MD, Ogden CL, Curtin LR. Prevalence and trends in obesity among US adults, 1999-2008. *JAMA.* 2010;303(3):235-241
50. Ogden CL, Carroll MD, Curtin LR, et al. Prevalence of overweight and obesity in the United States, 1999-2004. *JAMA.* 2006;295(13):1549-1555
51. Institute of Medicine. *The Health of Lesbian, Gay, Bisexual, and Transgender People: Building a Foundation for Better Understanding*; 2011. Available at: www.iom.edu/Reports/2011/The-Health-of-Lesbian-Gay-Bisexual-and-Transgender-People.aspx. Accessed November 5, 2012
52. Flegal KM, Carroll MD, Kit BK, Ogden CL. Prevalence of obesity and trends in the distribution of body mass index among US adults, 1999-2010. *JAMA.* 2012;307(5):491-497
53. Nelson TF, Gortmaker SL, Subramanian SV, Wechsler H. Vigorous physical activity among college students in the United States. *J Phys Act Health.* 2007;4:495-508
54. Ogden CL, Lamb MM, Carroll MD, Flegal KM. Obesity and socioeconomic status in adults: United States, 2005-2008. *NCHS Data Brief.* 2010;(50):1-8
55. Ogden CL, Lamb MM, Carroll MD, Flegal KM. Obesity and socioeconomic status in children and adolescents: United States, 2005-2008. *NCHS Data Brief.* 2010;(51):1-8
56. Elder GH. The life course as developmental theory. *Child Dev.* 1998;69(1):1
57. National Center for Education Statistics. Enrollment rates of 18- to 24-year-olds in degree-granting institutions, by type of institution and sex and race/ethnicity of student: 1967 through 2007. 2011. Available at: http://nces.ed.gov/programs/digest/d08/tables/dt08_204.asp. Accessed November 5, 2012
58. VanKim NA, Laska MN. Socioeconomic disparities in emerging adult weight and weight behaviors. *Am J Health Behav.* 2012;36(4):433-445
59. Scharoun-Lee M, Adair LS, Kaufman JS, Gordon-Larsen P. Obesity, race/ethnicity and the multiple dimensions of socioeconomic status during the transition to adulthood: A factor analysis approach. *Soc Sci Med.* 2009;68(4):708-716
60. Scharoun-Lee M, Kaufman JS, Popkin BM, Gordon-Larsen P. Obesity, race/ethnicity and life course socioeconomic status across the transition from adolescence to adulthood. *J Epidemiol Community Health.* 2009;63(2):133-139
61. Austin SB, Ziyadeh NJ, Corliss HL, et al. Sexual orientation disparities in purging and binge eating from early to late adolescence. *J Adolesc Health.* 2009;45(3):238-245
62. Austin SB, Ziyadeh NJ, Corliss HL, et al. Sexual orientation disparities in weight status in adolescence: findings from a prospective study. *Obesity.* 2009;17(9):1776-1782

63. Laska MN, Pelletier J, Larson NI, Story M. Interventions for weight gain prevention during the transition to young adulthood: a review of the literature. *J Adolesc Health*. 2012;50:324-333
64. Gow R, Trace S, Mazzeo S. Preventing weight gain in first year college students: an online intervention to prevent the "freshman fifteen." *Eat Behav*. 2010;11:33-39
65. Klem M, Viteri J, Wing P. Primary prevention of weight gain for women aged 25-34: the acceptability of treatment formats. *Int J Obes*. 2000;24:219-225
66. Callahan S, Cooper W. Changes in ambulatory health care during the transition to young adulthood. *J Adolesc Health*. 2010;46:407-413

Adolesc Med 023 (2012) 589–609

Environmental and Policy Strategies to Improve Eating, Physical Activity Behaviors, and Weight among Adolescents

Marlene B. Schwartz, PhD*

Deputy Director, Rudd Center for Food Policy and Obesity, Yale University

The epidemic of adolescent obesity remains 1 of the top public health concerns facing our country. Rates of adolescent obesity tripled between 1966 and 1999, rising from 4.6% to 15.5%.[1] As of 2008, adolescent obesity rates stabilized for girls at 17%, whereas boys' rates continued to rise significantly to 19.6%.[1] The fact that adolescent obesity rates continue to be so high, and are still rising for boys, should serve as a wake-up call for parents, physicians, advocates, and policy makers.

Although there are some environmental and policy strategies that have reached adolescents, many major efforts to protect youth have failed to adequately include this segment of the population. One reason adolescents have not been directly targeted by obesity prevention policy efforts is political feasibility. It is easier to convince people that protective policies are warranted when the beneficiaries are very young. In contrast, our society views adolescents as emerging adults, and gradually grants them the rights and responsibilities of adulthood. Efforts to limit access to or marketing of unhealthy foods and beverages are immediately countered with arguments that it is not sensible to consider an adolescent old enough to drive, but too young to be the target of marketing for unhealthy products.[2]

A second reason why there are fewer policies to protect adolescents is the belief that they need to learn to make their own nutrition decisions. The problem is that neurological, behavioral, and psychological studies reveal that adolescents are actually more likely to engage in sensation-seeking, emotion-driven, and impul-

*Corresponding author.
E-mail address: marlene.schwartz@yale.edu (M. B. Schwartz).

 ISSN 1934-4287

sive behavior than younger children because of the unique developmental changes occurring in their brains.[3-5] Research suggests that the prefrontal cortex, which controls impulses and uses cognitive strategies, does not fully develop until early adulthood.[3-6] Further, the emotional lability that is common among adolescents increases the risk of impulsive behavior.[7-10] Finally, adolescents' high brain plasticity makes them vulnerable to negative environmental input, like marketing.[3,6]

Many argue that providing nutrition education to adolescents leads to healthier behaviors. Unfortunately, research on the effectiveness of nutrition education has shown that while attitudes and intentions may change, actual eating behavior rarely does.[11] This is unsurprising in light of research on other types of teen-directed education, like sex, drug, and driver's education, which also suggest that education alone does not effectively reduce teens' risky behaviors.[12] Researchers believe that "logical reasoning" abilities reach adult levels by age 16, but psychosocial maturity does not peak until age 25, which is why many adolescents engage in risky behavior, even though they know it is unsafe or unhealthy.[5]

Table 1
Policies to improve nutrition and physical activity

	Nutrition	Physical Activity
Local School Wellness Policies	Strengthen standards for all competitive foods and beverages in schools Prohibit an "open campus" during lunch Restrict food use for fund-raising Conduct nutrition assessment with BMI screening Prohibit food marketing on school property	Increase time and quality of physical education Provide after-school intramural sports Support and promote walking/biking to and from schools by installing bike racks on campus Conduct physical activity assessment with BMI screening
City or State Action	Limit fast food and convenience stores around schools Ask convenience stores near schools to not sell unhealthy beverages and snacks to students before or after school Ask convenience stores and restaurants near schools to provide and promote competitively priced, healthy snacks and beverages Institute a sugary drink tax Set a limit on portion sizes for sugary drinks that can be sold in restaurants	Require complete streets and safety measures for safe routes to schools, libraries, and community centers Create joint use agreements so that schools can be used for physical activity Provide classes and programs specifically for adolescents at community athletic facilities
Federal	Recommend nutrition standards for all foods and beverages marketed to youth younger than age 16 Force energy drinks to follow the same labeling regulations required of other beverages	

Therefore, it is important to not only provide nutrition education, but to create policies that limit adolescent access to less healthy foods and beverages when they are not under the supervision of their parents.

There are many promising environmental policies that could help adolescents improve their nutrition and physical activity levels. This article begins with a detailed discussion of school-based nutrition and physical activity policies that are currently politically feasible, prominent in public discourse, and have substantial empirical support. Next is a discussion of the issue of food and beverage marketing directed at youth, which is currently quite controversial but of critical importance. Finally, the issue of sugary drinks is reviewed in detail because of the strong research linking these products to adolescent obesity.

SCHOOL-BASED FOOD AND BEVERAGE POLICIES

Why Adolescents Need Policies to Improve the Nutrition Environment

It is critical that advocates and policymakers do not fall into the trap of thinking that only younger children need to be protected from an unhealthy nutrition environment at school. Older children are more likely than younger children to be in the school building after school hours for extracurricular activities, providing frequent unsupervised opportunities to use their money to buy food from vending machines, fund-raisers, and school stores. Although it is reasonable to provide students with access to snacks after school to bridge the time between lunch and dinner, those snacks must positively contribute to the overall healthfulness of student diets.

School Wellness Policies

The Child Nutrition and Women, Infants, and Children Reauthorization Act of 2004 required all local education agencies participating in the United States Department of Agriculture (USDA) food programs to create a written school wellness policy by the 2006 to 2007 school year.[13] This legislation required that the policies include goals for nutrition education and physical activity; nutrition guidelines for food provided at school; assurance that all USDA requirements for school meals are met; a plan for measuring implementation for the policy and designation of a responsible party; and the creation of a committee that includes parents, students, food service workers, school board members, school administrators, and the public.

A substantial amount of advocacy and research has emerged in response to the requirement to create school wellness policies. School-health advocates have created materials to help districts write and improve their policies.[14,15] Researchers have developed a quantitative measure to assess policy comprehensiveness and strength, which has been used to document the relationship between policy strength and implementation.[16,17] Further, several states have done in-depth analyses of the components best addressed in their state policies and the predictors of actual implementation.[18-20] Each of these efforts underlines the importance of creating strong policies and having champions at the district level to ensure implementation.

Although there have been a number of successful environmental changes achieved because of school wellness policies, one problem that has not been solved is the significant disparity between younger and older students' nutrition environments. The prevalence of unhealthy foods and beverages remains much higher in middle and high schools than elementary schools, and research has documented that student diets and body mass index (BMI) deteriorate as a consequence of a less healthy school nutrition environment.[21-24]

There is research showing that middle and high school nutrition environments can be measurably improved if stronger nutrition standards are implemented.[22,25,26] Unfortunately, this remains uncommon. The largest national study of school wellness policies is an ongoing effort by Bridging the Gap, which collects a representative sample of policies each year and codes them on more than 100 items.[27,28] One of the key findings has been that there are much stronger policies at the elementary school level than the middle and high school levels.[27] Specifically, regulations of competitive foods and beverages are significantly more lenient in middle and high schools than in younger grades. For example, data from 2008 to 2009 indicate that 30% of elementary schools ban competitive foods from at least some locations (eg, vending machines), while only 11% of middle schools and 7% of high schools have comparably strong policies.[27]

An alternative to local school wellness policies is state competitive food laws, which mandate nutrition standards. Although it is more politically complicated to achieve a state law than a local district policy, state laws are also significantly more effective in making actual changes in the cafeteria and other school settings.[17] Recent work suggests that strong state competitive food laws are associated with a better BMI trajectory among middle school students.[29]

Open Campus Policies and Fast Food Surrounding Schools

Whether a school has an "open campus" (ie, students are allowed to go off school grounds during lunch) has the potential to significantly influence student diets. Nationally, about one-fourth of high schools have open campus policies; however, the prevalence of open campus policies is higher in California, where almost 50% of schools allow students to leave during lunch. Open campus policies put students at dietary risk because fast food restaurants often cluster around schools.[30,31] In Chicago, Illinois, there are 6 times more fast food restaurants within 1.5 km of schools, with 35% of schools having at least 1 fast food restaurant within a quarter mile and 80% within a half mile.[30] A study in Los Angeles, California, found similar results; 31% and 71% of high schools had at least 1 fast food restaurant within a quarter mile and a half mile, respectively.[31]

Access to fast food near school may also contribute to socioeconomic and racial health disparities.[31-33] Research suggests that schools with higher percentages of free meals have more food retail businesses nearby,[32] and fast food restaurant proximity to schools is more likely in low-income, high-commercial areas.[31] Further, schools with higher percentages of Hispanic and black students are more likely to be surrounded by food retail operations.[32,33] Although this is due in part to the fact that urban locations are more likely to have both fast food and Hispanic and black students, one study found that Hispanic adolescents are significantly more likely to attend schools clustered by food retail operations, regardless of location or income.[32]

There is evidence that young people who attend schools or reside near fast food restaurants and convenience stores have worse diets and greater risk of obesity.[34,35,36] One California study found that students in schools within a half mile of a fast food restaurant consumed more soda and fewer fruits and vegetables and were also more likely to be obese than students farther away.[37] This is not surprising, in light of a recent findings that in an average visit, adolescents purchase foods that contain between 800 and 1100 calories, typically from large and extra large French fries, soft drinks, large-sized burgers, and desserts.[38] Although people from all age groups go to fast food restaurants, this study also found that teens are more likely than other segments of the population to visit a fast food restaurant for an afternoon or evening snack and are more likely to order the highest-calorie, least nutritious items on the menu.[38]

It seems that fast food restaurants are uniquely attractive to teens. Therefore, strong policies to make them less obesogenic are needed. Although closed campus policies do not prevent students from frequenting nearby restaurants before or after school, they could effectively remove at least 1 time a day when students are exposed to unhealthy choices and promote participation in the National School Lunch program instead. Cities or states can consider policies that support creating and promoting other venues for teens to meet after school and in the evenings. These might include a teen lounge in the public library, community recreation centers, or religious buildings. At the same time, some of the harm associated with fast food restaurants and convenience stores could be alleviated if they limited sales of their least healthy products to students before and after school and instead developed, promoted, and competitively priced water and healthy snacks for their adolescent customers.

Federal School Food Regulations

As part of the Healthy, Hunger Free Kids Act of 2010, the USDA was charged with updating the National School Lunch and Breakfast nutrition standards. These standards were released in January 2012 and represent a significant step forward in promoting better nutrition at school.[39] Notably, although the standards set different portion sizes based on age, the nutrition standards are not more lenient for high school students.

The USDA is scheduled to release updated federal competitive food regulations in 2012. This is a significant policy change because the USDA has historically provided little oversight of food and beverages sold outside the school lunch program. As stated earlier, most state and local competitive food policies are more lenient for high schools than elementary and middle schools. Although the anticipated federal regulations will likely improve the high school nutrition environment substantially, it is possible that they will still permit less healthy food to be sold to adolescents than younger children. If this occurs, state and local policies must be strengthened to compensate for this gap in protection.

SCHOOL-BASED PHYSICAL ACTIVITY POLICIES

The transition from childhood to adolescence is characterized by not only deterioration in diet quality, but less physical activity as well. One in 4 high school students does not participate in any vigorous exercise weekly.[40] Adolescent girls are less likely to be physically active than adolescent boys, and students at highest risk for obesity are the ones who are least physically active. Black and Hispanic female adolescents are less physically active and perceive more barriers to physical activities than their white peers.[41] For example, although only 9% of whites reported not exercising outside because they feel unsafe in their neighborhood, 71% of blacks and 62% of Hispanic students reported this barrier.[42] At the same time, black female adolescents also reported less social support from teachers, family, friends, and males for physical activity.[43] Interestingly, black female adolescents reported more enjoyment with physical education classes, but not physical activity in general, than white females, suggesting that in-school physical education is a critically important strategy to protect these adolescent girls from inactivity.[43]

Physical Education

There are a number of hypotheses as to why physical activity drops so precipitously in adolescents, but one of the most likely reasons is that far fewer high schools offer or require physical education (PE) classes when compared with elementary and middle schools. One study found that although almost all middle schools require students to participate in PE, only 1 in 5 high schools have similar requirements.[44] Participation rates mirror the requirements; more than 90% of 8th graders participated in PE, compared to only 34% of 12th graders.[44] State-based data further support a close connection between the requirement of PE and amount of student physical activity.[45]

To address this problem, the National Association for Sports and Physical Education (NASPE) recommends that all elementary schools require 150 minutes per week of PE, and middle and high schools require 225 minutes per week.[46] To date, few school districts have adopted this policy and only 1 state, Illinois, has legislation that requires PE to be offered in grades K to 12. Official policies requiring PE are critical and have been shown to increase the likelihood of schools actually delivering the recommended number of minutes per week to students.[47]

Organizations such as NASPE have been advocating for federal and state legislation to put PE back in the curriculum, but there are a number of obstacles. The most frequently cited is that schools are preoccupied with standardized test scores and consequently feel they cannot afford to take time away from classroom academic instruction.[48,49] The research on this topic, however, is extremely clear; test scores do not suffer when students spend more time in PE.[48-50] Further, there is research documenting a positive relationship between student fitness and academic achievement.[50-53]

The field of PE has moved toward a greater focus on lifetime physical activities, such as yoga, rock climbing, and weight training, in addition to the traditional volleyball and flag football.[54-56] The focus on personal fitness and lifetime skills is likely to help students maintain their enjoyment and ability to stay active beyond high school and is particularly important for adolescents.[55,56] Local and state policies that require the inclusion of lifetime skills as part of the PE curriculum are needed to ensure that these changes are implemented throughout the country.

There are obstacles to stronger PE policies. In addition to concerns about taking time away from classroom instruction, districts are also wary of the costs of a high quality PE program. NASPE recommends hiring only PE teachers who are trained and certified and requiring that PE classes have appropriate teacher to student ratios. A potentially more affordable way to improve a district's PE program is using resources, such as SPARK (Sports, Play, and Active Recreation for Kids), which have been developed to train PE teachers to make the most of the time they have with students.[57]

Promoting Structured Physical Activity Outside of Physical Education

Extramural sports provide another school-based opportunity for adolescents to be physically active. High schools have more organized school sports teams than elementary or middle schools; however, these teams are usually selective and therefore only help the most talented athletes. One policy option to remedy this is to offer additional intramural sports for all students. One study found that students in schools offering numerous intramural sports had substantially more physical activity per week than students in schools offering only a few intramural sports.[58]

Safe Routes to School

Encouraging students to walk or bike to and from school is another physical activity promotion strategy that is gaining national momentum. There has been a well-documented decrease in the number of students walking or biking to school today compared to a generation ago.[59] Some of this decrease may be attributable to children living farther from their schools, but the rate of walking for students who live within a mile of school has decreased from 89% to 35%.[59] There is also evidence that as students get older they are less likely to walk or bike to school, with 1 study reporting that 20% of 8th graders walked or biked to school compared to fewer than 7% of 12th graders.[44]

Advocates can work with the national Safe Routes to School (SRTS) initiative, which provides federal funding for infrastructure, education, encouragement, and enforcement measures for safe walking and bicycling routes to school.[59] In 2010, the SRTS provided $821 million to all 50 states, reaching more than 10,400 schools and potentially 4.8 million children.[59] Funds are most used for safety measures like improving sidewalks and calming traffic near schools.[59] Strategies to promote walking and biking to school can be included in district wellness policies, as well as city and state policies that address transportation. The SRTS Local Policy Guide provides many examples of how advocates have worked to promote active student transportation in their communities.[60] Once schools are accessible, communities can build on this by creating safe routes from schools to other buildings such as libraries and community centers.

Joint Use Agreements

Another policy option to increase physical activity is encouraging school buildings to remain open and available for community activities, such as basketball in the gym or soccer on the playing fields. Currently, only 29% of schools open up their facilities outside normal school hours.[61] School districts are frequently concerned about costs, vandalism, security, and liability in case of injury. Joint use agreements have been widely recommended as a way to address these concerns.[62] This formal agreement between schools and another government entity allows schools to share or even fully allocate the costs and responsibilities of opening their facilities. ChangeLab Solutions offers guidance to creating and implementing joint use agreements.[62] This solution is particularly appealing to low-income and minority neighborhoods, where there are often fewer facilities for physical activity.[62] One study found that opening up school facilities increased the number of children who played and were physically active after school by 84%.[63]

School wellness policies can address participation in joint use agreements, as well as other community programs aimed at adolescents, such as Girls on the Run.[64] Another school policy is to remove food as a fund-raiser and suggest active fund-raisers, such as bike-a-thons, fun runs, or organized walks where students get sponsors. These fund-raisers provide all students (not just the athletes) with opportunities to be physically active, while also contributing to an important cause.

Measuring Body Mass Index in Schools

Measuring student body mass index (BMI) is associated with 2 distinct policies: BMI surveillance and BMI screening.[65] BMI surveillance refers to the practice at the state or district level of tracking student BMI in the aggregate and assessing changes in the population as a whole. The American Heart Association, the American Academy of Pediatrics, and the Centers for Disease Control and Prevention support this practice as an appropriate way to monitor trends in childhood obesity rates. More than a dozen states have legislation that requires districts to track BMI and report the data back to the state government for surveillance. The effort put into tracking BMI has illuminated the slow but steady progress in reducing childhood obesity in Arkansas, Mississippi, and New York City.[66-68]

BMI screening is a different and more controversial policy than surveillance. Screening involves measuring BMI in school and then notifying parents about their child's weight status, usually by sending a health information packet home. The rationale is that some parents may not realize that their children are overweight; therefore, school systems should screen for obesity, just as they screen for vision or hearing problems, to help inform parents of a potential health risk. Although there is some evidence that parents of overweight children are well aware of the problem,[69] other studies suggest that many parents do not realize that their children are overweight.[70] One explanation may be that families who live in communities with particularly high rates of obesity find it more difficult to assess their child's status because it is not dissimilar from their peers. Some data suggest that sending BMI screening feedback to parents may increase parental awareness of their child's health.[70]

An argument in favor of using BMI for screening is that it is relatively easy and inexpensive to measure reliably. When examining large numbers of people, BMI tracks closely with percent body fat; however, like all screening measures, BMI produces both false positives and false negatives. BMI false positives are most likely to occur with children who are very muscular. BMI false negatives occur when a child is not overweight but consumes a very poor diet and is not physically active and therefore is still at increased risk of health problems in the future.

An argument against screening for only BMI is that it may send a negative and misleading message to adolescents that weight should be the primary, and sole, concern in regard to health. This could undermine efforts to emphasize a healthy lifestyle of moderate physical activity and a healthy diet and promote unhealthy attempts to lose weight through extreme dieting, laxatives, and other dangerous weight-loss tactics. One study found that parents with overweight children who were concerned about their children's weight (after receiving information about their child's health status) were very likely to plan weight-control strategies for their children, but were not more likely to adopt the preventive lifestyle behaviors described in the health education materials.[71]

Similarly, BMI surveillance may foster negative body image and preoccupation with weight, particularly among female adolescents. Given that an estimated 60% of female adolescents and 30% of male adolescents report body dissatisfaction, this is a serious concern.[72] Body dissatisfaction increases the risk of disordered eating, depression, and other psychological and physiological damage. Perceived pressure from parents, peers, and society are the main source of body dissatisfaction among adolescents[72] and thus a BMI report may cause greater body dissatisfaction among overweight children, and potentially even among healthy weight children. Research confirms that overweight children have lower self-esteem than children of healthy weight and further found that the self-esteem of these children significantly decreased after a school BMI report.[73]

To increase the likelihood that BMI reporting leads to productive family and individual behavior changes, it should always be combined with a comprehensive assessment of dietary quality and fitness level. Completing a 24-hour food recall assessment and a standardized, comprehensive physical fitness assessment would provide more detailed and useful information. Specific feedback could be provided to the family about what dietary changes would be most important (eg, remove sugary drinks, increase fiber through more fruits and vegetables), rather than a general suggestion to eat more healthfully. Similarly, there are several components to fitness, including strength, cardiovascular health, and flexibility. By assessing each of these, students could learn what their personal fitness strengths and weaknesses are and receive tailored recommendations on how to improve. This strategy would also prevent the problem of false positive BMI scores for muscular adolescent athletes. Ideally, a school wellness policy could require that this type of multicomponent assessment be done through schools so that all youth would be able to access this information.

POLICIES TO LIMIT FOOD MARKETING TO YOUTH

Recent data on the changes in marketing trends over the past several years suggest that the food industry is shifting its strategy away from marketing on child-targeted television (ie, shows with an audience of ≥35% children aged 2-11) to adolescent-targeted shows. Although advertising to children peaked in 2004 and has since declined, the number of food and beverage advertisements targeting adolescents has steadily increased and showed a sharp 11% rise from 2007 to 2008.[74] In 2010, $948 million was spent on the marketing of sugary drinks and energy drinks, and adolescents saw 50% more advertisements than younger children.[75] To better reach adolescents, food and beverage companies are increasingly turning to social media and other online marketing strategies.

Our Youth Are "Children" Until Age 15

The food industry is fiercely protecting its ability to market to adolescents. One strategy was to create a self-regulatory body through the Better Business Bureau called the Children's Food and Beverage Advertising Initiative (CFBAI) that sets nutrition standards for marketing to children younger than age 12.[76] When the federal interagency working group suggested in 2011 that children up to age 17 should be considered a protected group,[77] the CFBAI responded:

> "We allow adolescents, but not children, to drive, hold jobs, pay taxes, get married and enlist in the services (at age 17 with permission) and we sometimes hold them criminally liable for their actions. Though adolescents' brains continue to develop throughout the second decade of life, their cognitive capacities are far more advanced than those of children."[78]

The flaw in the logic of this argument is that we do not allow 12-, 13-, 14-, or even 15-year-olds to do any of the activities listed (drive, pay taxes, get married, or enlist in the armed services). A far more reasonable cut-off for marketing to youth is younger than 16 years, not younger than 12 years. Furthermore, the argument that adolescent brain development is more advanced than that of children is irrelevant—the question should be whether adolescents have cognitive capacities comparable to adults. Here, the answer is clear: Compared to adults, adolescents are more apt to engage in high-risk behavior and seek immediate gratification,[3,79,80] which makes them more vulnerable to marketing.

If the food industry is unwilling to extend protection to children between 12 and 15 years, alternative strategies are needed to protect this group. Federal regulation is unlikely, but middle and high schools can set policies to eliminate all food and beverage marketing from campus. Parents can protest teen-directed marketing practices and demand greater regulation of social media and other online sites that target adolescents. The voices of physicians are especially important in these efforts because they can speak to the unique vulnerabilities of young adolescents and argue that this is an important health issue.

THE UNIQUE PROBLEM OF SUGARY DRINKS

When it comes to unhealthy foods and beverages, sugary drinks are in a class by themselves. Regular soft drinks represent the single largest source of added sugar in the American diet[81] and the consumption of these and other sugar-sweetened beverages is associated with poor overall nutrition, rising obesity rates, and a heightened risk for diabetes.[82-85] Adolescent consumption of sugary drinks is a serious problem; sugary drinks represent the greatest single source of calories for adolescents, making them a clear target for calorie reduction efforts.[86]

A combination of many strategies is needed to break adolescents of the habit of drinking sugary beverages. Physicians who work with adolescents have the opportunity to educate their patients about the low nutritional value and high caloric nature of these beverages and encourage consumption of water and low-fat milk instead. Further, physicians are trustworthy advocates for strong policies to protect teens from excess exposure to sugary drinks. These policies can include local school wellness policies, state and federal competitive food regulations, and local or state policies to restrict the sale or serving size of sugary beverages in public venues.

Industry Self-Regulation of Beverages Sold in Schools

In 2004, the American Beverage Association (ABA) entered into an agreement with The Alliance for a Healthier Generation to follow specific nutrition standards for beverages sold in schools. Elementary and middle schools were supposed to receive only 100% juice and water. The high school standards required that 50% of nonmilk beverages were water and no- or low-calorie options, although up to 50% of the beverages could remain the same as they were before.[87]

In 2010, the ABA announced that this program was a tremendous success, resulting in excellent compliance by bottlers and an 88% decrease in the number of calories shipped to schools.[87] A closer look at the results presented in the ABA's final report, however, paints a less impressive picture.[87] Although elementary schools are only supposed to have juice and water, a full 57% of the beverages still being sold in 2010 are noncompliant, including a substantial amount of diet sports drinks and carbonated drinks. The high school standards are significantly more lenient, so even though schools are compliant, 69% of the beverages they are offering do not meet the elementary/middle school standards.[87]

Although the beverage industry touts this program as evidence of the power of self-regulation, the national data likely overestimate the effect of this program because they include districts that are now compelled by state law to limit what is sold in their schools. For a true test of the effectiveness of self-regulation, one would need to combine the data from all of the states and cities that have legislation prohibiting the sale of sugary drinks in schools and compare them to districts in states with no legislation.

Sports Drinks

Although purchases of full-calorie soda have been decreasing over the past few years, the consumption of sports drinks has increased.[88] Sports drinks have similar amounts of sugar and calories as soft drinks, but are perceived as healthy. One study of adolescents found that unlike soda consumption, sports drink consumption was correlated with consumption of healthy foods, suggesting that sports drinks are considered part of a healthy diet.[89] Another study found that

27% of parents believed sports drinks were healthy for children, and 40% believed Gatorade was healthy.[75]

Efforts to market sports drinks to adolescents are extensive and effective. In 2010, companies used a variety of social media to promote sports drinks and featured many famous athletes.[75] Ads for Gatorade were among the top 5 most viewed ads by youth in 2010.[75] Marketing emphasizes the health halo of these products, evidenced by the finding that 40% of ads for sports drinks feature nutrition-related claims.[75] The beverage industry is invested in maintaining a healthy image so that it can justify why these sugary drinks are still available in high schools.

The ABA explains that sports drinks are needed in high schools because [they] "provide a functional benefit necessary for students to add energy and absorb fluids efficiently . . . the calories contained in sports drinks, largely through carbohydrates, are needed to fuel working muscles of active students."[87] This position is countered by the American Academy of Pediatrics, who state that "water, not sports or energy drinks" should be the principal source of hydration for adolescents, and regular consumption of sports drinks should be "avoided or restricted" to "a specific and limited function for child and adolescent athletes."[90] They go on to explain that sports drinks should only be used when there is a need for rapid replenishment of carbohydrates and/or electrolytes . . . during prolonged, vigorous sports participation or other intense physical activity."[90] In light of the data presented earlier that this level of physical activity is not occurring in school, there is no justification for providing these products in this setting.

Energy Drinks

Energy drinks are one of the most concerning additions to the sugary drink environment. As the name implies, energy drinks are marketed as a method to stay alert and thus are appealing to and often used by adolescents, who are often chronically sleep-deprived. Similar to sports drinks, consumption of energy drinks has rapidly increased in the past 10 years. From 2005 to 2006, energy drink sales increased by more than 50% and have continued to increase over the years, with a 15% increase between 2008 and 2010.[91-93]

Adolescents are among the most targeted and frequent consumers of energy drinks.[94] According to 1 survey, approximately 30% of adolescents reported consumption of energy drinks, while another study found that almost 1 in 2 adolescents regularly consumed energy drinks.[95,96] Adolescents list sports performance, peer group pressure, and attractive packaging as the top reasons for consuming energy drinks.[97] The growth in consumption is undoubtedly linked to the growth in marketing; in 2010, energy drinks had the second highest advertising expenditure among nonalcoholic drinks, totaling to $164 million.[75] Also in 2010, the most viewed television advertisements among adolescents were those for 5-Hour Energy.[75]

Other strategies used to market energy drinks include sponsorships of music and other events frequented by adolescents and the use of celebrities and extreme sports to promote their products.[98]

Most energy drink companies claim a health benefit from their products, despite minimal evidence supporting these claims.[99] Because of their classification as natural dietary supplements, energy drink manufacturers are not held to the same government regulation standards as are other beverage manufacturers. Companies do not need FDA approval; instead, the company is responsible for determining that the product is reasonably safe, but they do not need to list nutrition facts or ingredient amounts.[100] One major concern is that there is no caffeine limit for sports drinks as there is for soft drinks.[100] Companies exploit the lack of limits by putting large amounts of caffeine in their products; Monster Energy, Red Bull, and Rockstar surpass the FDA caffeine limit for soft drinks by 170%, and Spike Shooter exceeds the limit by 600%.[101] Disappointingly, one-half of all energy drinks do not even reveal their caffeine content (as they are exempt from labeling regulations), so the amount of caffeine is completely unknown to the consumer.[93]

Although caffeine is safe in moderation, there is reason to worry that the high concentrations of caffeine in energy drinks pose a health risk for adolescents. One study found that 40% of teenagers who consumed caffeine exceeded recommended limits.[102] Excess caffeine can cause health problems like nausea, palpitations, insomnia, anxiety, dehydration, and irritability,[103] and large doses of caffeine can cause seizures, muscle spasms, myocardial arrhythmias, vomiting, and fertility problems.[102,104] Among children and adolescents, regular caffeine consumption has been associated with depression and difficulty in concentrating.[97,105] There is a greater risk of serious cardiovascular, renal, neurologic, and psychiatric side effects when energy drinks are consumed with alcohol.[103,106]

Policies to Reduce Sugary Drink Consumption

There are various regulatory changes that are needed regarding energy drinks, including requiring full disclosure of ingredients and caffeine content, and requiring warning labels about possible negative health effects. Policies requiring ID for the purchase of these beverages should also be considered to limit consumption of energy drinks by adolescents.

One policy to reduce consumption of all sugary drinks, including not only energy and sports drinks, but also soft drinks, fruit drinks, and sweetened teas, is to tax them. This strategy is controversial, but also has the potential to be the most effective policy to reduce adolescent consumption. Taxes on both tobacco and alcohol have shown that increasing the price of these goods reduces levels of consumption.[107-109] For cigarettes, taxes have been found to have the most profound effect on consumption among children. Several economic studies have shown that a 10% increase in the real price of cigarettes reduces consumption in the general population by between 3% to 5%, but by between 6% to 7% among children.[110] These findings suggest that taxing sugary drinks could be particularly effective at combating obesity among young people. In addition to affecting consumption, the revenue raised by a sugary drink tax could be used to support nutrition or other health-related initiatives, such as healthier school lunch programs. The revenue that could be generated is significant. An estimate generated by the Rudd Center for Food Policy and Obesity Revenue Calculator reveals that introducting a national sales tax of 1 cent per ounce for sugar-sweetened beverages would raise $13 billion in 2013.[111]

CONCLUSION

Although adolescents have more advanced logical reasoning abilities than younger children, they are a vulnerable segment of the population that needs to be protected from obesogenic environments. If obesity were caused by lack of knowledge or faulty reasoning, one could argue that adolescents need to learn and use skills to protect their health. However, there is abundant evidence that obesity is not caused by lack of knowledge, lack of reasoning ability, or failure of personal responsibility.[112] Obesity is caused largely by an environment that promotes poor diet and physical inactivity,[113] and most adults have difficulty maintaining a healthy weight. To expect adolescents to overcome the current environment is unreasonable.

Our society must be restructured to promote, rather than hinder, healthful diets and physical activity. There are a number of public places where adolescents study and play, and in each, there are opportunities to create an environment that promotes good nutrition and physical activity. School wellness policies are a powerful, yet underused, tool to improve our nation's high schools. Local policies can state that competitive foods must be healthy, vending machines cannot sell sugary drinks, and fund-raisers should support increased physical activity instead of promoting sweets. Local wellness policies can also state that physical education classes need to help adolescents learn lifetime physical activity skills, and schools must provide ample opportunities for students to practice these skills.

In addition to local school wellness policies, city and state governments are important partners. The best progress to date in changing school food and measurably changing BMI trajectories has occurred because states have passed strong legislation, or cities have adopted strong policies to make changes such as limiting consumption of sugary drinks and requiring competitive foods to meet nutrition standards.

Federal government policy changes are fewer and farther between, but have tremendous effect. As the USDA works to improve the regulations for all of the government food programs, the voices of physicians are welcome. The national debate on food marketing to children will likely emerge again, and when it does, advocates need to stand up for the protection of adolescents.

Physicians are a critical part of the solution to childhood obesity in the United States. Parents and the general public trust physicians to prioritize childhood safety and well-being; this makes members of the health care system extremely powerful advocates. Physicians can work as individuals or part of a professional organization and connect with other advocacy groups to form coalitions. Many states have already created such alliances and would welcome the opportunity to work with local physicians. There are political and economic challenges to changing policies at the local, state, and federal level. A collaborative effort that engages everyone who cares about adolescent health is needed to overcome the obstacles and create an environment where adolescents can thrive.

ACKNOWLEDGEMENTS:

The author would like to thank Kathryn Strangfeld for her assistance in the research for this paper.

References

1. Ogden CL, Flegal KM, Carroll MD, Johnson CL. Prevalence and trends in overweight among US children and adolescents, 1999-2000. *JAMA*. 2002;288(14):1728-1732
2. The Legal Pulse. Five Questions for CFBAI's Elaine Kolish on Self Regulation of Advertising. *Washington Legal Foundation Advocate for Freedom and Justice.* 2011
3. Pechmann C, Levine L, Loughlin S, Leslie F. Impulsive and self-conscious: adolescents' vulnerability to advertising and promotion. *American Marketing Association.* 2005;24(2):202-221
4. Byrnes JP. The development of decision-making. *J Adolesc Health.* 2002;31:208-215
5. Steinberg L. Risk taking in adolescents - new perspective from brain and behavioral science. *Curr Dir Psychol Sci.* 2007;16(2):55-59
6. Johnson SB, Blum RW, Giedd JN. Adolescent maturity and the brain: the promise and pitfalls of neuroscience research in adolescent health policy. *J Adolesc Health.* 2009;45:216-221
7. Tercyak K, Goldman P, Smith A, Audrain J. Interacting effects of depression and tobacco advertising receptivity on adolescent smoking. *J Pediatr Psychol.* 2002;27(2):145-154
8. Whalen C, Jamner L, Henker B, Delfino R. Smoking and moods in adolescents with depressive and aggressive dispositions: evidence from surveys and electronic diaries. *Health Psychol.* 2001;20(2):99-111
9. Tice DM, Bratslavsky E, Baumeister RF. Emotional distress regulation takes precedence over impulse control: if you feel bad, do it! *J Pers Soc Psychol.* 2001;80(1):53-67
10. Shiv B, Fedorikhin A. Heart and mind in conflict: the interplay of affect and cognition in consumer decision making. *J Consum Res.* 1999;26(3):278-293
11. Carson DE. Changes in obesity-related food behavior: A nutrition education intervention to change attitudes and other factors associated with food-related intentions in adolescents: an application of the theory of planned behavior. 2011. *Dissertation Abstracts International: Section B: The Sciences and Engineering.* 2011;71(8-B)
12. Steinberg L. Risk-taking in adolescence: what changes and why. *Ann N Y Acad Sci.* 2004;1021:51-58

13. United States House of Representatives. Child Nutrition and WIC Reauthorization Act of 2004. Vol 108-4981. Washington, D.C.; 2004
14. Action for Healthy Kids. Wellness Policy Tool. 2011. Available at: http://www.actionforhealthykids.org/for-schools/wellness-policy-tool/. Accessed April 6, 2012
15. National Alliance for Nutrition and Activity. Model School Wellness Policies. 2005. Available at: http://www.schoolwellnesspolicies.org/. Accessed April 6, 2012
16. Schwartz MB, Lund AE, Grow HM, et al. A comprehensive coding system to measure the quality of school wellness policies. *J Am Diet Assoc.* 2009;109(7):1256-1262
17. Schwartz MB, Henderson KE, Falbe J, et al. Strength and comprehensiveness of district school wellness policies predict policy implementation at the school level. *J School Health.* 2012;82(6):262-267
18. Belansky ES, Cutforth N, Delong E, et al. Early effects of the federally mandated Local Wellness Policy on school nutrition environments appear modest in Colorado's rural, low-income elementary schools. *J Am Diet Assoc.* 2010;110(11):1712-1717
19. Probart C, McDonnell ET, Jomaa L, Fekete V. Lessons from Pennsylvania's mixed response to federal school wellness law. *Health Aff (Millwood).* 2010;29(3):447-453
20. Kubik MY, Lytle LA, Farbakhsh K. School and district wellness councils and availability of low-nutrient, energy-dense vending fare in Minnesota middle and high schools. *J Am Diet Assoc.* 2011;111(1):150-155
21. Kubik MY, Lytle LA, Hannan PJ, Perry CL, Story M. The association of the school food environment with dietary behaviors of young adolescents. *Am J Public Health.* 2003;93(7):1168-1173
22. Cullen KW, Watson K, Zakeri I. Improvements in middle school student dietary intake after implementation of the Texas Public School Nutrition Policy. *Am J Public Health.* 2008;98(1):111-117
23. Cullen KW, Eagan J, Baranowski T, Owens E, de Moor C. Effect of a la carte and snack bar foods at school on children's lunchtime intake of fruits and vegetables. *J Am Diet Assoc.* 2000;100(12):1482-1486
24. Kubik MY, Lytle LA, Story M. Schoolwide food practices are associated with body mass index in middle school students. *Arch Pediatr Adolesc Med.* 2005;159(12):1111-1114
25. Cullen KW, Watson KB. The impact of the Texas public school nutrition policy on student food selection and sales in Texas. *Am J Public Health.* 2009;99(4):706-712
26. Schwartz MB, Novak SA, Fiore SS. The impact of removing snacks of low nutritional value from middle schools. *Health Educ Behav.* 2009;36(6):999-1011
27. Chriqui JF, Schneider L, Chaloupka FJ, et al. *School District Wellness Policies: Evaluating Progress and Potential for Improving Children's Health Three Years after the Federal Mandate. School Years 2006–07, 2007–08 and 2008–09.* Chicago, IL: Bridging the Gap Program, Health Policy Center, Institute for Health Research and Policy, University of Illinois at Chicago; 2010
28. Turner L, Chaloupka FJ, Sandoval A. *School Policies and Practices for Improving Children's Health: National Elementary School Survey Results: School Years 2006–07 through 2009–10.* Chicago, IL: Bridging the Gap Program, Health Policy Center, Institute for Health Research and Policy, University of Illinois at Chicago; 2012
29. Taber DR, Chriqui JR, Perna FM, Powell LM, Chaloupka FJ. Weight status among adolescents in states that govern competitive food nutrition content. *Pediatrics.* 2012;130(3)
30. Austin SB, Melly SJ, Sanchez BN, Patel A, Buka S, Gortmaker SL. Clustering of fast-food restaurants around schools: a novel application of spatial statistics to the study of food environments. *Am J Public Health.* 2005;95:1575-1581
31. Simon PA, Kwan D, Angelescu A, Shih M, Fielding JE. Proximity of fast food restaurants to schools: do neighborhood income and type of school matter? *Prev Med.* 2008;47(3):284-288
32. Sturm R. Disparities in the food environment surrounding US middle and high schools. *Public Health.* 2008;122(7):681-690
33. Kwate NO, Loh JM. Separate and unequal: the influence of neighborhood and school characteristics on spatial proximity between fast food and schools. *Prev Med.* 2010;51(2):153-156
34. Davis B, Carpenter C. Proximity of fast-food restaurants to schools and adolescent obesity. Disparities in the food environment surrounding US middle and high schools. *Am J Public Health.* 2009;99(3):505-510

35. Laska MN, Hearst MO, Forsyth A, Pasch KE, Lytle L. Neighbourhood food environments: are they associated with adolescent dietary intake, food purchases and weight status? *Public Health Nutr.* 2010;13(11):1757-1763
36. Galvez MP, Hong L, Choi E, Liao L, Godbold J, Brenner B. Childhood obesity and neighborhood food-store availability in an inner-city community. *Acad Pediatr.* 2009;9(5):339-343
37. Davis B, Carpenter C. Proximity of fast-food restaurants to schools and adolescent obesity. *Am J Public Health.* 2009;99:505-510
38. Harris JL, Schwartz MB, Brownell KD. *Fast Food FACTS.* New Haven, CT: Yale Rudd Center for Food Policy and Obesity; 2010
39. Food and Nutrition Service. Nutrition standards in the national school lunch and school breakfast programs. In: USDA, ed. Vol 77. Washington, D.C.: Federal Register; 2012:4088-4167
40. Eaton DK, Kann L, Kinchen S, et al. *Youth Risk Behavior Surveillance - United States, 2009.* Center for Disease Control and Prevention- Department of Health and Human Services; June 4, 2009
41. Kubik MY, Lytle L, Fulkerson JA. Fruits, vegetables, and football: Findings from focus groups with alternative high school students regarding eating and physical activity. *J Adolesc Health.* 2005;36(6):494-500
42. Fahlman MM, Hall HL, Lock R. Ethnic and socioeconomic comparisons of fitness, activity levels, and barriers to exercise in high school females. *J Sch Health.* 2006;76(1):12-17
43. Grieser M, Neumark-Sztainer DR, Saksvig BI, Lee J, Felton GM, Kubik M. Black, Hispanic, and white girls' perceptions of environmental and social support and enjoyment of physical activity. *J Sch Health.* 2008;78(6):314-320
44. Johnston LD, Delva J, OMalley PM. Sports participation and physical education in American secondary schools: current levels and racial/ethnic and socioeconomic disparities. *Am J Prev Med.* 2007;33(4 Suppl):S195-208
45. Agazzi H, Armstrong K, Bradley-Klug KL. BMI and physical activity among at-risk sixth- and ninth-grade students, Hillsborough County, Florida, 2005-2006. *Prev Chronic Dis.* 2010;7(3): 1-9
46. Activity NAfSaP. Physical Education Guidelines. 2012. Available at: http://www.aahperd.org/naspe/standards/nationalGuidelines/PEguidelines.cfm. Accessed July 3, 2012
47. Slater SJ, Nicholson L, Chriqui J, Turner L, Chaloupka F. The impact of state laws and district policies on physical education and recess practices in a nationally representative sample of US public elementary schools. *Arch Pediatr Adolesc Med.* 2012;166(4):311-316
48. Trost SG, Mars H. Why we should not cut P.E. *Edu Leadership.* 2009/2010;67(4):60-65
49. Trost SG. *Active Education: Physical Education, Physical Activity and Academic Performance.* Available at: http://www.activelivingresearch.org/activeeducation. Accessed November 8, 2012
50. Sallis JF, McKenzie TL, Kolody B, Lewis M, Marshall S, Rosengard P. Effects of health-related physical education on academic achievement - SPARK. *Res Q Exerc Sport.* 1999;70(2):127-134
51. Chomitz VR, Slining MM, McGowan RJ, Mitchell SE, Dawon GF, Hacker KA. Is there a relationship between physical fitness and academic achievement? Positive results from public school children in the northeastern United States. *J Sch Health.* 2009;79(1):30-37
52. Grissom JB. Physical fitness and academic achievement. *J Exerc Physiol.* 2005;8(1):11-25
53. Kwak L, Kremers SP, Bergman P, Ruiz JR, Rizzo NS, Sjostrom M. Associations between physical activity, fitness, and academic achievement. *J Pediatr.* 2009;155:914-918
54. Virgilio, SJ. The changing face of physical education. *Curriculum Rev.* 2009;48(7)
55. Schachter R. The new phys ed. *Instructor.* 2011;120(6):39-42
56. Warner L. A place for healthy risk-taking. *Edu Leadership.* 2009/2010;67(4)
57. McKenzie TL, Sallis JF, Rosengard P. Beyond the stucco tower: design, development, and dissemination of the SPARK physical education programs. *Quest.* 2009;61:114-127
58. Fuller D, Sabiston C, Karp I, Barnett T, O'Loughlin J. School sports opportunities influence physical activity in secondary school and beyond. *J Sch Health.* 2011;81(8):449-454
59. National Center for Safe Routes to School. *How Children Get to School: School Travel Patterns From 1969 to 2009.* 2011. Available at: http://www.saferoutesinfo.org/program-tools/NHTS-school-travel-1969-2009. Accessed October 3, 2012

60. Cowan D, Hubsmith D, Ping R. *Safe Routes to School Local Policy Guide.* 2011. Available at: www.saferoutespartnership.org/sites/default/files/pdf/local_policy_guide_2011.pdf. Accessed November 5, 2012
61. *Healthy People 2020- Phsyical Activity Objectives.* Washington, DC: U. S. Department of Health and Human Services; 2010
62. Kappagoda M, Ogilvie RS. *Playing Smart: Maximizing the Potential of School and Community Property through Joint Agreements.* Available at: http://americanindianhealthyeating.unc.edu/wp-content/uploads/2011/05/Playing_Smart-National_Joint_Use_Toolkit_FINAL_20120309.pdf. Accessed November 8, 2012
63. Farley TA, Meriwether RA, Baker ET, Watkins LT, Johnson CC, Webber LS. Safe play spaces to promote physical activity in inner-city children: results from a pilot study of an environmental intervention. *Am J Public Health.* 2007;97(9):1625-1631
64. Girls on the Run. 2012. Available at: http://www.girlsontherun.org/. Accessed August, 2012
65. American Heart Association. *Policy Position Statement of Body Mass Index (BMI) Surveillance and Assessment in Schools*; 2009
66. *Assessment of Childhood and Adolescent Obesity in Arkansas: Year Four (Fall 2006-Spring 2007).* Little Rock, AR: Arkansas Center for Health Improvement; 2007
67. *Year Three Report- Assessing the Impact of the Mississippi Healthy Students Act.* Jackson, MS: Center for Mississippi Health Policy; 2012. Available at: http://www.mshealthpolicy.com/assessing-the-impact-of-the-mississippi-healthy-students-act-on-childhood-obesity-2/. Accessed November 8, 2012
68. New York City Obesity Task Force. *Reversing the Epidemic: The New York City Obesity Task Force Plan to Prevent and Control Obesity.* New York: NY, Office of the Mayor; 2012
69. Neumark-Sztainer DR, Friend SE, Flattum CF, et al. New moves-preventing weight-related problems in adolescent girls a group-randomized study. *Am J Prev Med.* 2010;39(5):421-432
70. Chomitz VR, Collins J, Kim J, Kramer E, McGowan RJ. Promoting healthy weight among elementary school children via a health report card approach. *Arch Pediatr Adolesc Med.* 2003;157:765-772
71. Ikeda JP, Crawford PB, Woodward-Lopez G. BMI screening in schools: helpful or harmful? *Health Educ Res.* 2006;21(6):761-769
72. Presnell K, Bearman SK, Stice E. Risk factors for body dissatisfaction in adolescent boys and girls: a prospective study. *Int J Eat Disord.* 2004;36(4):389-401
73. Hesketh K, Wake M, Waters E. Body mass index and parent-reported self-esteem in elementary school children: evidence for a causal relationship. *Int J Obes Relat Metab Disord.* 2004;28(10):1233-1237
74. Harris JL, Weinberg ME, Schwartz MB, Ross C, Ostroff J, Brownell KD. *Trends in Television Food Advertising- Progress in Reducing Unhealthy Marketing to Young People?* New Haven, CT: Yale Rudd Center; 2010
75. Harris JL, Schwartz MB, Brownell KD, et al. *Sugary Drinks FACTS: Food Advertising to Children and Teens Score.* Rudd Center for Food Policy and Obesity. New Haven, CT: Yale University; 2011
76. Better Business Bureau Children's Food and Beverage Advertising Initiative. *Food and Beverage Products That Meet Participants' Approved Nutrition Standards*; 2011
77. Interagency Working Group. *Preliminary Proposed Nutrition Principles to Guide Industry Self-Regulatory Efforts*; 2011
78. Better Business Bureau Children's Food and Beverage Advertising Initiative. *General Comments and Comments on the Proposed Nutrition Principles and Marketing Definitions*; 2011
79. Steinberg L. Risk taking in adolescence: new perspectives from brain and behavioral science. *Cur Dir Psychol Sci.* 2007;16(2):55-59
80. Pollay RW, Siddarth S, Siegel M, et al. The last straw? Cigarette advertising and realized market shares among youths and adults, 1979-1993. *J Market.* 1996;60(April):1-16
81. Welsh JA, Sharma AJ, Grellinger L, Vos MB. Consumption of added sugars is decreasing in the United States. *Am J Clin Nutr.* 2011;94(3):726-734
82. Babey S, Jones M, Yu H, Goldstein H. *Bubbling Over: Soda Consumption and Its Link to Obesity in California.* Los Angeles, CA: UCLA Center for Health Policy Research and California Center for Public Health Advocacy; 2009

83. Chen L, Appel L, Loria C, Lin P, Champagne C, Elmer P. Reduction in consumption of sugar-sweetened beverages is associated with weight loss: the PREMIER trial. *Am J Clin Nutr.* 2009;89(5):1299-1306
84. Vartanian L, Schwartz MB, Brownell KD. Effects of soft drink consumption on nutrition and health: A systematic review and meta-analysis. *Am J Public Health.* 2007;97(4):667-675
85. Malik V, Schulze M, Hu F. Intake of sugar-sweetened beverages and weight gain: a systematic review. *Am J Clin Nutr.* 2006;82(4):274-288
86. Reedy J, Krebs-Smith SM. Dietary sources of energy, solid fats, and added sugars among children and adolescents in the United States. *J Am Diet Assoc.* 2010;110(10):1477-1484
87. *Alliance School Beverage Guidelines Final Progress Report.* American Beverage Association; 2010
88. Story, M, Klein, L. *Consumption of Sports Drinks by Children and Adolescents: A Research Review;* June 2012. Available at: http://www.healthyeatingresearch.org/images/stories/her_research_briefs/RRSportsDrinkFINAL6-2012.pdf. Accessed July 3, 2012
89. Ranjit N, Evans MH, Byrd-Williams C, Evans AE, Hoelscher DM. Dietary and activity correlates of sugar-sweetened beverage consumption among adolescents. *Pediatrics.* 2010;126(4):e754-761
90. Committee on Nutrition; Council on Sports Medicine. Sports drinks and energy drinks for children and adolescents: are they appropriate? *Pediatrics.* 2011;127(6):1182-1189
91. Fuhrman E. *Rush of Energy.* Beverage Industry. 2006. Available at: http://www.bevindustry.com/articles/rush-of-energy. Accessed July 3, 2012
92. Dinuzio J. Wary of energy drinks in an adrenaline sport. *The New York Times*; 2012. Available at: http://www.nytimes.com/2012/01/08/sports/pro-water-in-snowboarding-culture-heavy-on-energy-drinks.html. Accessed November 9, 2012
93. Harris JL, Schwartz MB, Brownell KD. *Sugary Drink FACTS.* Rudd Center for Food Policy and Obesity. New Haven, CT: Yale University; 2011
94. Higgins JP, Tuttle TD, Higgins CL. Energy beverages: content and safety. *Mayo Clin Proc.* 2010;85(11):1033-1041
95. O'Dea JA. Consumption of nutritional supplements among adolescents: usage and perceived benefits. *Health Educ Res.* 2003;18(1):98-107
96. Press A. Teens Abusing energy boosting drinks, doctors fear. *Fox News.* 2006. Available at: http://www.foxnews.com/story/0,2933,226223,00.html. Accessed July 3, 2012
97. Luebbe AM, Bell DJ. Mountain Dew or mountain don't?: a pilot investigation of caffeine use parameters and relations to depression and anxiety symptoms in 5th and 10th-grade students. *J Sch Health.* 2009;79(8):380-387
98. Kovacic WE, Harbour PJ, Leibowitz J, Rosch JT. *Marketing Food to Children and Adolescents: A Review of Industry Expenditures, Activities, and Self-Regulation.* Washington, DC: Federal Trade Commission; 2008
99. Heneman K, Zidenberg-Cherr S. *Nutrition and Health Info Sheet: Energy Drinks.* University of California; 2007
100. US Food and Drug Administration. Overview of Dietary Supplements. 2009. Available at: http://www.fda.gov/Food/Dietarysupplements/ConsumerInformation/default.htm. Accessed November 6, 2012
101. Center for Science in the Public Interest. Caffeine Content of Food & Drugs. 2007. Available at: http://www.cspinet.org/new/cafchart.htm: table_coffees. Accessed July 3, 2012
102. Thomson B, Scheiss S. *Risk Profile: Caffeine in Energy Drinks and Energy Shots.* Available at: http://www.foodsafety.govt.nz/elibrary/industry/Risk_Profile_Caffeine-Science_Research.pdf. Accessed November 8, 2012
103. Babu KM, Church RJ, Lewander W. Energy drinks: the new eye-opener for adolescents. *Clin Pediatr Emerg Med.* 2008;9:35-42
104. Rath M. Energy drinks: what is all the hype? The dangers of energy drink consumption. *J Am Acad Nurse Pract.* 2012;24(2):70-76
105. O'Connor E. A sip into dangerous territory. *Am Psychol.* 2001;32(6). Available at: http://www.apa.org/monitor/jun01/dangersip.aspx
106. Wolk BJ, Ganetsky M, Babu KM. Toxicity of energy drinks. *Curr Opin Pediatr.* 2012;24(2):243-251

107. Andreyeva T, Long MW, Brownell KD. The impact of food prices on consumption: a systematic review of research on the price elasticity of demand for food. *Am J Public Health.* 2010;100(2):216-222
108. Wagenaar AC, Salois MJ, Komro KA. Effects of beverage alcohol price and tax levels on drinking: a meta-analysis of 1003 estimates from 112 studies. *Addiction.* 2009;104(2):179-190
109. Yen ST, Lin B-H, Smallwood DM, Andrews M. Demand for nonalcoholic beverages: the case of low-income households. *Agribusiness.* 2004;20(3):309-321
110. Chaloupka F. Macro-social influences: the effects of prices and tobacco control policies on the demand for tobacco product. *Nicotine Tob Res.* 1999;1(1):S77-81
111. Friedman RR, Brownell KD. Sugar Sweetened Beverage Taxes: An Updated Policy Brief. Rudd Center for Food Policy and Obesity, New Haven, CT; Yale University; 2012
112. Brownell KD, Kersh R, Ludwig DS, et al. Personal responsibility and obesity: a constructive approach to a controversial issue. *Health Affairs.* 2010;29(3):379-387
113. Brownell KD, Horgen KB. *Food Fight: The Inside Story of the Food Industry, America's Obesity Crisis, And What We Can Do About It.* New York: McGraw-Hill; 2004

Adolesc Med 023 (2012) 610–630

Advances in Methodologies for Assessing Dietary Intake and Physical Activity among Adolescents

Amy L. Yaroch, PhD*[a,c], Carmen Byker, PhD[b], Courtney A. Pinard, PhD[a,c], Teresa M. Smith, MS[a,c]

[a]*Gretchen Swanson Center for Nutrition, 505 Durham Research Plaza, Omaha NE 68105*
[b]*Department of Health and Human Development, Montana State University, 222 Romney Gym, Bozeman MT 59718*
[c]*Department of Health Promotion, Social and Behavioral Health, University of Nebraska Medical Center, 984355 Nebraska Medical Center, Omaha NE 68198*

Overweight, poor diet, and inadequate physical activity (PA) affect adolescent physical, social, and emotional health in addition to increasing risks for chronic illnesses that were previously only diagnosed in adults, such as type 2 diabetes, cardiovascular disease, anemia, and dyslipidemia.[1] The prevalence of overweight or obesity among American adolescents has reached epidemic proportions with 33.6% of youth ages 12 to 19 years having a body mass index (BMI) at or greater than the 85th percentile for age and sex.[2] An energy imbalance and subsequent health problems occur as a result of behavioral choices—either when excess energy is ingested or not enough energy is expended—resulting in obesity.[3] With less than 1 in 10 adolescents meeting the daily fruit or vegetable recommendations,[4] this and similar poor dietary habits can be attributed to behavioral and environmental factors.[5] Alternatively, adolescents sometimes succumb to social pressures to skip meals (in particular, breakfast), intending to improve physique through altered eating patterns and experimentation with alternative or fad diets.[6] In today's society, maintaining a healthful diet is difficult for adolescents because food environments (eg, school and home) increasingly promote the availability, access, and allure of less healthful foods and sedentary behaviors—together these factors are commonly referred to as an obesogenic environment.[7] Referred to as Generation Z, the Net Generation, or the Multitasking Generation, adolescents of today are characterized by their frequent use of technology for communication, work, and

*Corresponding author.
E-mail address: ayaroch@centerfornutrition.org (A. L. Yaroch).

 ISSN 1934-4287

free time activities. This poses a challenge as the use of computers, video games, and other electronic devices can contribute to a sedentary lifestyle[8] and potentially increase exposure to marketing[9] of less healthful foods.

To address these types of risks for chronic diseases related to poor diet and physical inactivity, intervention should occur early and often. Adolescence is a particularly important period during which to intervene, and physicians can play a key role in promoting healthy behaviors. A nutrient-dense diet is essential for adolescents, as rapid physiological changes demand increased levels of vitamins and minerals, protein, and energy.[7] In a time during the lifespan where several bodily changes are occurring, increased participation in PA (eg, competitive sports) places extra demand on adolescent nutrient requirements. The dietary and PA habits formed during adolescence may also carry forward into adulthood.[10] The authority of the physician and the relationships developed with patients present an ideal opportunity to counsel adolescents about diet and PA. In their Guidelines for Adolescent Preventive Services (GAPS), the American Medical Association (AMA) articulates "adolescents should receive health guidance annually about dietary habits, including the benefits of a healthy diet, and ways to achieve a healthy diet and safe weight management" and "adolescents should receive health guidance annually about the benefits of PA and should be encouraged to engage in safe physical activities on a regular basis."[11]

Assessing dietary intake and PA status is an essential first step to helping adolescent patients adopt lifelong health behaviors and weight management strategies.[12] To facilitate the assessment of diet and PA and subsequently promote healthy weight management and obesity prevention, physicians need a "toolbox" of assessment strategies. Given the variation in health care settings with regard to resources, structure, and goals, it is useful to have a wide range of diet and PA assessment strategies from which physicians can choose the methods most applicable to them and their adolescent patients. This article describes existing methodologies and examines advancements in methods for assessing dietary intake and PA among adolescents. Advancements in methodologies are described with regard to their utility to the physician, focusing first on diet and then PA. Recommended strategies for monitoring patient diet and PA status are provided, with consideration of the potential needs, resources, and abilities in a health care setting.

WHY MEASURE DIET AND PHYSICAL ACTIVITY?

It is important to assess dietary and PA behaviors to help youth achieve recommended guidelines and promote good health. Individualized assessment results can provide a platform for educating adolescents about making lifestyle choices that decrease health risks for chronic diseases, many of which have dietary and PA behaviors as their determinants. Each method of dietary and PA assessment has advantages and limitations that are outlined in Table 1 (diet assessment methods) and Table 2 (PA assessment methods). The tables also include an

Table 1
Subjective Dietary Assessment Methods

Method	Main Advantages	Main Limitations	Resources*	Select Recent Advances
Gold Standard Methods				
24-Hour Dietary Recall *A structured interview in which a trained professional or automated system asks the respondent to list everything they ate and/or drank during the previous 24 hours*[13]	Automated as alternative to interviewer-administered Information captured after eating behaviors occur, introducing less bias Free software available	Cognitive influences may interfere with accurate reporting At least 3 recalls are needed to measure typical diet Moderate respondent burden	\$-\$\$\$\$ 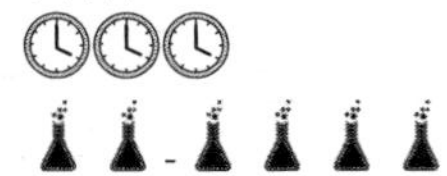	*ASA24*[14] *PACE+*[15]
Diet Record *Written account of actual food and beverages consumed during a specified time period, usually for 3, 5, or 7 days*[13]	More quantitatively accurate when compared to other methods Foods recorded as consumed More accurate portion sizes compared to other methods	Requires literate and motivated respondents High respondent burden	\$\$\$ 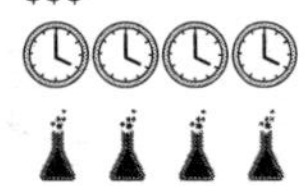	*DIFR*[16] *HEST*[17,18]
Other Subjective Methods				
Diet History *Report on past diet, usually conducted by a trained dietitian who provides cognitive support*[13]	Assesses usual meal patterns and details of food intake Can estimate effects of foods consumed together Provides cognitive support for respondents	Higher respondent and interviewer burden Difficult for respondents who "graze" Trained personnel typically needs to administer	\$\$\$ 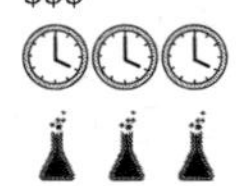	

Food Frequency Questionnaires (FFQs) *Tool used to collect consumption frequency for a specified list of food and beverage items consumed within a reference time period*[13]	Can be used to rank individuals based on reported intake Can be self-administered Typically lower cost and less respondent burden	Only rank level information Intake tends to be overestimated with longer FFQs and underestimated with shorter FFQs Serving size and foods in mixtures difficult to capture	$-$$ 🕒-🕒🕒 ⚗-⚗⚗	*FFQ W82*[19] *Adolescent FFQ*[20] *Web-based FFQ for food group intake*[21]
Dietary Screeners *Brief tools useful in situations when quantitative accuracy and total dietary intake are not needed*[13]	Useful when time and resources are limited Determine if individuals warrant additional assessment Captures patterns of intake	Does not assess total diet Only gives snapshot information	$ 🕒 ⚗	*Fast food and beverage consumption*[22] *NYPANS*[23]

*Cost, time, and materials needed to administer the method of assessment are represented by:
Cost = $ to $$$$; inexpensive to very expensive
Time = 🕒 to 🕒🕒🕒🕒; not time intensive to very time intensive
Materials = ⚗ to ⚗⚗⚗⚗; not resource intensive to very resource intensive
Note: The table is organized so that the tools listed first are considered to have higher validity and reliability, and those further down the list may have greater feasibility because of lower cost and need for resources and materials.

Table 2
Physical Activity Assessment Methods

Method	Main Advantages	Main Limitations	Resources*	Select Recent Advances
Objective Methods				
Accelerometers *Devices that measure accelerations produced by body movement and provide output of minutes in sedentary, light, moderate, and vigorous activity; steps; or activity counts, in up to 3 axes*[24]	Objective assessment Small and unobtrusive Can capture the intermittent activity patterns characteristic of adolescents	Variability because of use of different brands, placement (eg, hip), and specific activities performed Lack of sensitivity to certain types of activity Costly	$$$$ 🕒🕒🕒 ⚗⚗⚗⚗	Mathematical models to distinguish between specific types of activities[25]
Heart Rate Monitoring *Monitoring devices that allow measurement in real time or recording of heart rate for later study. The output is typically time spent in beats per minute (BPM) range*[26]	Unobtrusive Low participant and investigator burden Inexpensive for smaller studies relative to other objective methods	Does not provide robust assessment of sedentary or light activities Emotions, stimulants, and drugs can change heart rate May mask sporadic activity	$$$ 🕒🕒 ⚗⚗⚗	
Pedometers *Simple electronic devices used to estimate mileage walked or the number of steps taken over a period of time*[24]	Objective assessment Most inexpensive objective method Easy to obtain	Only detects total counts or steps; cannot assess the intensity or pattern of activities performed Lack of sensitivity to certain types of activity	$-$$ 🕒🕒 ⚗⚗	Native applications on smartphones that incorporate pedometry[27]
Global Positioning System (GPS) *A satellite-based system that can provide information on a person's location, neighborhood context, mode of transportation, and speed of locomotion*[28]	Can help advance our understanding of PA through technology	Complexity of data collection, processing, and analysis High equipment costs and erroneous signals Limited to assessment of outdoor activities with "visible" sky	$-$$$ 🕒🕒🕒 ⚗⚗⚗	Now embedded in some cell phones
Subjective Methods				
Direct observation *Systematic observation guided by a checklist or other recording tool to collect real time PA levels*[24,29-31]	Appropriate for adolescents who have difficulty with reporting and other techniques Captures sporadic play and activities that may not be detected by other methods	High observer burden Potential reactivity of study respondents	$$ 🕒🕒🕒🕒 ⚗⚗⚗	

Self-report Surveys *Paper/pencil or Web-based surveys that require respondents to recall information on PA levels*[24,32-43]	Inexpensive across a large number of respondents Low administrative burden	Sporadic nature of children's activity makes it difficult to recall Social desirability bias Decreased ability to measure "usual" PA surveys	\$-\$\$ 🕓 - 🕓🕓🕓 ⚗ - ⚗⚗	*IPAQ*[44] PAQ-A[38,39] *NYPANS*[23]
Interview *Researcher or physician administered interviews that ask respondents to recall PA levels*[31]	Inexpensive across a large number of respondents Low investigator burden Interview method may improve a respondent's cognition and accuracy	Sporadic nature of adolescent's activity makes it difficult to recall Social desirability bias Decreased ability to measure "usual" PA	\$\$ 🕓🕓🕓 ⚗⚗⚗	
Diary *A self-report method that asks respondents to report PA in real time*[31]	Inexpensive across a large number of respondents Low investigator burden	High participant burden Low accuracy in report of children and adolescents	\$\$ 🕓🕓🕓🕓 ⚗⚗⚗	
Ecological Momentary Assessment (EMA) *Through electronic surveys delivered on mobile phones, respondents can report their activity type and their physical and social context*[45-47]	Assesses full range of settings in which adolescents are physically active Reduces distortion caused by recall bias Capitalizes on technology familiar to Generation Z adolescents	Costly Nonresponse because of frequent prompts Participant burden	\$\$\$ 🕓🕓🕓 ⚗⚗⚗⚗	

*Cost, time, and materials needed to administer the method of assessment are represented by:
Cost = \$ to \$\$\$\$; inexpensive to very expensive
Time = 🕓 to 🕓🕓🕓🕓; not time intensive to very time intensive
Materials = ⚗ to ⚗⚗⚗⚗; not resource intensive to very resource intensive
Note: The table is organized so that the tools listed first are considered to have higher validity and reliability, and those further down the list may have greater feasibility because of lower cost and need for resources and materials.

estimation of time, resources, and equipment needed to conduct each technique, as well as a brief outline of novel approaches available.

CRITERION STANDARDS FOR OBJECTIVE DIET AND PA ASSESSMENT

The criterion standard measures of diet and PA include doubly labeled water and indirect calorimetry.[48,49] These 2 laboratory methods are resource intensive and are often used to validate less intensive methods. The doubly labeled water technique tracks carbon dioxide and water produced during PA, in comparison to calories consumed, to calculate differences between isotope elimination rates. This technique can be carried out on a wide range of individuals over lengthy periods, usually between 4 and 21 days, capturing habitual energy consumption and expenditure patterns. The measure has been considered a criterion standard for more than 30 years; however, it is also typically cost prohibitive and the materials (eg, isotopes) are difficult to obtain. Indirect calorimetry is a technique that provides accurate estimates of energy expenditure from measures of carbon dioxide production and oxygen consumption during rest and steady-state exercise. Indirect calorimetry is carried out on an individual basis, which makes it fairly time-consuming (eg, 1-5 hours). Although some health care settings may have access to indirect calorimetry equipment, it may be time prohibitive, in addition to incurring a high participant burden. Therefore, these methods are not necessarily recommended for use by physicians, but they are described here because they are the criterion standard measures in both diet and PA assessment.

SUBJECTIVE DIETARY INTAKE ASSESSMENT METHODS

Subjective (or self-report) dietary intake assessments are more feasible than the criterion standard measures described earlier and can be tailored to physician and patient needs. Traditional methodologies for assessing dietary intake are highly developed and tested, but can be resource intensive with results that may not represent average intake. Novel methods are available, but may not be as well developed or tested. However, novel methods are potentially less resource intensive with a focus on specific patient needs. Although several assessment methods exist, each fills a particular niche in understanding patient diet. The physician should first decide what type of dietary information they think is optimal or feasible to collect (eg, caloric and nutrient intake, specific food groups, recent or long-term intake, etc.) and then choose the appropriate tool. Traditional approaches include 24-hour dietary recalls, diet records, diet histories, food frequency questionnaires (FFQs), and dietary screeners. Novel methods and advances tend to be adaptations of the traditional methods and fit within these categories. Table 1 may be used to help navigate the nuances of each method and its appropriateness for health care setting use.

Subjective Dietary Assessment Methods: Gold Standards

The 24-hour dietary recall is a structured interview where a trained professional or automated program guides the respondent to list all foods and beverages consumed during the previous 24 hours. This method requires a moderate amount of time to complete (eg, 20-30 minutes per recall) but involves less participant burden when compared to other comprehensive methods, such as the diet history or diet record[13] because it only requires the respondent to recall foods and drinks consumed in the past day. Because the tool collects information in reference to a specific day, reported intake may or may not be representative of normal dietary patterns because of day-to-day variability in diet. Therefore, at least 3 recalls are recommended to obtain estimates of usual individual-level intake, increasing burden on respondents and physicians.[50]

The Automated Self-Administered 24-Hour Recall (ASA24) is a Web-based 24-hour dietary recall that guides respondents through several audio and visual prompts.[14] The computer program asks respondents about meals consumed in the past 24 hours; contains probes for foods and beverages consumed between meals; and obtains details about each food and beverage (eg, serving size and preparation method), forgotten items, and usual intakes. Adolescents with higher literacy levels should be able to complete the ASA24. Further, ASA24 data can be collected in English and Spanish and are available for use free of charge for researchers, physicians, and others.

Diet record is a method where the respondent provides a written account of actual foods and beverages consumed during a specified time period, usually for 3, 5, or 7 days.[13] The diet record works best for highly motivated, literate populations because it requires respondents to record all the foods and beverages and amounts typically consumed over several days, making it time intensive and burdensome, particularly for adolescents.[13] There is also an additional burden on physicians who need to plan appropriate strategies to administer, collect, and review diet records.

The digital image-based food record (DIFR) is a novel diet record in which photographs are taken of food and beverage items before and after eating. Analysts then view the photos and use visuals aids to help judge portion size and estimate the amount of food and beverage that was consumed.[16] The DIFR has been found to produce reliable results similar to a traditional diet record. Adolescents may prefer the DIFR[16] because it uses interactive technology. Although this method was developed and assessed in a researcher-administered setting, physicians may adapt it for a clinical setting by encouraging adolescents to take pictures of their meals and snacks (before and after), using a camera or phone, and bring photos in for a follow-up session.

The Healthy Eating Self-Monitoring Tool (HEST) is a computer-mediated diet record designed to assess fruit and vegetable intake.[17,18] It guides respondents through 3 screens to record fruit, juice, and vegetable intake. Respondents could complete the HEST while in the waiting room or with the assistance of the physician. The tool has been assessed for criterion validity among black adolescents, and it was determined to be a viable alternative to a traditional diet record.[17,18]

Subjective Dietary Assessment Methods: Other Methods

Diet history is a tool that asks the respondents to report usual food intake over an extended period of time. A trained professional typically conducts an interview to provide cognitive support to probe for food preparation methods and intake patterns. This method can be highly burdensome to the respondent, as well as resource intensive[13] because the respondent must cognitively recall foods and drinks eaten over several days in the past.

Food frequency questionnaires (FFQs) assess frequency of consumption of foods and beverages from a specified list of food/beverage items for a specified time period. They can be interviewer- or self-administered by various modes (scannable response form, paper and pencil, Internet, etc.).[13] Variations of FFQs have been developed to assess dietary intake among adolescents and most have shown reasonably good validity and/or reliability estimates.[20,51-53] However, this method only grossly represents usual dietary intake because it has substantial error associated with it. The FFQ provides minimal information when compared to the gold standard methods, but it has the added advantage of relatively low participant burden[13] and administration can be computerized, making this a more feasible approach for assessing major dietary patterns in adolescents.[54,55] Koldziejcyk et al reviewed child and adolescent FFQ studies published from 2001 to 2010 and found higher validity estimates compared with the referent method when portion sizes were not assessed, a shorter span of time was measured, the FFQ contained 20 to 60 items, and the FFQ was not administered to a parent as proxy.[56]

The FFQW82 is a self-administered 82-item FFQ that assesses intake frequency and portion size over a 1-month period from a list of pictured foods and can be completed in 30 mintues.[19] The FFQW82 was recently adapted for an adolescent population and was determined to be reliable and valid for estimating energy and nutrient intake compared with a diet record when evaluated among Japanese females ages 12 to 13 years.[19]

A novel, self-administered, Web-based FFQ used for measuring average consumption for 15 food groups during the past month was recently evaluated by conducting a cross-sectional validation, and it was found that the assessment was valid and reliable in an adolescent population from Belgium (ages 12 to 18 years).[21] Web-based assessments are useful because they can be accessed quickly from several locations and are delivered in a way that is familiar to Generation Z.

Dietary screeners are brief surveys that typically obtain information about patterns of behaviors or focus on a particular food group (such as fruits and vegetables, fast foods, various types of beverages, etc.). They do not estimate calories and nutrient values but rather obtain gross level estimates of intake for a particular food/beverage or food group. Screeners can be useful when patterns of dietary behaviors are of interest, but limited time or funds are available. There are a few select dietary screeners that have recently been found to be reliable or valid for adolescent populations.[22,57-59]

The Dietary Screener Questionnaire is a 26-item dietary screener that was developed for use in conjunction with the National Health and Nutrition Examination Survey (NHANES) to assess frequency of consumption in the past month of selected foods and beverages, including intakes of fruits and vegetables, dairy/calcium, whole grains/fiber, added sugars, red meat, and processed meat.[60] This dietary screener allows important dietary groups to be assessed in a short amount of time. This screener has been further modified for high school-aged students for the National Youth Physical Activity and Nutrition Study (NYPANS).[23] The dietary screener portion consists of 16 items, making it easy to administer for general information on dietary patterns.

PHYSICAL ACTIVITY ASSESSMENT METHODS

As described earlier for dietary assessment, assessment of PA also varies. The methodologies differ in the output (eg, Metabolic Equivalent of Tasks [METs], energy expenditure, steps, heart rate, minutes of activity, or general scores of activity level), the cost and other administration needs, and the advantages and limitations. Each method also has varying levels of validity and reliability. The selection of a given method to assess PA depends on the type of information sought, planned use of data, and acceptable burden (eg, respondent, cost, staff resources, etc.); Table 2 may be used to help navigate the nuances of each method and its appropriateness for health care setting use. Traditional approaches have been categorized here as *Objective Monitoring Tools* and *Subjective Measures*. Unlike dietary assessment, novel methods and advances of PA tend to be completely new technologies that cannot be considered adaptations of traditional methods, thus they are discussed next in separate categories.

Objective Monitoring Tools for PA Assessment

Objective monitoring tools include instruments such as pedometers, accelerometers, and heart rate monitors. These methods provide some level of objectivity, but still have bias associated with their use. For example, all monitoring tools are limited in the types of activity that they can capture and may not be considered ideal for capturing the sporadic nature of youth PA. Further, because the devices must be worn, respondents may choose not to wear them and in other cases may be unable to wear the tool during performance of certain activities (eg, swimming).[27]

Accelerometers are small, unobtrusive instruments worn on the trunk and/or limbs that monitor the intensity of body mass movements in up to 3 planes. Those that capture movement in 2 or 1 plane(s) are more limited in their ability to detect movement associated with activities such as swimming and biking.[61] Accelerometers are considered the most accurate of the monitoring tools and are used extensively, particularly in small and medium-sized research studies. Accelerometers are relatively expensive, making them less feasible for physicians to give to patients to obtain PA estimates. One novel advance made with the use of accelerometers is the use of mathematical models to distinguish between 2 activities that produce similar total acceleration over time, but have different energy costs.[25]

Heart rate monitors are small, unobtrusive instruments that measure electrical activity of the heart. Instrument refinements over the past 20 years have resulted in heart rate monitors that can record and store data in 15-second to 1-minute time intervals, for up to several days, and can be downloaded to a computer.[26] Heart rate monitors are slightly lower in cost than accelerometers; however, values can be influenced by emotions and stimulants.[26]

Pedometers are small, belt-mounted devices primarily used for quantifying the daily number of counts (eg, steps) accumulated. Total daily steps can be compared to current PA recommendations and classifications (eg, adolescents obtaining 10,000-11,700 steps/day also meet the recommendations for moderate-to-vigorous PA).[62] Pedometers are the least cost-prohibitive of the monitoring tools, but are limited to capturing 1 dimension of movement, so are not suited for activities such as swimming and biking.[27]

Subjective Tools for PA Assessment: Direct Observation

Direct observation includes measurement tools that guide observers through a standardized approach to monitoring PA levels. This method has been most used in school settings to monitor the PA levels of groups of children or adolescents (eg, a researcher could develop a protocol to observe PA levels during physical education courses).[29] The benefit of direct observation includes the ability to garner more contextually rich data in the setting in which the activity occurs,[30] as well as having a more reliable and valid report of PA when compared to self-report methods.[24] The drawback is the potential reactivity of adolescents in response to being observed (eg, adolescents may perform more PA in response to being observed), as well as increased time and burden on the observer(s).[31]

Subjective Tools for PA Assessment: Surveys, Interviews, and Diaries

PA surveys are practical, subjective recall instruments that vary in detail, type of activity assessed, reference periods, administration mode, required completion time, targeted population, and how respondents are classified.[24] However, because of their subjective nature, these instruments are inherently limited by factors such as recall error, social desirability or gender bias, floor and ceiling effects, misinterpretation of terminology, and the failure of some surveys to quantify the totality of PA dimensions and contexts.[24,32] Despite these limitations, a plethora of surveys exist and many have already been successfully tested in comparison to criterion standards and accelerometry in children and adolescents.[33-35] Additionally, surveys can be used in conjunction with objective monitoring tools to obtain more complete information on PA among adolescents. Some advantages to using self-report surveys include their low cost, applicability to a wide range of ages, ability to collect data from a large number of respondents, suitability for multiple modes of administration (eg, face-to-face, mailed, etc.) and adaptability to fit the needs of a particular population or research question.[36,37] Two PA surveys to note include the International Physical Activity Questionnaire (IPAQ) and Physical Activity Questionnaire for Adolescents (PAQ-A).[38,39] The IPAQ has been used extensively to assess PA across countries, as well as age, sex, and other sociodemographic factors.[39] The PAQ-A has been validated in numerous adolescent populations.[40-42] In addition, the NYPANS, mentioned earlier for diet, also includes 10 items assessing PA behaviors. So when combined, the NYPANS diet and PA screeners are easy to administer to obtain general information on both dietary and PA patterns.[43]

The interview format is similar to the self-report survey, except that the researcher asks the respondent a series of questions about their PA level. The benefit of an interview over a self-report format is that probing may improve the adolescent's cognition and accuracy.[31] Another survey option is a proxy report, which allows parents or teachers to report on the PA level of the adolescent. Proxy report may be most appropriate for younger children and adolescents with disabilities, but it is subject to the bias of the proxy person reporting because they might not know all the PA behaviors that occurred for the child or adolescent.[31]

The diary method of assessing PA is similar to the diet record method for assessing dietary patterns, but requires the respondent to record PA that they are engaging in throughout the day. Few studies have utilized the diary method for calculating PA among youth. However, those that have tested the validity among youth have been found to be useful for assessing total energy expenditure when activity is reported accurately.[31] However, because of the relatively high participant burden and challenges with accuracy in reporting in real world settings, the diary method may not be as feasible for use by physicians.[31]

Advances in PA Methodology

Most of the novel methods and advances in PA assessment described next capitalize on new technologies and cannot be considered adaptations of traditional methods. Although many have not been tested among adolescents, Generation Z may appreciate the advancements of methods in recent years given the utilization of familiar communication technology.

Ecological momentary assessment (EMA) is a novel method that involves respondents recording information on smartphones and other devices after receiving prompts. EMA has been applied to several fields, including psychopharmacology, eating disorders, and more recently to PA assessment.[45,46,63,64] Through electronic surveys delivered on the display screen of mobile phones or other network-connected devices, adolescents can report where and with whom they are currently engaging in PA, as well as how they perceive those settings. For example, an adolescent might receive a prompt 2 to 4 times daily asking them to report their current activity level, social context, physical context, and perceived characteristics (eg, safety, positive or negative attributes) of that location. Benefits of EMA include its ability to assess a full range of settings in which adolescents may be physically active and reduce distortion caused by recall bias by simultaneously capturing a behavior and the factors that may influence it.[46,47]

Global positioning system (GPS) involves a satellite-based system that can provide information on a person's location, neighborhood context, mode of transportation, and speed of locomotion,[28] and is often integrated into a smartphone. The major benefit of monitoring PA in youth using GPS technology is that adolescents may already carry a smartphone, and GPS provides an objective assessment of their activity.[28] However, the technology relies on "visible sky" and may be limited by other smartphone related issues (eg, power loss, erroneous signal).[28]

ADVANCES IN COMBINED DIET AND PA ASSESSMENT

Patient-centered Assessment and Counseling for Exercise plus Nutrition (*PACE+*) is a novel, computer-based dietary and PA program with an innovative measurement component that was developed for adolescents and adults. The *PACE+* program provides an interactive FFQ administered in the clinic waiting room.[15] Patients complete an individualized health behavior screener that is sent to the physician before the appointment, who can then tailor the message to the patient to encourage healthier eating, PA, or other lifestyle behaviors. The *PACE+* program was tested in health care settings in 2006 and found to be acceptable by participants.[15,65] In addition to *PACE+*, kiosks have been used in waiting rooms to assess both diet and PA behaviors, and tailor weight management messages based on participant response.[66,67] This integrated method of assessment may be more of a "one-stop shop" that physicians may want to consider implementing in their practice.

TOOLS FOR THE PHYSICIAN

Figure 1 summarizes how to select a dietary assessment method for the diagnosis and prevention of a variety of diet-related conditions among adolescents. Specifically, when more detailed information is needed for diet-related concerns such as food allergies or sensitivities, digestive diseases, and in some cases for weight and obesity, gold standard measures such as multiple 24-hour dietary recalls and diet records are recommended for their ability to generate more discrete information about caloric intake, as well as macro- and micronutrient intakes. Whereas for other situations such as obesity and chronic disease prevention, other subjective methods to assess diet may be more appropriate to determine dietary patterns for a respondent (eg, intakes of certain food grouping such as fruits and vegetables or sugar-sweetened beverage intake) rather than assessing the comprehensive diet.

Another tool is covered in Figure 2, which describes each of the dietary and PA assessment methodologies in terms of resource intensity, validity and reliability, feasibility of administration, and specificity of the assessment. Not surprisingly, methods that generally have higher validity and reliability are also typically more time-intensive and costly. Methodologies that generally have lower validity and reliability associated with their use also tend to be more feasible to implement in a wider range of settings/populations, and can have greater specificity in terms of food groups or types of PA to be assessed. For example, if a physician is

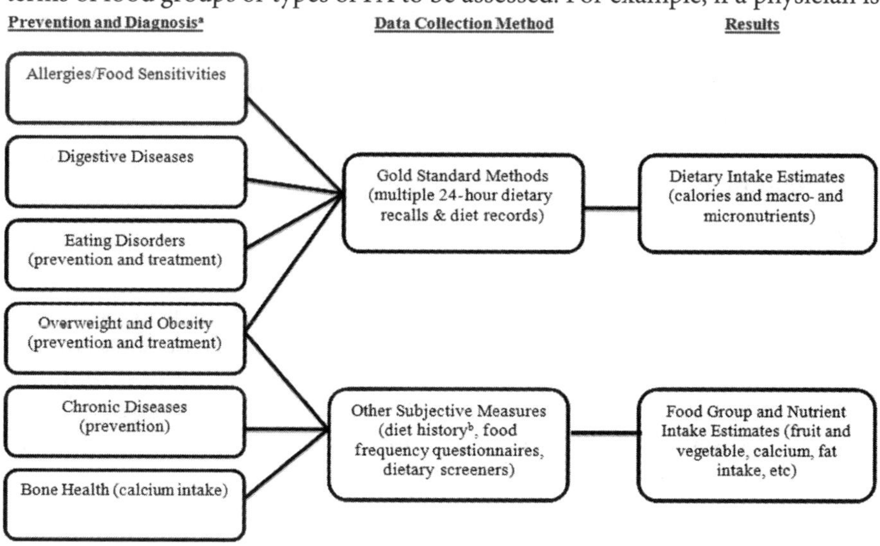

Fig 1. Diagnosis and Prevention of Diet-Related Diseases in the Adolescent Population. [a]Categories adapted from USDA National Agricultural Library Diet and Disease Food and Nutrition Information Center. Available at: http://fnic.nal.usda.gov/diet-and-disease.
[b]Note: Diet History does provide some quantitative information but is not considered as valid and reliable as the gold standard methods. Other subjective measures such as Food Frequency Questionnaires and Dietary Screeners provide rank order and other less specific estimates.

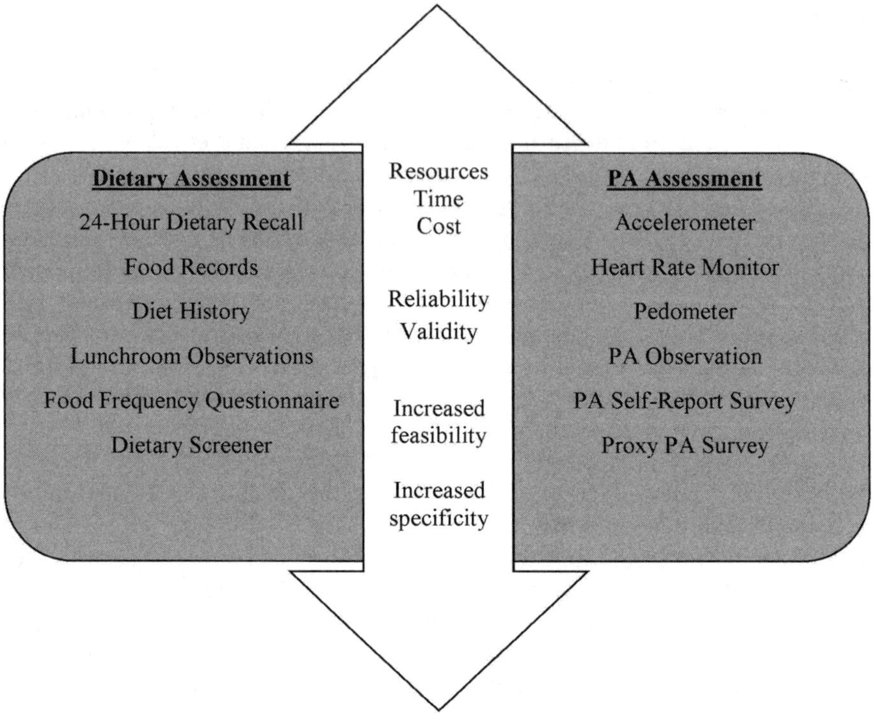

Fig 2. Considerations when choosing diet and/or physical activity (PA) assessment methods

actively conducting research or evaluating a program, they may want to choose a more comprehensive diet or PA assessment method with stronger validity and reliability. Alternatively, if the intent is to assess dietary or PA patterns for patient counseling, they may prefer a simple, short method to administer.

DISCUSSION

The purpose of this article is to describe the various methods for assessment of diet and PA among adolescents and to highlight advances in both fields. Numerous techniques exist to measure diet and PA, requiring varying levels of resources for administration, taking into account both physician and participant burden. These methods are described with regard to major advantages and limitations, resource intensiveness, and advances for dietary methods (see Table 1) and PA methods (see Table 2). The gold standards for diet and PA assessment are recommended first, with the caveat that they require more resources and time. Physicians may want to use these comprehensive methods when considering food allergies, drug interactions, PA implications, and other factors important to patient care. However, acknowledging time and money constraints in the health care setting, more comprehensive measures may not be feasible, but screeners or other self-report measures for diet and PA may still yield useful information for the physician and patient, especially with regard to the prevention or treatment of chronic diseases.

Monitoring and achieving behavior change and subsequent healthy weight management is difficult at best, no matter the tool, research angle, or robustness of the investigation. Contento et al found that a minimum of 12 to 15 hours of education begins to change behavior.[68] Therefore, longer time frames are needed to make and observe some of these changes, so physicians may want to consider evaluating some more short-term outcomes (eg, self-efficacy, knowledge, social support)[69] or recommending patients in serious need of treatment to consult with a specialist (eg, registered dietitian or personal trainer). Although there are several choices for prevention, diagnosis, and treatment in the PA and diet arenas, the physician should find methods appropriate to the health care setting and patient needs.

For PA, objective and subjective tools are beneficial for tracking the prevention and treatment of weight-related and chronic diseases correlated with inactivity. Traditional heart rate monitors, pedometers, and accelerometers capture movement for several activities, but may not be time- or cost-effective for the physician. There are several self-report measures that can capture the patient's PA status while at the clinic, but bring potential reporting biases. Direct-observation of PA may be out of the scope of the physician, but they can recommend tools for parents to track their adolescent's PA status. Although not scientifically tested, smartphone applications (usually using GPS technologies) exist that capture movement for patients that own such devices and can be recommended for use in conjunction with PA goals.

Physicians looking for technological advancements for tracking dietary and PA behaviors may want to consider the myriad smartphone applications or native applications (apps) that are currently available and continue to emerge on a daily basis. Although these apps are typically not theory driven or evidence-based,[70] physicians are encouraged to search for apps that they think would be useful for their patients.[71] Some of these apps have costs associated with their use, while others are free, and they are available for variety of smartphones (e.g., BlackBerry, Android, iPhone). These apps can be optimized when they are used alongside clinical supervision. Although it is outside of the scope of this article to review a comprehensive list of apps, we have listed some that may be appropriate for use among adolescents, along with their descriptions, in Table 3. In addition, with regard to technology, along with the more traditional kiosks,[72] iPads and other tablets present new opportunities to obtain both diet and PA self-report information in office waiting rooms as they become more ubiquitous and less costly.[66,67] To capitalize on the versatility and applicability of tablet and kiosk technology, physicians may implement screeners and other less comprehensive diet and PA assessment methodologies via these technologies in waiting rooms. However, self-report measures could also be administered fairly easily in paper and pencil format, if technologies are not an option.

Table 3
Select Smartphone Applications

Name	Description	Physical Activity	Dietary Intake
Fooducate[73]	Adolescent uses phone to scan the barcode of foods and is given recommendations for alternative healthier food options		X
MyFitnessPal[74]	A self-report diet and PA journal that tracks calories and nutrients and offers a companion Web site	X	X
Weight Watchers[75]	Available for *Weight Watchers* members with portions available for nonmembers; allows the user to track dietary intake, PA, and body weight	X	X
SmartDiet[76]	Analyzes daily nutrient intake and patterns of daily exercise and has been shown to assist in weight loss in obese adults	X	X
MapMyFitness[77]	Offers the ability to track running, cycling, walking, or hiking routes using the built-in GPS of associated smartphones	X	
FitnessBuilder[78]	Allows the user to find workouts and fitness plans, build their workouts, and track and share their workouts	X	
iTreadmill[79]	Uses a "Dial-Pacer," which uses advanced signal processing to accurately monitor motion and measure parametrics, acting as a pedometer	X	

CONCLUSIONS

Although many advances have emerged to assess diet and PA among adolescents, new or modified methods are still warranted because practical, easy to administer methods typically have low validity or reliability, or have not been formally evaluated. Physicians are encouraged to incorporate some level of assessment into their practice, whether for the purpose of engaging in collaborative and robust research or simply to aid in the counseling and translation of recommendations on diet and PA to adolescents. By using assessment of diet and PA as a platform for prevention, diagnosis, and treatment of related disorders, positive health outcomes can be promoted for the adolescent into adulthood.

ACKNOWLEDGEMENTS

The authors would like to thank Frank Perna, EDD, PhD, and Genevieve Dunton, PhD, for their contribution of research resources to our manuscript.

References

1. Daniels S. The consequences of childhood overweight and obesity. *Future Child.* 2006;16(1):47-67
2. Ogden CL, Carroll MD, Kit BK, Flegal KM. Prevalence of obesity and trends in body mass index among US children and adolescents, 1999-2010. *JAMA.* 2012;307(5):483-490

3. Centers for Disease Control and Prevention. Obesity and Overweight for Professionals: Causes and Consequences. Available at: http://www.cdc.gov/obesity/causes/index.html. Accessed March 29, 2012
4. Kimmons J, Gillespie C, Seymour J, Serdula M, Blanck HM. Fruit and vegetable intake among adolescents and adults in the United States: percentage meeting individualized recommendations. *Medscape J Med.* 2009;11(1):26
5. Spiotta RT, Luma GB. Evaluating obesity and cardiovascular risk factors in children and adolescents. *Am Fam Physician.* 2008;78(9):1052-1058
6. Rampersaud GC, Pereira MA, Girard BL, Adams J, Metzl JD. Breakfast habits, nutritional status, body weight, and academic performance in children and adolescents. *J Am Diet Assoc.* 2005;105(5):743-760; quiz 761-762
7. Committee on Prevention of Obesity in Children and Youth. *Preventing Childhood Obesity: Health in the Balance.* Koplan JP, Liverman CT, Kraak VA, eds. Washington, DC: The National Academies Press; 2005
8. Utter J, Neumark-Sztainer D, Jeffery R, Story M. Couch potatoes or french fries: are sedentary behaviors associated with body mass index, physical activity, and dietary behaviors among adolescents? *J Am Diet Assoc.* 2003;103(10):1298-1305
9. Harris JL, Pomeranz JL, Lobstein T, Brownell KD. A crisis in the marketplace: how food marketing contributes to childhood obesity and what can be done. *Annu Rev Public Health.* 2009;30:211-225
10. Lee YS. Consequences of childhood obesity. *Ann Acad Med Singapore.* 2009;38(1):75-77
11. American Medical Association. Guidelines for Adolescent Preventive Services (GAPS). Available at: http://www.ama-assn.org/ama/pub/physician-resources/public-health/promoting-healthy-lifestyles/adolescent-health/guidelines-adolescent-preventive-services.page. Accessed April 18, 2012
12. Patrick K, Norman GJ, Calfas KJ, et al. Diet, physical activity, and sedentary behaviors as risk factors for overweight in adolescence. *Arch Pediatr Adolesc Med.* 2004;158(4):385-390
13. Thompson FE, Byers T. Dietary assessment resource manual. *J Nutr.* 1994;124(11 Suppl):2245S-2317S
14. Subar AF, Kirkpatrick SI, Mittl B, et al. The Automated Self-Administered 24-Hour Dietary Recall (ASA24): a resource for researchers, clinicians, and educators from the national cancer institute. *J Acad Nutr Diet.* 2012;112(8):1134-1137
15. Patrick K, Calfas KJ, Norman GJ, et al. Randomized controlled trial of a primary care and home-based intervention for physical activity and nutrition behaviors: PACE+ for adolescents. *Arch Pediatr Adolesc Med.* 2006;160(2):128-136
16. Matthiessen TB, Steinberg FM, Kaiser LL. Convergent validity of a digital image-based food record to assess food group intake in youth. *J Am Diet Assoc.* 2011;111(5):756-761
17. Di Noia J, Contento IR, Schinke SP. Criterion validity of the Healthy Eating Self-monitoring Tool (HEST) for black adolescents. *J Am Diet Assoc.* 2007;107(2):321-324
18. Di Noia J, Contento IR. Criterion validity and user acceptability of a CD-ROM-mediated food record for measuring fruit and vegetable consumption among black adolescents. *Public Health Nutr.* 2009;12(1):3-11
19. Watanabe M, Yamaoka K, Yokotsuka M, Adachi M, Tango T. Validity and reproducibility of the FFQ (FFQW82) for dietary assessment in female adolescents. *Public Health Nutr.* 2011;14(2):297-305
20. Marchioni DM, Voci SM, Lima FE, Fisberg RM, Slater B. Reproducibility of a food frequency questionnaire for adolescents. *Cad Saude Publica.* 2007;23(9):2187-2196
21. Matthys C, Pynaert I, De Keyzer W, De Henauw S. Validity and reproducibility of an adolescent web-based food frequency questionnaire. *J Am Diet Assoc.* 2007;107(4):605-610
22. Nelson MC, Lytle LA. Development and evaluation of a brief screener to estimate fast-food and beverage consumption among adolescents. *J Am Diet Assoc.* 2009;109(4):730-734
23. Centers for Disease Control and Prevention. National Youth Physical Activity Nutrition Study (NYPANS). Available at: http://www.cdc.gov/healthyyouth/yrbs/nypans.htm. Accessed April 20, 2012
24. Kohl III HW, Fulton JE, Caspersen CJ. Assessment of physical activity among children and adolescents: a review and synthesis. *Prev Med.* 2000;31(2):S54-S76

25. Bassett DR Jr, Rowlands A, Trost SG. Calibration and validation of wearable monitors. *Med Sci Sports Exerc*. 2012;44(1S):S32-S38
26. Butte NF, Ekelund U, Westerterp KR. Assessing physical activity using wearable monitors: measures of physical activity. *Med Sci Sports Exerc*. 2012;44(1 Suppl 1):S5-S12
27. Trost SG. Objective measurement of physical activity in youth: current issues, future directions. *Exerc Sport Sci Rev*. 2001;29(1):32-36
28. Wiehe SE, Carroll AE, Liu GC, et al. Using GPS-enabled cell phones to track the travel patterns of adolescents. *Int J Health Geogr*. 2008;7:22
29. Bocarro JN, Kanters MA, Cerin E, et al. School sport policy and school-based physical activity environments and their association with observed physical activity in middle school children. *Health Place*. 2012;18(1):31-38
30. McKenzie TL. 2009 C. H. McCloy Lecture. Seeing is believing: observing physical activity and its contexts. *Res Q Exerc Sport*. 2010;81(2):113-122
31. Sirard JR, Pate RR. Physical activity assessment in children and adolescents. *Sports Med*. 2001;31(6):439-454
32. Dollman J, Okely AD, Hardy L, Timperio A, Salmon J, Hills AP. A hitchhiker's guide to assessing young people's physical activity: deciding what method to use. *J Sci Med Sport*. 2009;12(5):518-525
33. Goran MI, Hunter G, Nagy TR, Johnson R. Physical activity related energy expenditure and fat mass in young children. *Int J Obes Relat Metab Disord*. 1997;21(3):171-178
34. Trost S, Ward D, McGraw B, Pate R. Validity of the Previous Day Physical Activity Recall (PDPAR) in the fifth-grade children. *Pediatr Exerc Sci*. 1999;11(4):341–348
35. Sallis JF, Buono MJ, Roby JJ, Micale FG, Nelson JA. Seven-day recall and other physical activity self-reports in children and adolescents. *Med Sci Sports Exerc*. 1993;25(1):99-108
36. Haskell WL. Physical activity by self-report: a brief history and future issues. *J Phys Act Health*. 2012;9 Suppl 1:S5-10
37. Chinapaw MJM, Mokkink LB, van Poppel MNM, van Mechelen W, Terwee CB. Physical activity questionnaires for youth: a systematic review of measurement properties. *Sports Med*. 2010;40(7):539-563
38. Kowalski KC, Crocker PRE, Faulkner RA. Validation of the physical activity questionnaire for older children. *Pediatr Exerc Sci*. 1997;9(2):174-186
39. The IPAQ group. International physical activity questionnaire. Available at: https://sites.google.com/site/theipaq/. Accessed April 2, 2012
40. Crocker PR, Bailey DA, Faulkner RA, Kowalski KC, McGrath R. Measuring general levels of physical activity: preliminary evidence for the Physical Activity Questionnaire for Older Children. *Med Sci Sports Exerc*. 1997;29(10):1344-1349
41. Kowalski KC, Crocker PRE, Kowalski NP. Convergent validity of the physical activity questionnaire for adolescents. *Pediatr Exerc Sci*. 1997;9(4):342-352
42. Janz KF, Lutuchy EM, Wenthe P, Levy SM. Measuring activity in children and adolescents using self-report: PAQ-C and PAQ-A. *Med Sci Sports Exerc*. 2008;40(4):767-772
43. Centers for Disease Control and Prevention. CDC - YRBSS - NYPANS - Adolescent and School Health. Available at: http://www.cdc.gov/healthyyouth/yrbs/nypans.htm. Accessed March 29, 2012
44. Alomari MA, Keewan EF, Qhatan R, et al. Blood pressure and circulatory relationships with physical activity level in young normotensive individuals: IPAQ validity and reliability considerations. *Clin Exp Hypertens*. 2011;33(5):345-353
45. Dunton GF, Jamner MS, Cooper DM. Assessing the perceived environment among minimally active adolescent girls: validity and relations to physical activity outcomes. *Am J Health Promot*. 2003;18(1):70-73
46. Dunton GF, Whalen CK, Jamner LD, Henker B, Floro JN. Using ecologic momentary assessment to measure physical activity during adolescence. *Am J Prev Med*. 2005;29(4):281-287
47. Dunton GF, Kawabata K, Intille S, Wolch J, Pentz MA. Assessing the social and physical contexts of children's leisure-time physical activity: an ecological momentary assessment study. *Am J Health Promot*. 2012;26(3):135-142

48. Schutz Y, Weinsier RL, Hunter GR. Assessment of free-living physical activity in humans: an overview of currently available and proposed new measures. *Obes Res.* 2001;9(6):368-379
49. Seale JL, Conway JM, Canary JJ. Seven-day validation of doubly labeled water method using indirect room calorimetry. *J Appl Physiol.* 1993;74(1):402-409
50. Johnson RK. Dietary intake - how do we measure what people are really eating? *Obesity.* 2002;10:63S-68S
51. Shatenstein B, Amre D, Jabbour M, Feguery H. Examining the relative validity of an adult food frequency questionnaire in children and adolescents. *J Pediatr Gastroenterol Nutr.* 2010;51(5):645-652
52. Papadopoulou SK, Barboukis V, Dalkiranis A, Hassapidou M, Petridou A, Mougios V. Validation of a questionnaire assessing food frequency and nutritional intake in Greek adolescents. *Int J Food Sci Nutr.* 2008;59(2):148-154
53. Roumelioti M, Leotsinidis M. Relative validity of a semiquantitative food frequency questionnaire designed for schoolchildren in western Greece. *J Nutr.* 2009;8(1):8
54. Baghurst KI, Record SJ. A computerised dietary analysis system for use with diet diaries or food frequency questionnaires. *Community Health Stud.* 1984;8(1):11-18
55. Ambrosini GL, O'Sullivan TA, de Klerk NH, Mori TA, Beilin LJ, Oddy WH. Relative validity of adolescent dietary patterns: a comparison of a FFQ and 3 d food record. *Br J Nutr.* 2011;105(4):625-633
56. Kolodziejczyk JK, Merchant G, Norman GJ. A systematic review: reliability and validity of child/adolescent food frequency questionnaires that assess foods and/or food groups. *J Pediatr Gastroenterol Nutr.* 2012;55(1):4-13
57. Di Noia J, Contento IR. Use of a brief food frequency questionnaire for estimating daily number of servings of fruits and vegetables in a minority adolescent population. *J Am Diet Assoc.* 2009;109(10):1785-1789
58. Magarey A, Golley R, Spurrier N, Goodwin E, Ong F. Reliability and validity of the Children's Dietary Questionnaire; a new tool to measure children's dietary patterns. *Int J Pediatr Obes.* 2009;4(4):257-265
59. Li L, Levy-Milne R. Vegetable and fruit intake and factors influencing their intake. *Can J Diet Pract Res.* 2008;69(4):213-217
60. Centers for Disease Control and Prevention. Dietary Screener in the NHANES 2009-10. Available at: http://riskfactor.cancer.gov/studies/nhanes/dietscreen/. Accessed April 20, 2012
61. Ward DS, Evenson KR, Vaughn A, Rodgers AB, Troiano RP. Accelerometer use in physical activity: best practices and research recommendations. *Med Sci Sports Exerc.* 2005;37(11 Suppl):S582-588
62. Adams MA, Caparosa S, Thompson S, Norman GJ. Translating physical activity recommendations for overweight adolescents to steps per day. *Am J Prev Med.* 2009;37(2):137-140
63. Moskowitz DS, Young SN. Ecological momentary assessment: what it is and why it is a method of the future in clinical psychopharmacology. *J Psychiatry Neurosci.* 2006;31(1):13-20
64. Smyth J, Wonderlich S, Crosby R, Miltenberger R, Mitchell J, Rorty M. The use of ecological momentary assessment approaches in eating disorder research. *Int J Eat Disord.* 2001;30(1):83-95
65. Patrick K, Sallis JF, Prochaska JJ, et al. A multicomponent program for nutrition and physical activity change in primary care: PACE+ for adolescents. *Arch Pediatr Adolesc Med.* 2001;155(8):940-946
66. Norman GJ, Zabinski MF, Adams MA, Rosenberg DE, Yaroch AL, Atienza AA. A review of eHealth interventions for physical activity and dietary behavior change. *Am J Prev Med.* 2007;33(4):336-345
67. Van den Berg M, Schoones J, Vliet VTP. Internet-based physical activity interventions: a systematic review of the literature. *J Med Internet Res.* 2007;9(3):e26
68. Contento I, Balch GI, Bronner YL, et al. The effectiveness of nutrition education and implications for nutrition education policy, programs, and research: a review of research. *J Nutr Edu.* 1995;27
69. Shaikh AR, Yaroch AL, Nebeling L, Yeh MC, Resnicow K. Psychosocial predictors of fruit and vegetable consumption in adults: a review of the literature. *Am J Prev Med.* 2008;34(6):535-543

70. Rabin C, Bock B. Desired features of smartphone applications promoting physical activity. *Telemed J E Health*. 2011;17(10):801-803
71. Azark R. Smartphone apps for your practice. *CDS Rev*. 2011;104(7):12-13
72. Kroeze W, Werkman A, Brug J. A systematic review of randomized trials on the effectiveness of computer-tailored education on physical activity and dietary behaviors. *Ann Behav Med*. 2006;31(3):205
73. Fooducate LTD. Fooducate | eat a bit better. Available at: http://www.fooducate.com/. Accessed April 2, 2012
74. MyFitnessPal LLC. Free Calorie Counter, Diet & Exercise Journal | MyFitnessPal.com. Available at: http://www.myfitnesspal.com/. Accessed April 2, 2012
75. Weight Watchers International Inc. WeightWatchers.com: Weight Watchers mobile. Available at: http://www.weightwatchers.com/templates/Marketing/Marketing_Utool_1col.aspx?pageid=1163301. Accessed April 16, 2012
76. Lee W, Chae YM, Kim S, Ho SH, Choi I. Evaluation of a mobile phone-based diet game for weight control. *J Telemed Telecare*. 2010;16(5):270-275
77. MapMyFITNESS Inc. Map Fitness Training and Track Fitness Workouts | MapMyFITNESS. Available at: http://www.mapmyfitness.com/. Accessed April 2, 2012
78. PumpOne LLC. FitnessBuilder. Available at: https://www.fitnessbuilder.com/plus. Accessed April 2, 2012
79. iTreadmill. iTreadmill for iPod Touch & iPhone. Available at: http://www.itreadmill.net/iTreadmill/Home.html. Accessed April 2, 2012

Adolesc Med 23 (2012) 631–636

Note: Page numbers of articles are in **boldface** type. Page references followed by "*f*" and "*t*" denote figures and tables, respectively.

A

B

 ISSN 1934-4287

O

P

R

S